ASIAN AMERICANS

RECONCEPTUALIZING CULTURE, HISTORY, AND POLITICS

Edited By
Franklin Ng
California State University
Fresno

A ROUTLEDGE SERIES

STUDIES IN ASIAN AMERICANS
RECONCEPTUALIZING CULTURE, HISTORY, AND POLITICS
FRANKLIN NG, *General Editor*

Hmong American Concepts of Health, Healing, and Conventional Medicine

Dia Cha

Routledge
New York & London

Published in 2003 by
Routledge
29 West 35th Street
New York, NY 10001
www.routledge-ny.com

Published in Great Britain by
Routledge
11 New Fetter Lane
London EC4P 4EE
www.routledge.co.uk

Routledge is an imprint of the Taylor & Francis Group
Printed in the United States of America on acid-free paper.

Copyright © 2003 by Taylor & Francis Books, Inc.

10 9 8 7 6 5 4 3 2

Library of Congress Cataloging-in-Publication Data

Cha, Dia.
   Hmong American concepts of health, healing, and conventional medicine / by Dia Cha.
      p. cm. — (Asian Americans)
Includes bibliographical references and index.
   ISBN 0-415-94495-3 (hardcover : alk. paper)
   1. Hmong Americans—Medicine. 2. Transcultural medical care—United States. 3. Health attitudes—United States.
   [DNLM: 1. Attitude to Health—ethnology—Asia, Southeastern. 2. Attitude to Health—ethnology—United States. 3. Asian Americans—Asia, Southeastern. 4. Asian Americans—United States. 5. Delivery of Health Care—Asia, Southeastern. 6. Delivery of Health Care—United States. 7. Medicine, Oriental Traditional—Asia, Southeastern. 8. Medicine, Traditional Oriental—United States. W 85 C426h 2003] I. Title. II. Series.
   RA418.5.T73C48 2003
   362.1—dc21   2002156762

To my parents
Chong Ze Cha (Ntxoov Zeb Tsab)
and
See Lo (Xis Lauj)
for their love, inspiration, and motivation

Contents

Acknowledgments

I AM INDEBTED TO, AND HAVE BEEN SUBSTANTIALLY ENRICHED BY, THE MANY informants who took the time to share with me their personal experiences and their knowledge of Hmong traditional medicine and medical techniques; out of respect for their privacy, and to honor commitments of confidentiality, I will not name them here. My indebtedness is particularly profound to that handful of Hmong healers who spent so many long hours responding to my inquiries into the arcana of traditional Hmong medicine. Our knowledge and understanding of Hmong concepts of health, healing, and illness, and the Hmong experience with conventional medicine, have been immeasurably enhanced thanks to their trust and their openness in sharing their knowledge and experience.

I would like to extend my profuse thanks to Mrs. Chong Ze Her for her assistance in transcribing some of the focus group interview sessions in Hmong. Without her assistance, this work, in its present form, would have been impossible.

In addition, this research project would not have been possible without the good will and cooperation of the Hmong American Association of Colorado, Inc., and the Lao-Hmong American Coalition. Leaders of those two organizations not only took time out from busy schedules to allow me to interview them, but also very kindly referred their members to me for additional interviews. I want to thank them all profoundly for their support of this research project, and for sharing their ideas and insights.

Further and heartfelt thanks are due to my thesis chairman, mentor, and much-admired role model, Dr. Robert A. Hackenberg, without whose constant encouragement and unwavering patience I would never have been able to complete this undertaking; together with the entire thesis committee; Drs. Lauren Clark, Craig R. Janes, Darna L. Dufour, Lane R. Hirabayashi, and Deward E. Walker.

I am also very grateful to my friend, Dr. Norma Livo, for her support and admiration, and for taking the time to read this manuscript and offer her insightful comments.

My special thanks are extended to Dr. Evelyn Hu-Dehart, Chair of the Department of Ethnic Studies, University of Colorado, Boulder, Colorado, for taking the time to read this book and for her unbounded kindness in supporting and encouraging me in my pursuit of an academic career. She has seemed consistently to know my potential better than I, myself do, and has been an invaluable quide in directing me toward the light at the end of the tunnel.

I would like to take this opportunity to extend to the faculty and staff of the Ethnic Studies Department at St. Cloud State University my very special thanks for their constant support and their warm friendship; and especially to Dr. Robert C. Johnson, my mentor, and to Karen DeRung and Deborah Schlumberger for their generous clerical assistance. With my involvement in this department, and its wonderfully kindhearted personnel, I count myself fortunate—even as I find myself personally enriched to a profound degree.

Steve Carmen, my oaken staff, has been of immeasurable assistance. His kindheartedness, his patience, his encouragement, his support, his unwavering friendship, his professionalism, and his virtually numberless hours of hard work on my behalf have inspired in me an eternal gratitude.

In concluding, I would be remiss were I to omit mention of my loving and astoundingly patient husband, Kao Xiong, whose loyalty and commitment I deeply appreciate, and to my mother, See Lo; thank you both for your steadfast encouragement, support, and assistance with household and other family duties, that I might have more time to give to my studies.

Dia Cha
St. Cloud, Minnesota

Foreword

THIS BOOK EXAMINES HMONG AMERICAN CONCEPTS OF HEALTH, healing and illness; the varieties of Hmong diagnosticians and healers who utilize traditional techniques and methodologies, and the nature of Hmong interactions with conventional health care professionals. In addition, it identifies specific factors that either obstruct or enable conventional health care delivery to Hmong Americans, particularly with reference to Colorado.

Since the late 1970s, when Hmong refugees began to immigrate to the United States, it has been well documented that Hmong Americans have experienced many instances of the "clash of cultures" with conventional health care professionals due to differing perceptions of appropriate health treatment procedures.[1] The literature indicates that many Hmong Americans exhaust all avenues of traditional healing practice before consulting with conventional health care professionals.[2] When the Hmong finally do consult with conventional medical professionals, many physicians are unable to diagnose any disease or to prescribe appropriate medicines to relieve symptoms.[3] In consequence, these health care providers label such symptoms "somatization," which is defined as the claim to experience physical symptoms without identifiable organic pathological explanation.[4]

It is a common belief that the use of traditional or alternative medicines, and somatic symptoms, are associated with people who have lower socioeconomic status than mainstream Americans, are less educated, are from rural backgrounds, and belong to ethnic groups that discourage expression of emotional distress.[5]

Elizabeth Lin et al. have estimated that, "thirty to ninety percent of patient visits to primary care clinics have psychosomatic origins." In the United States, patients who demonstrate somatization constitute the most frequent users of medical care programs and facilities, and tend to become a major burden on the health care system.[6]

According to Lin et al., patients with somatization account for fifty per cent of ambulatory care costs in this country.[7] The same study found that somatization is a major health problem among Asian refugees and immigrants as a whole. The study indicated that, "[Asian] refugees had a higher rate of somatization (42.7 per cent) than immigrants (27.1 percent)." Refugees with somatic symptoms tended to consult primary care physicians more than immigrants.[8]

The above statements assume that, 1) Hmong patients; Asian refugees; Asian immigrants; and people who have large families and low income, lower levels of education, and belong to an ethnic group, tend to avail themselves more frequently of non-biomedical medicines, be more dissatisfied with conventional medicines and be associated more frequently with somatization than mainstream Americans; 2) the conventional health care system has not been able to effectively treat the health symptoms of this population; and, 3) patients with somatic problems engender a high percentage of ambulatory care costs and have become a major burden on the conventional medical health care system. The above literature, written from the conventional perspective, recognizes the existence of those somatic problems that have been troubling patients in the system, but seems to place these patients at fault for seeking health care treatments that are not commensurate with their symptoms. However, the writer seeks to demonstrate that, 1) the "somatic" symptoms of which Hmong patients have complained when consulting conventional health care professionals may be viewed as a culturally defined syndrome rather than as somatized, and, 2) the use of traditional medicines or alternative health treatments is wide spread among people of different economic classes, gender, age, and educational levels. Moreover, the use of traditional Hmong medicines and medical practices is not on the verge of disappearing, as is commonly believed.

The Colorado Hmong community consists of twelve clans. Some clans have over a thousand members, while some have only one or two families. The author held a meeting in May, 1999, at which all clan representatives attended. The author then presented the nature of the anticipated research to them. The majority of these clan representatives were supportive of the project and were willing to assist with the research by referring their clan members to the author for interviews. These leaders were asked to provide a list of their members as contacts for interviews. The author asked the clan representatives to consider the issues of gender and age differences, socioeconomic status, and educational level when making references. Only those who wished to share their experiences and views were interviewed, and, if those who were first contacted refused to be interviewed, others were chosen from the list, to comprise a total sample population of forty individuals (all pertinent forms are reproduced as appendices). Interviews took from about forty-five minutes to three or four hours, and were conducted at the interviewees' homes and at public library study and/or conference rooms.

Methods of data collection included focus group discussions, in-depth interviews, one-on-one interviews, and participant-observations during ceremonies conducted by shamans, at healing rituals, clinic or hospital visits, and in the course of massage sessions. The research design included qualitative open-ended questionnaires used during both the focus group discussions and in-depth interviews. Eighteen Hmong American health care providers, leaders, interpreters, and patients were included in the focus group discussions. One focus group interview was conducted among a group of four Hmong male community leaders. Two focus group interviews were conducted with Hmong health care providers and interpreters working in the health system. One of these two interviews mixed both male and female participants, while one had only female participants. The fourth focus group was conducted with a group of four female and one male Hmong patients. Nine individual in-depth interviews were conducted with seven Hmong traditional healers: two shamans, three massage therapists, and two herbalists (refer to Appendix for detailed information on informants). One shaman and one massage therapist were each interviewed twice with in-depth interview technique.

Quantitative questionnaires formed the basis of a health history survey, for which forty Hmong American healers, patients, and community members were interviewed using a one-on-one structured interview technique. The health history survey included questions of self-reported demographic information, Hmong categories of illness encountered, types of Western medicines utilized, and Hmong American concepts of health and healing, together with their associated practices (see Appendix). A consent form was explained to the interviewees, and they were required to sign it before an interview took place (see Appendix). If the interviewee was not literate, the author translated orally all of the instruments to him in the Hmong language. The interviewees were Hmong adult women and men who were both patients and healers. Data collection for this research project ran from May, 1999, to February, 2000. Data analysis occurred from March to May, 2000, with the dissertation being written from June to November, 2000.

HMONG AMERICAN CONCEPTS OF HEALTH, HEALING, AND CONVENTIONAL MEDICINE

Chapter I

The Impact of Christianity and Refugee Resettlement on Hmong Society and Health Care

THE IMPACT OF CHRISTIANITY ON HMONG SOCIETY AND HEALTH CARE

IT HAS BEEN DOCUMENTED THAT CATHOLIC MISSIONARIES INTRODUCED Christianity to the Hmong, or Miao, of China as early as 1863.[1] Additional documentation shows that Protestant missionary work began with the Hmong in the Yunnan and Guizhou regions shortly prior to the turn of the century.[2] Christian missionaries came to Laos during the 1940s, but mass conversions did not occur until the late 1940s to early 1950s, due to interruptions caused by constant political instability in the region.[3] It is widely believed that Catholic missionaries have been more sympathetic and successful in converting the Hmong to Christianity than Protestant, who have maintained a "radical intolerance" of traditional Hmong religious beliefs and practices.[4] The successful mass conversions of Hmong to Christianity have tended to occur during periods when Hmong experienced extreme hardship, economic deprivation, and political instability.[5] Christianity has been presented to many poor Hmong families as an alternative to traditional beliefs, with their associated practices, which affords relief from expensive ritual or kinship obligations.[6] As a result, Hmong Christians often expect a "supreme force to intervene in their favour," as many were drawn into the Christian fold by the "Saviour aspects" of Christianity.[7]

The effect that Christianity has had on Hmong society has been, 1) to provide the opportunity for Hmong children in Laos, Thailand and China to attend school and become literate; 2) to enable the development of messianic movements in contemporary Hmong society; and, 3) to widen the gap between the Hmong and those dominant peoples, such as the Chinese, Lao, Thai, and other non-Christian ethnic groups, of the nations in which the Hmong have, throughout history, resided. Together, these sociocultural consequences of religious affiliation have contributed to the marginalization of the Hmong, and this marginalization has increased with increasing membership in Christian sects.[8]

Christianity represents a threat to Hmong communal harmony and health care, in that devotion to the Christian faith tends to weaken the importance of maintaining the traditions of lineage and of clan solidarity, and sometimes results in conflict between non-Christian and Christian kinsmen.[9] Ironically, the Christian messages embraced by some Hmong are not always those espoused by their Western missionaries. Rather, Christian ideas are occasionally modified to fit the Procrustean bed of Hmong cultural expectations, and have come thereby to reflect Hmong social values and traditional religious beliefs.[10]

Lineage and clan solidarity are endangered by the message that all men are brothers, and that one's family, therefore, is inclusive of both relatives and all Christians. This places an obligation upon a Hmong Christian, in cases wherein aid of any sort is a necessity, to help his Christian non-relatives to the same extent as his non-Christian relatives. When a member of each of these groups needs assistance at the same time, this obligation, born of the Christian ideal, is difficult to fulfill.[11]

The most serious problem arising between the minority Christian Hmong and the majority Non-Christian Hmong is the refusal of some Hmong Christians to join in on common ritual obligations toward relatives, especially in connection with spiritual healing and funerary rites.[12] In these instances, animal sacrifices are standard practice, something which many Christian Hmong will not countenance. These Christian Hmong, moreover, will not eat the meat of sacrificed animals, believing, at best, that animal sacrifice is irrational and wasteful, and "therefore sinful behaviour;" at worst, that such meat has been offered to and touched by the devil. Elderly Hmong parents who have sons or daughters who have converted to Christianity are, in many instances, greatly disturbed because, should they become ill, their children will not seek spiritual healers to treat them. Should they die, their children will neither sacrifice chickens, pigs, and cows, nor perform certain funerary rituals believed necessary to ensure the elders' safe journey to and reception in the ancestors' world. In life, if the elder Hmong, in maintaining their traditional animist religion, sacrifice animals in the performance of a major ceremony, their Christian children may not join the feast, let alone assist at the rite. One Hmong Christian center in the Philippines is even said to distribute cassette tapes in a campaign against animal sacrifice.[13]

Christian missionaries have targeted Hmong spiritual healers, such as soul callers, shamans, and *Khawv Koob* or magic healers, because they believe that the practices of these people are a form of devil worship.[14] Once these healers agree to become Christians, their altars and healing paraphernalia are burned or dismantled.[15] All Hmong who have converted to Christianity are strongly discouraged from commissioning the very common soul calling, as well as being enjoined from resorting to any shaman's ceremonies or allowing magic (*Khawv Koob*) when they are sick. In place of these spiritual healing techniques, prayer is counseled.

THE IMPACT OF REFUGEE RESETTLEMENT ON HMONG SOCIETY AND HEALTH CARE

THE HMONG DIASPORA

The Hmong are refugees whose immediate origins may be traced to the highlands of Laos. During the course of the Vietnam War, they supported the US armed forces, and, by the end of that conflict in 1975, thousands of Hmong had been uprooted from their villages, while one-third of their erstwhile population of 300,000 had been killed. It has been documented that the Hmong suffered ten times the casualties of their American sponsors.[16] To make matters worse, after the American withdrawal, the new communist regime in Laos embarked upon a course of persecution of the thousands of Hmong who had supported the United States, and many of these were forced to flee to Thailand where they were placed in refugee camps.[17] Ultimately, while some of these refugees returned to Laos or took up a surreptitious residence in Thailand, hoping, perhaps, to eventually become Thai citizens, a significant number resettled in the West.[18]

Since 1975, the Hmong Diaspora has spread throughout the world.[19] Today, there are Hmong living in the Asian nations of China, Burma, Laos, Thailand, and Vietnam, and in such Western nations as Canada, Australia, France, French Guyana, and Argentina, with some 300,000 Hmong in the United States.[20]

According to the U.S. Census of 2000, the states which have the largest Hmong American communities in America are California (65,095), Minnesota (41,800), Wisconsin (33,791), and North Carolina (7,093).[21] However, it should be noted that many Hmong American community leaders believe the census of 2000 undercounted, to a considerable extent, the Hmong American population. At variance with the official tally, they estimate that California is host to approximately 95,000 Hmong Americans, Minnesota 70,000, Wisconsin 50,000, and North Carolina 20,000. Smaller Hmong American communities, numbering from a few hundred to a few thousand, are located in Arkansas, Colorado, Texas, Oklahoma, Iowa, Nebraska, Nevada, Montana, Washington, Oregon, South Carolina,

Georgia, Florida, Washington DC, Connecticut, Rhode Island, New York, Michigan, Illinois, Massachusetts, Pennsylvania, Idaho, Ohio, Indiana, Alaska, and Virginia.[22]

CULTURE

Hmong culture is characterized by a patrilineal, patrilocal, and exogamous kinship system, and the Hmong practice polygyny and levirate. The main social structure in traditional Hmong society is the clan (*Xeem*) system.[23] Originally, there were twelve clan names, used in a manner similar to Chinese or Western surnames. Although the exact number of Hmong clan names currently in use is not known, the literature provides a range of from fifteen to twenty-one.[24] Each clan has many lineages, and each lineage has many families, and the Hmong show significant social attachment to their family, their lineage (*Kwv Tij*), and their clan (*Xeem*).[25] In truth, the whole fabric of Hmong social organization is woven together on the basis of descent lines rather than locality, and, even in contemporary America, the majority of Hmong still organize their allegiances and many of their activities based on the clan and lineage system.[26]

Above the level of clan, the Hmong consist two main groups; White Hmong and Blue (or Green) Hmong (*Hmoob Dawb* and *Hmoob Lees*).[27] Two main characteristics separate these groups; a different dialect of the language, and different traditional costumes worn by either gender. The linguistic differences are not such a barrier as might be supposed, however, for although the two dialects are different in some respects, they are mutually intelligible, and, inasmuch as there are other sub-regional differences in traditional costume and accent, the demarcation between the White and the Blue Hmong is not particularly sharp.[28] It has been argued by some Western scholars that sub-regional differences dictate separation of the Hmong into such additional cultural groupings as the Green/Blue, the Black, and the Armband or the Striped Hmong, but the Hmong themselves do not recognize such categories.[29]

The Hmong male exists at the center of Hmong society, with women taking a decidedly secondary position. Hmong males learn, practice, and transmit their oral traditions and ritual observances from one generation to the next.[30] Hmong parents are expected to live with their sons, while these sons and their wives, the parents' daughters-in-law, are expected to care for the parents during their old age.[31] If they have more than one son, parents are expected to live with the youngest son and his family. Sons are, in addition, charged with making sacrifice on behalf of the parents when they die, and to the ancestors. As a consequence of these many duties, obligations, and offices of power, males are considered superior to females in Hmong society, an attitude which still pervades Hmong American families, despite the fact that many have converted to Christianity, and, in consequence, no longer need, in fact decline to perform, the various rites and rituals customarily associated with the passages of Hmong life.[32]

CHANGES IN GENDER ROLES, PROTECTION, AND SOCIAL STATUS

Although the Hmong in America retain many of their traditions, there are aspects in the lives of Hmong Americans that have undergone significant change. Before the Vietnam War era, both Hmong men and Hmong women raised animals and worked in the fields, planting rice, corn, and vegetables for family consumption. Both genders engaged in the same activities relative to providing for the family's basic needs. During the war, traditional subsistence practices shifted to a wage-labor based cash economy, and Hmong men became the main income earners as soldiers. As the war continued, men were sent away to fight, while women constantly moved from place to place with their children and the family elders. Such movement prevented women from engaging in agricultural activities, and, as a result, rendered them even more dependent on the income of the male family members.[33]

In this situation, the nature both of women's and of men's daily activities shifted. Men were neither providing for nor protecting their families; rather, they were protecting their political factions and their country. This new role, unique, as it was, to the Hmong male, gave men prestige, political power, and authority. Women continued, as always, to assume the responsibilities inherent in caring for dependent family members. In this, their responsibilities had not changed; but the resources over which they formerly had control were removed by circumstance, and the tasks they performed did not yield them the prestige, power, and authority enjoyed by men. This had the effect of gradually lowering women's status and self-esteem.[34]

As the war came to an end, a great many Hmong found themselves in refugee camps and in the West. Families were no longer required to move constantly, yet they no longer engaged in subsistence agriculture. This freed women from many of the labor-intensive duties that were routine in a village setting, including, but not limited to; rice pounding; the planting, weeding, harvesting, and threshing of rice; feeding and otherwise caring for livestock; and collecting firewood. Indeed, most of the former economic and domestic activities of Hmong women on the farm of Laos disappeared. As a result, most moved from barter to cash economies, having changed their primary occupation from subsistence rice farming to income-generating handicrafts in the refugee camps or to wage earning labor positions in the United States. In addition, many Hmong men have been forced to take up occupations previously designated "solely women's work." These include sewing, tailoring, food marketing, and child rearing. As the camps offered them limited earning opportunities, Hmong men no longer provided at least fifty percent of the family's basic needs. Instead, women, via the medium of their embroidery and other handicrafts, became the primary income earners, and, once settled in the United States, many of these same Hmong women began to work outside the home to contribute at least fifty percent of the family income. In this manner, and with few options available, camp life and life in America pressed Hmong men into accepting women as income-earners, as well as into helping with traditionally female-related household tasks.[35]

These shifts in the nature of their respective activities and responsibilities have forced Hmong men and Hmong women to face corresponding shifts in their relative financial status and degree of control over family earnings. Within Hmong households in Laos, for example, it is the prerogative of the husband to decide who holds family savings, and whether or not his wife is to be involved in financial decisions. In the refugee camps and in the United States, by contrast, that authority is opening up, and Hmong women have achieved a measure of equality.

However, the Hmong woman's enhanced economic position has not automatically translated into greater social status.[36] It remains the case that professional Hmong American women receive less respect than professional Hmong American men, and little support in their efforts to promote either themselves or issues of importance to them. Politically, their voices are little heard in the community. A professional Hmong American woman may express a brilliant idea at a community meeting, but her idea will be as if unheard until a Hmong man expresses the same idea. Then, and only then, will anyone applaud.

Despite changes in their economic status relative to Hmong women, Hmong men continue to regard themselves as superior to their women in dealing with public affairs and in communicating with outsiders. No Hmong women, for example, sat on any of the governing committees in the refugee camps of Thailand. All clan representatives in Colorado are men, and no clan has ever elected a woman to represent it. As a result, Hmong women subconsciously and repeatedly degrade themselves, and surrender any self-confidence they might have in the sphere of public affairs. When this lack of self-confidence becomes pervasive throughout a community, even the strongest and most educated women will accept inferior status. Even when women are recruited to participate in leadership roles, they often decline, saying, "We don't know enough," or, "Men know better, let them serve the community." With such pervasive beliefs even in the face of a heightened economic importance, Hmong women perpetuate the inferior position they have traditionally held in relation to Hmong men, and thus their social status has remained largely unchanged in Hmong society.[37]

In America, the impact of these changing and increasingly ambiguous gender roles, with the concomitant shift in responsibility, social status, and the formation and maintenance of spheres of power, has been to aggravate a variety of social, family, and health related problems. Both those Hmong who accept, and those who reject, these changing roles experience some levels of distress. Those who embrace these shifts are forced to endure the disapproval of family members, which may lead to tension or open conflict. Those who reject the changes find themselves losing the respect and trust of those who embrace such change. When these crucial issues are suppressed for an extended period, the result is often an emotional blowup, if not outright violence. This is attested in unpleasant fashion by recent cases of Hmong youth violence, and by episodes of domestic violence, all of which feature prominently in the media. In general, it may be said that Hmong men, and most members of older generations, wish to preserve traditional Hmong culture; while Hmong women, and Hmong of younger generations, wish to foster those changes which serve to alter the face of modern Hmong life.

In the early 1990s, this conflict led to the very strong yearning to return to Laos which characterized many Hmong men, and Hmong elders of both genders, interned in Thai refugee camps. At the same time as this desire increased in that segment of the population, Hmong women and Hmong youth, eager to avail themselves of opportunities for education and other features of modern life they viewed as desirable, developed an equally strong wish to settle in the West.[38]

It will be clear from the foregoing that the series of cultures referred to down the ages as "Hmong" have been influenced by, and are themselves a product of, changes resulting from many past experiences of geographic and cultural dislocation. In other words, we may say that what the Hmong described above are seeking either to retain or to modify is not a fixed, calcified "traditional culture," but a culture that has evolved over many centuries of Hmong migration. On a more temporally localized level, we can see that Hmong culture, as it currently exists, is very different from that even of the pre-Vietnam War period in the ways people make a living, in the gender division of labor, in politics, and in social mores and the parameters of social interaction.[39] Furthermore, unless alternative approaches are explored to help the Hmong deal with the widespread sense of dislocation created by their changing traditions, we may anticipate in the Hmong American community an increase in social stress, in a variety of social problems, in violence—both potential and actual—and in health problems.

One of the most serious dilemmas faced by modern Hmong Americans is what may be called the "two-way cultural pull," whereby one fraction of the population wants to change fast and soon, while the other segment wants to hold onto a romanticized vision of cultural tradition that allows them to revel in a fanciful notion of the glorious past. On the one hand, Hmong youth and others who are changing too fast find no commonality with and receive no understanding from family members. They turn to friends who may not have their best interests at heart; who may even exert an influence upon them which, in extreme cases, leads to violent crime, or drug or alcohol addiction. On the other hand, the elderly and certain former leaders who want to preserve a static Hmong culture—and the authority over others they once exerted—may find themselves abandoned to nostalgic recollections of the past and impossible hopes for the future. A male Hmong informant in Colorado describes these people as follows: "Most of the older Hmong people are nostalgic for their homeland. They miss their country of origin. They think of it all the time. Many of them wish they could return to Laos and live there just like the old days. When they think too much, they seem to be a little crazy (*Vwm Ntsuav*). They think of how their lives used to be, and how much easier everything was. When they think a lot about these things, they become more confused and unhappy with life in the US. When they want something so much and don't get it, they feel irritation with every little thing that occurs surrounding them. Their children and wives attempt to communicate with them, but they cannot respond in a friendly manner. The major issue facing these older Hmong generations is that they have lost their social status upon becoming refugees. They lose their power or control. Their lives are better in the United States, in that they have plenty of food to eat, clothes to wear, and good places to live. But they don't have anything—like the Americans say—'burning inside of them,' that makes them feel in control of their own lives. If they don't have this, then they don't have the ability, hope and strength to make anything happen, even though they may want to do so much in this country.

"A lot of the older people, especially Hmong males, feel that they have lost respect from their friends and outsiders. They've lost their social standing and social status. People don't respect and honor them anymore. Even though they may have a lot of money, good appetite, and a good night's sleep, if they don't have something that they used to have, like having or being influential political leaders (*Nom Tswv*), they are being treated just like ordinary people when they step out of their houses and their community. Because they cannot bring back the power, prestige, and authority that they used to have, they are silently longing for this pristine dream, which can sometimes make them very angry (*Chim Heev*). When someone says something disrespectful to older Hmong people, especially the former military class, they will become very angry and say something like, 'I used to be an influential political leader (*Nom Tswv*), too. Why do you have the guts to say such a thing to me?' It is best to approach these people with friendly conversation, agree with everything they say, and never challenge their opinions; otherwise, they will become angry immediately when someone disagrees with them. When dealing with these people, one has to go along with whatever they want; otherwise, even if one's view is right, they will say it is not right.

"Most of the older Hmong men don't want to give up their former military titles. They want to hold on to their titles for the rest of their lives, even though they are no longer officially holding such titles. They have become refugees in foreign lands. They are no longer majors, captains, colonels, but they do not want to give up their power, authority, and responsibility. They still expect other people to treat them as if they are still in those positions. They cannot accept the fact that, since they are strangers in a foreign country, they have to start all over like children, who must learn everything—from the English language to sociocultural issues to work force regulations, and so on. They cannot live the same kind of lifestyle that they used to live in Laos. They cannot expect their wives to treat them like royalty, as they did in Laos. The Hmong women now have to work outside of the home in order to support the family. Most of them have full time jobs. However, when they arrive home from work, they are expected to carry out the same traditional housewives' duties as before they became refugees. They have no time to rest, or for themselves. If their husbands do not make any changes, and expect too much from them, they will eventually say words the husbands don't want to hear. When the women are expressing what they consider the truth of their daily lives, their husbands don't want to know or hear it.

"All of these social changes can create tremendous stress and mental health problems in the family, especially for the Hmong males who seem to have lost control of their social status, power and authority. The situation will become even worse as the children become more Americanized and become disrespectful of their parents. Hmong parents worry about their teenagers dropping out of school, getting drunk, or becoming addicted to drugs, running away from home and joining gangs (*Ua Laib*). When the Hmong men, women, and children do not see eye-to-eye on issues affecting their families, more stress, anger, and problems will develop in the families."

HMONG LIFE IN THE UNITED STATES

As the United States began to admit Hmong refugees in the late 1970s, three major government policies played intersecting roles in disrupting Hmong social organization and social and economic support systems.[40] First, the United States Immigration and Naturalization Service (INS) declined to recognize a number in excess of eight members per refugee family. In setting this figure, INS representatives interviewed Hmong family members in refugee camps, then divided many Hmong extended families, in which three or four generations resided together in a household, into smaller nuclear families; nuclear families were then allowed to migrate together as a unit, but extended families were not.[41] This policy effectively broke up the traditional Hmong extended family, fracturing, as it did so, the Hmong clan system, prevalent in the traditional Hmong village in Laos, by which many members of the same clan live closely together to provide social and economic support to each other in times of stress or difficulty.[42] Second, was what might be called the INS policy of "scattering." As Hmong immigration into the United States began, it was thought by INS officials that dispersal of Hmong families across the breadth of the nation would aid speedy assimilation into American society.[43] Naturally enough, the Hmong knew nothing about American culture, society, food, beliefs, or values, and most Americans knew nothing about the Hmong.[44] The result of scattering, therefore, was to place Hmong refugees in the most unfamiliar environment they had ever experienced in their lives, to "sink or swim" among all of the well-documented difficulties and with all of the comparable culture shock historically expressed by other, previous, immigrant groups.[45] There was, as well, a widely felt impact on the public service sectors and overburdened health facilities of many smaller American communities across the country.[46]

In time, many Hmong families chose to move away from their sponsoring communities, and this movement, known as secondary migration, which quickly became widespread, inevitably led to increased distance from, and, thus, decreased access to, designated resources for those families.[47] At last, the United States government was forced to reconsider the philosophy behind its scattering policy, and Hmong families were allowed to resettle where they had relatives.[48]

Third, American policies with regard to the disbursal of public welfare support funds impose constraints on kinship organization, indirectly encouraging people from an extended family to live alone. For example, grandparents living separately from a son's or daughter's household receive more monthly income than if all lived together; however, these same grandparents, living alone, may be able neither to drive nor to speak English. This will, of necessity, force them to bear an additional burden of physical, emotional, and psychological distress.[49]

The three aforementioned policies, operating in tandem with the Law of Unintended Consequences, have exerted in the direction of the breakdown of the extended family, with its social and economic support systems; the increased dependency of a large number of Hmong families on public assistance; and the isolation of many Hmong refugees at precisely the time they were overwhelmed with changes in their lives. Exacerbating the many stresses induced by the above policies, the majority of Hmong refugees came to America with little or no formal education, a great sense of post-war loss (e.g. of loved ones, homeland, social status, and material possessions), little exposure to urban life, few skills appropriate to the urban workforce, and a set of cultural beliefs and practices vastly different from those of most Americans,[50] and many of these same refugees eventually became psychiatric patients.[51] As a consequence of all of this, and in a fashion similar to patients whose doctors have prescribed the wrong medication, many Hmong Americans are reluctant to trust government authority and government policy. Especially suspect is any policy for which the claim is made that it will improve life.

EMPLOYMENT AND INCOME

In the late 1970s and early 1980s, at least sixty to eighty percent of Hmong refugees living in the three states of largest Hmong concentration—California, Minnesota, and Wisconsin—were receiving some form of public assistance.[52] In California, as an example, the percentage of Hmong completely dependent on public assistance was 81.1 percent, while the average Hmong family income was nine thousand dollars.[53] Since then, welfare dependency has declined to some extent. Westermeyer et al. conducted a longitudinal study of the psychosocial adjustment of one hundred Hmong refugees in Minnesota. The study indicated that the proportion of Hmong subjects on welfare has declined from fifty-three to twenty-nine percent.[54] Waters et al. cited a study conducted for the Wisconsin Policy Research Institute, revealing a nineteen percent decline in the number of Hmong on welfare.[55] In 1994, Yang and Murphy conducted a study in Minnesota using 1990 US Census data. This study found that in 1990, sixty-five percent of Hmong adults in Minnesota were not in the labor force, thirty percent were employed, and five percent were unemployed. The same study also showed that more than half of Hmong households had an annual income of less than fifteen thousand dollars, women headed twenty-four percent of Hmong households, and the average income of the women heads of household was $6,397. Mills and Yang found that, as of 1990, the median income of a Hmong family in California was $15,978, with forty-seven percent of Hmong households in California below the federal poverty line.[56]

According to Mills and Yang, many Hmong in California engage in farm labor, while others have received some form of training in wage-labor skills.[57] One positive trend revealed by Yang and Murphy's study is that Hmong in Minnesota are employed in nearly all sectors of the workplace and have made significant strides in moving from the welfare recipient to the wage-labor sectors.[58]

In Colorado, meanwhile, the percentage of employed Hmong is higher than that in Minnesota and California, with at least ninety-five percent of Hmong in Colorado working.[59] Those who are unemployed and dependent on public assistance are either disabled or single parents with dependent children. The majority of the employed Hmong adults in Colorado work in manufacturing companies in suburban Denver/Boulder. To make ends meet, many of these work two jobs, or interchange day and night shifts between spouses so that one can care for the children at all times. Interestingly, Westermeyer at al. found that Hmong adults who are employed experience more physical distress and anxiety than those who do not work.[60] This seems to be the result of a lack of familiarity with the workplace, of difficulties in negotiating language barriers, and of the sometimes harsh demands of low-wage, manual labor.

EDUCATION

It has been estimated that about eighty percent of Hmong adult refugees entering the United States are illiterate.[61] The percentage of Hmong who lacked English proficiency in 1982 was ninety, while the percentage of those Hmong literate in English in 1987 was thirty-four.[62] Yang and Murphy found that, among Hmong living in Minnesota, thirty percent of Hmong males and fifty-seven percent of Hmong females aged eighteen or older had no education, while twenty-four percent of Hmong males and eighteen percent of Hmong females had a high school diploma.[63] With regard to college education, one study indicated that two percent of each gender has four years, and only two percent of Hmong males and one percent of Hmong females have completed post-graduate studies.[64] The same study also revealed the positive sign that thirty percent of Hmong adults were in school, a percentage that the researchers, Yang and Murphy, believe to be larger than at any time in Hmong history. However, the same study showed that, among the Hmong in Minnesota, which is considered to be the most advanced Hmong American population in pursuing formal education, claiming the largest number of Hmong professionals and intellectuals, nearly half of Hmong adults have little or no English proficiency. In 1995, Jambunathan and Stewart published a study of pregnancy and childbirth among Hmong women in Wisconsin which showed that seventy-four percent of the fifty-two women sampled did not speak English. Mills and Yang write that, among the Hmong in California, only eighteen percent have a high school education, while about sixty percent have failed to achieve fifth grade level.[65]

Having lived in the Colorado Hmong community for sixteen years, the author believes that community may be behind the Minnesota Hmong community with regard to advancement in education. In 1989, the Hmong

Youth Association of Colorado conducted an informal, state-wide telephone survey throughout the Hmong clan system. Their results showed that, of the approximately three thousand Hmong questioned, there were but twenty-four Hmong males and one Hmong female who had finished four years of college. Although it is thought that the number of Hmong in Colorado entering institutions of higher education has increased recently, no reliable study can be cited.

In sum, all literature on the general subject of Hmong education levels indicates that a majority of Hmong American adults are not proficient in English; have a low level of education; have low socioeconomic status; and need the assistance of a cultural broker or translator when interacting with mainstream American service providers such as health care professionals. Hmong adults who are not able to express their feelings or opinions to service providers cannot provide basic needs for their families; must rely on other people to translate or to fill out forms for them; and, in consequence of these facts, experience tremendous anxiety, emotional distress, and depression.[66]

COMMUNITY AND SOCIAL SERVICE PROGRAMS

The Hmong population of Colorado is smaller than that of either Minnesota or California; with a total of six, it also has fewer social programs than those other states, each of which can boast over ten Hmong non-profit organizations with full-time staff, plus mainstream social service agencies. This difference reflects the various policies and approaches each state has created to integrate refugees into mainstream American society. The Hmong in California and Minnesota have cultural and service-oriented programs to assist them in exploring a variety of opportunities, ranging from education to employment to health care services. Due to a different atmosphere and the smaller size of the Hmong community there, however, Colorado has evolved very limited resources to support the Hmong, who, for various reasons, have not been able to unite themselves in their requests for assistance. Nevertheless, owing, perhaps, to intense media focus on cases of gang-related activities among Hmong teenagers, most particularly the case of six young Hmong males who raped a Caucasian woman in Boulder, the Hmong American Association of Colorado, Inc., a non-profit organization, employs two staff to serve the Hmong community. Those few social and community service agencies in Colorado which have Hmong staff are; the Colorado Refugee and Immigrant Service Program, the Asian Pacific Development Center, the Boulder County Mental Health Center, the Boulder County Community Action Program, the San Juan Health Clinic in Boulder, and the Denver Medical Center in

Denver. Four of these agencies have existed for over ten years, providing some services specifically to Hmong and Asian clients.

Still, in dealing with state agencies and non-governmental service organizations, Hmong adults in Colorado who are not fluent in English most frequently must request family members to translate for them. These family members will only rarely have been trained in the specific language ("jargon") of, or with specific reference to, the subculture of the service with which they seek to interact, and are, for the most part, lacking in knowledge of legal or medical terms and concepts.[67] Such interactions are thus not executed with the degree of understanding on either side which would enable the transfer of information on the one hand, and a sound decision on the other. This is particularly true in health care service situations. Hmong patients usually do not know what will take place until after a specific service has been rendered, and instances are documented in which this has led to unsatisfactory results, while creating distrust toward conventional health care professionals and institutions and fostering untold anxiety in Hmong patients and their families.[68]

PSYCHOSOCIAL ISSUES

Scholarly investigations of psychopathology among Southeast Asian refugee populations and among Asian Americans indicates that the highest rates of psychopathologic symptoms are to be found among Hmong and Cambodian refugees.[69] In standardized tests, fifty-five percent of the Hmong of California had high depression scores, eighty-six percent had high anxiety scores, and fifty percent had high psychosocial dysfunction scores.[70] Also in California, Gong-Guy estimated the percentage of Hmong who require inpatient mental health services at twenty percent; needing outpatient mental health services at thirty-five percent.[71] Joseph Westermeyer has conducted extensive research on the subject of Hmong psychiatric, psychosocial, and substance abuse issues. In the course of this research, he has identified four reliable predictors of psychiatric disorder among the Hmong and other Southeast Asian refugees.[72] For the span of a decade, from 1976-1986, he and others also conducted an epidemiological study of the Hmong in Minnesota. The results of this study reinforce the first of Westermeyer's four indicators; i.e., that those Hmong who came to the United States without any prior language training are more apt than others to develop psychiatric disorders. Ironically, people who received English-as-a-Second-Language (ESL) training after arriving in this country showed neither an improvement in mental health, nor a lower rate of psychiatric symptoms.[73] Westermeyer thus argued that people who attend ESL classes are not those who feel a need for language skills in order to better adapt to the workplace or to further their socialization, but, on the contrary, those who are unable to find jobs and those who are lonely. Moreover, if refugees simply attend ESL classes while having no other form of social interaction with English speaking people, they manage to learn only a few English words; even after years of study, they cannot engage in a "limited social conversation."[74] Among the one hundred two Hmong clients that Westermeyer followed for the space of a decade, more than half were unable to make friends with any non-Hmong. At all events, there can be no doubt that the circumstances which both suggest to the new arrival in America the value of, and surround the attainment of fluency in, the English language create tremendous stress within the Hmong adult population.[75]

The second predictor of psychiatric disorder in Hmong American populations has to do with the level of expectation upon first coming to this country. Those Hmong who expect to continue to "live their lives as before, to achieve wealth, or have a calm, peaceful life" were more at risk of becoming psychiatric patients than those who came with the expectation that they would work hard, study, and struggle.[76]

The third predictor of mental illness has to do with the nature of being dependent on public assistance; that is to say, Hmong refugees who have been on welfare are more likely to become psychiatric patients. These people have less self-esteem and less self-confidence than those who are economically self-sufficient, and exhibit a high degree of anxiety; occasionally even to the extent that they are fearful to leave the house to seek a job or go to school. The welfare system, in this way, creates an additional layer of isolation from mainstream American society. Westermeyer, in fact, feels that, in addition to the foregoing, the system has played a major role in creating and fostering dependency by rewarding precisely those refugees who are in the worst social position, and thus militates against those impulses which might be expected to lead to any improvement in that position.[77]

The fourth of Westermeyer's predictors of psychiatric disorder has to do with the "continuous in-country migrations in search of a mythical location like the country-of-origin," which are common among refugees, particularly the Hmong, who have historically resorted to migration as a means of dealing with problems. Such a migration pattern increases rates of unemployment, leads to high levels of psychiatric distress, and inhibits integration into and acculturation within mainstream American society.[78]

All of Westermeyer's predictors can be found in Colorado's Hmong community. The majority of adult Hmong refugees who came to the region had no command of English. Those who attend English classes have not made significant progress, and certainly have not mastered the language. Since America is often spoken of as a sort of "promised land;" that is, a nation of enormous potential for the individual, most Hmong refugees did not expect their new life to be difficult or financially disadvantaged. Those whose circumstances necessitate the receipt of disability income and/or Aid to Families with Dependent Children (AFDC) are often troubled by a deep-seated sense of shame, and are thus reluctant to leave the home to learn English, to find jobs, or to interact with mainstream service providers. In search of opportunity, many Hmong move in and out of Colorado according to economic conditions. An availability of jobs will attract job seekers, while a dearth of jobs will force many Hmong residents to move elsewhere in search of wages. This does nothing to ameliorate social problems in the Hmong community, and as community instability rises with economic instability, a few Hmong will move to other parts of the country simply to avoid family conflicts, something which further worsens social conditions.

In this fashion, many Hmong parents and elders are overwhelmed by the pace of change in their lives, their families, and their communities. Certainly, a new life in a new land has not come without a price. However, despite the challenges and hardships, many Hmong in Colorado have made tremendous progress in achieving a substantial level of material well-being and a standard of living which is commensurate with that of their neighbors, and is unquestionably greater than that which they have ever before enjoyed. Possessions such as comfortable homes, late model cars, and expensive, "hi-tech," luxury consumer electronics are all within reach of substantial numbers of these Hmong immigrants.

Yet other aspects of their lives, including general health and the education of children, have suffered. There is endemic physical distress, widespread emotional detachment, and, not infrequently, complete alienation. The many changes in life and living encountered by the Hmong have resulted in a variety of unpleasant and uncomfortable physical symptoms, such as carpal tunnel syndrome, various sorts of nerve and muscle pains, loss of appetite, sleeplessness, and indigestion. They have, as well, resulted in those family dysfunctions which can lead parents to divorce, children to the exhibition of emotional difficulties, and teens to fail in their studies, drop out of school, join youth gangs, and/or become involved with drug and alcohol abuse. Conventional health care professionals may label these symptoms "somatization," but the Hmong and their traditional healers will view these problems differently.

Chapter II

The Hmong Health System: A Literature Review

Among works available which treat Hmong health related beliefs and healing traditions, the works of the French anthropologist Jacques Lemoine,[1] Hmong American health administrator Bruce Thowpaou Bliatout,[2] English anthropologist Robert Cooper,[3] Thai anthropologist Nusit Chindarsi,[4] American freelance writer Ann Fadiman,[5] Thai-Australian Senior Lecturer Pranee L. Rice,[6] and Hmong American M. D. Xoua Thao[7] are the best, most original, and most thorough treatments. Other scholars touch on these considerations, but either provide only a few sentences, paragraphs, or pages; or simply cite the above works. Of such scholars, noteworthy are Adler,[8] Ensign,[9] Long,[10] O'Connor,[11] Quincy,[12] Her,[13] Henry,[14] Spring,[15] Waters et al.,[16] Nuttall and Flores,[17] Barrett et al.,[18] Warner and Mochel,[19] Westermeyer,[20] and Yang.[21]

HMONG ANATOMIC PERCEPTION: THE LIVER DEFINES A PERSON'S CHARACTER AND HEALTH CONDITIONS

The Hmong believe the liver to be the center of human emotion and the organ which regulates these emotions, just as Westerners associate the heart with these functions.[22] In Hmong tradition, the liver, therefore, may be expected to play a large role in health, mental stability, and overall personality. In fact, liver imagery figures large in those Hmong linguistic traditions which have evolved to describe the human character and health status. For example, the Hmong label a bad person "ugly liver;" *Siab Phem* in Hmong. A good person is called "white liver;" *Siab Dawb*. When a person is startled or badly frightened, his liver may "drop," rendering him "dropped liver," or *Poob Siab*.[23] This latter event can also cause the soul to

19

"fall down," or leave the body, which, in turn, may act to cause illness in the frightened person.[24]

HMONG COSMOLOGY

The Hmong traditional religion is generally considered a variety of animism, which may be said to incorporate a worship of ancestors, together with the belief that everything has a soul and that this soul transmigrates or "reincarnates."

To the Hmong, the realm of sentient beings is divided into two worlds, or *Ceeb*: *Yaj Ceeb* is the world inhabited by the living, and *Yeeb Ceeb* is the world of deceased ancestors and supernatural. Cooper draws parallels between *Yaj Ceeb* and the Chinese world of *Yang*, the world of light, where human beings, material objects, and nature coexist.[25] He compares *Yeeb Ceeb* to the Chinese world of *Yin*, the dark side of creation, where the spirits thrive. Symonds and Rice iterate similar concepts, referring to *Yaj Ceeb* as the world of light that consists of the living, and *Yeeb Ceeb* as the world of darkness which is associated with death and spirits.[26] According to Cooper, the Hmong believe that, long ago, people and spirits were able to meet and interact, but that latterly these two worlds, *Yaj Ceeb* and *Yeeb Ceeb*, have "become divided, and only the shaman may, with impunity, venture into the Otherworld and return safely."[27] Symonds and Rice, however, in seeming contradiction, assert that these two worlds of light and darkness are interconnected in such a way that souls and spirits can easily travel back and forth.[28]

HMONG GODS

Described in the literature are several supreme beings who inhabit the Hmong spirit world. Rice conducted research among Hmong refugees in Australia.[29] Her informants refer to a deity named *Huab Tais Ntuj*, who is the creator and ruler of the world. He is the king of heaven and governs everything in the universe, including people and animals. While he can see what human beings are doing on earth, he usually does not interfere.

Another deity, known as *Saub*, is believed to be one of *Huab Tais Ntuj's* lieutenants. It is believed that *Saub* provided the first seeds and made the first hen to lay eggs. According to legend, after the great flood receded from earth, it was *Saub* who told the surviving Hmong sister and brother to cut their shapeless baby into pieces and spread them all over the land, which formed the twelve original Hmong clans.[30]

Cooper claims that *Saub* is a kind deity who has become disinterested in human affairs for a while; nevertheless, he may "be appealed to in times of need,"[31] and is associated with fertility and reproduction.[32] The Hmong believe that *Saub* existed when humans were created, and that today he lives far away in the upper reaches of the Otherworld. As to this, Symonds states that *Saub* has wives, and, together, they live in heaven, rarely interacting with human beings.[33]

While *Saub* may be of a kindhearted disposition, Cooper reports that there are two Lords of the Otherworld who are fearful, dreaded figures.[34] The first of these is *Ntxwj Nyug*, "who judges the souls of the dead and determines an appropriate animal, vegetable, or human form of reincarnation."[35] *Ntxwj Nyug* lives on top of a mighty mountain and guards the gates through which the souls of the dead must pass before arriving at the village of the ancestors. *Ntxwg Nyug* enjoys great feasts, and keeps a great herd of heavenly cattle for this purpose which consists of the reincarnated souls of those judged deserving of punishment.[36]

The second fearful Lord of the Otherworld is *Nyuj Vaj Tuam Teem*, who "issues licenses for rebirth from behind a great writing desk, seated on a magnificent and terrifying throne."[37] *Nyuj Vaj Tuam Teem* and *Ntxwg Nyug* in tandem control the nature and extent of human life and death. As a correlative of this fact, when a person's lease of life has expired, the shaman is the only person who can intervene. To do so, he will attempt to negotiate with *Ntxwg Nyug* to extend its term.[38]

SPIRITS OR DAB

Apart from the spirits of departed ancestors and such major personalities as *Saub* and *Ntxwg Nyug*, the Hmong *Yeeb Ceeb* consists of many different spirits (*Dab*). Ovesen categorizes these spirits as follows: the spirits of the household; the spirits of medicine; the nature spirits; and the shaman's spirit helpers.[39] Cooper separates these four categories of spirits into two groups which he calls *Dab Nyeg* and *Dab Qus*.[40] The *Dab Nyeg* include household spirits, or *Dab Qhuas*, comprised of the spirit of the main household post, the spirit of the pillars, the spirit of the loft, the spirit of the cooking hearth, the spirit of the ritual hearth, the spirit of the bedroom, and the spirit of the front door; and the *Xwm Kab*.[41] The household members worship these spirits according to their clan customs. The *Xwm Kab*, discussed at length elsewhere, is considered to be the most important spirit of the house, since it protects family members and ensures the wealth of the household. The *Xwm Kab's* altar is made of a rectangular sheet of joss paper, hung on the wall opposite the front door. A chicken or a large pig is sacrificed to the *Xwm Kab* at the New Year celebration, and the feathers or hair, and blood, of the sacrificed animal is daubed on the altar.[42]

Herbalists and magic healers, *Khawv Koob*, worship the spirits of medicine known as *Dab Tshuaj*. When called upon, these spirits assist Hmong healers to exorcise the dangerous and evil spirits known as *Vij Sub Vij Sw*, which are held responsible for causing illness. Ovesen states that the *Vij Sub Vij Sw* are evil nature spirits, while Cooper refers to them as spirits of disaster and accident.[43] Hmong informants in Colorado agree with Cooper that the *Vij Sub Vij Sw* are spirits of disaster and accident. In a traditional herbalist's house, an altar for the spirit of medicine is set next to the *Xwm Kab's* altar.[44] However, some Christian Hmong herbalists now dispense their medical lore and treatments without an altar.

The spirits referred to as *Dab Qus* include these *Vij Sub Vij Sw* and those spirits which inhabit wild and uncultivated places. The Hmong, particularly in Asia, believe the *Dab Qus* are nature spirits, which, while not inherently malevolent, will both attack if disturbed and capture any wandering human soul they encounter.[45]

SOULS PLAY A VITAL ROLE IN HEALTH, HEALING, AND ILLNESS

Bliatout and Rice et al. note that the Hmong believe an individual has three main souls.[46] One soul occupies the head area, one the region of the torso, and one the leg area. When a person dies, one soul stays at the grave to watch over the site, one goes to heaven to join the ancestors, and one soul may reincarnate as either a human or other variety of being. Chindarsi, Fadiman, Westermeyer, and Quincy disagree on the number of souls possessed of an individual, since their informants provided them with inconsistent reports.[47] Some Hmong informants averred there were three souls, while others stated a belief in five or eight or thirty-two.

In fact, in every instance in which a scholar has inquired of a number of Hmong how many souls a person has, responses have been inconsistent. Some reply that a person has only one soul; others say two; still others state they do not know. Occasionally, informants will be quite startled, as if they have never before considered the matter. The same problem occurs when Hmong are asked about the number of a shaman's spirit helpers. It is a distinction between the Hmong and many of their Western interviewers that the Hmong have always adopted a casual attitude toward exact figures, and we may even say, with some justification, that the Hmong do not conceptualize things in the same way as do Westerners. Certainly there are those aspects of life in which precise knowledge is paramount to someone born and educated in the West, while, to a Hmong, a vague notion will suffice.

At all events, and whatever their number, all of a person's souls must remain in harmony with the body in order to maintain good health, and, should the person lose one or more of his souls, he will experience a variety of illnesses. Extending this belief somewhat, it is additionally held that greater the number of souls he loses, the more serious his illness will become. Moreover, the longer the soul or souls are separated from the body, the less treatable will be the illness.[48] When a soul has been wandering for some time, it may become lost permanently. It may be reincarnated. It may be transformed into something else. In such cases, wherein a soul cannot find its owner, or has been reincarnated or transformed, the owner will become seriously ill, and death will inevitably follow in short order.[49]

With such an emphasis on the status of the souls, it will be apparent that the Hmong perception of health and healing includes both the physical and the spiritual well being of an individual.[50] If a person receives a physical injury, the resulting wound, whether superficial or deep, can be treated with herbal medicines. The herbalists responsible for this sort of treatment, as well as Hmong traditional massage therapists and Hmong acupuncture specialists, are healers who deal with the physical aspects of an illness.[51] However, when a person falls ill it is considered a different matter, and a spiritual healer—such as a shaman, egg reader, or soul caller—will be consulted.[52] Every Hmong clan will, in all likelihood, number a few of these healers in its membership; every Hmong village or community be the residence of several.[53]

At the conclusion of this section it should be noted that the above presentation of Hmong cosmology, with its discussion of the universe, of gods, of spirits, and of souls, is, to some extent, shaped and colored by such modern developments as large scale conversions to Christianity; significant levels of Hmong immigration to the West—with the resulting exposure to Western philosophies and cosmologies, both ancient and modern; and the Western interpretations of Hmong customs and beliefs which have crept into the scholarly literature.

Certainly there is room for demur and debate. According to one Hmong healer and informant, for example, prior to contact with the West, and, most particularly, with Christianity, the Hmong view of the Otherworld and of *Ntxwg Nyug* were neither as dark and forbidding, nor as well defined, as the they are currently, and the number and diversity of the gods, spirits, and souls identified above must be seen as representing a fragmentation of Hmong tradition which has occurred over time. This fragmentation has been the result of, 1) the lack, until quite recently, of a system of writing, and thus of a benchmark historical record; 2) the lack, among Hmong leaders, of a consensus with regard to Hmong culture, beliefs, and customs; and, 3) misinterpretations of established ways by Hmong and non-Hmong alike.

According to this informant, in fact, to the Hmong there is only one god. Owing to the aforementioned lack of benchmark historiography, the name of this god down the years has been altered, subjected to change, and even lost. There exist now a plethora of names by which the Hmong divinity is known: *Huab Tais Ntuj, Saub, Ntxwg Yug, Tus Tswv Tsim Neeg, Pog Yawm Txwv Koob, Nkawm Niam Txiv Dab Pog* or *Nkawm Niam Txiv Kab Yeeb.* Yet, according to this healer, although these names are many, each refers to some aspect of that single celestial entity who created and still protects the Hmong people.

In the same vein, and with regard to the many spirits described above, this Hmong healer argues that belief in their existence is not common to all Hmong, and that, among those Hmong who accept them, their significance varies among clans and lineages. To employ a metaphor, the multiplicity of beliefs in such matters represents the countless leaves, flowers, and small branches on the tree of traditional Hmong life; a tree which has been transplanted countless times. Nonetheless, this healer believes that most Hmong, in particular those who are not very familiar with their own cultural history, take the position that there are many spirits (*Dab*). The most important of these will be presented in chapter four.

TRADITIONAL HMONG HEALTH TREATMENT TECHNIQUES
THE FIRST SHAMAN: SIV YIS

Siv Yis was sent to earth a long time ago by *Saub*, at a time when illness and death were rising as a judgment and a scourge on the part of *Ntxwg Nyug*.[54] *Saub* (alternatively *the Saub*) gave *Siv Yis* the power to cure disease, and in this *Siv Yis* was singularly successful, until, one day, he himself died and embarked on his return to the *Yeeb Ceeb* to live with the *Saub*. At the half way point on his climb up the celestial ladder which connects the two worlds, *Siv Yis* dropped his instruments, which tumbled and fell all the way back to earth. The people who picked up these precious utensils became the first shamans, and began to cure those afflicted with illness.[55]

HMONG SHAMANISM

A shaman (*tus ua neeb*) oversees the clan's mental, spiritual, and physical well being,[56] and serves as an intermediary between the physical and spiritual worlds.[57] The shaman's field of expertise is the prevention of disease and, if unsuccessful, its treatment; and the shaman's methodology involves donning a veil and entering a trance state in order to perform a variety of elaborate ceremonies.[58] The intent of these ceremonies is to communicate with spirits and to recruit their assistance in the elimination of pathology.[59]

In a novitiate parallel to that of the priesthood, the aspiring shaman must make radical changes in his life. He must fulfill all of the duties and responsibilities associated with shamanism, and observe all of the rules associated with his calling. These rules are many, and not a few of them are demanding. For example, his food must be washed, well stored, and properly prepared—no raw food is permitted him;[60] other Hmong may not touch his head; and he may not walk under a clothes drying rack or any other sort of pole, for this latter risks offending the spirits who accompany him wherever he goes.[61]

Although both male and female may become shamans, there tend to be more males who take up this calling.[62] Long observes that, owing to a shortage of men as the result of the Vietnam War, increasing numbers of women have lately become shamans and, of necessity, the Hmong have come to accept these women.[63]

According to Jacques Lemoine and others, Hmong shamanism is a particular psychotherapeutic methodology; it is a way of healing, not a religion.[64] Lemoine argues that a shaman is not a ritualist; however, many Christian missionaries disagree, and prefer to categorize Hmong shamanism as a "form of devil worship."[65] Perhaps as a result of this, missionaries generally target shamans specifically in their efforts to "spread the word of God." Many American Christian churches and Christian families have sponsored Hmong refugees who, immediately they arrive in the United States, are obligated to convert to Christianity and both eschew shamanism and forego any consultation with shamans.[66] This fact notwithstanding, many Christian Hmong will secretly consult shamans if their illness is prolonged and if prayer does not help.[67] Lemoine, Adler, Tapp, and Westermeyer believe that this attitude has contributed to the psychological distress that Hmong refugees often experience in their resettlement in the West.[68]

By custom, if a shaman engages in ritual activities, such as those traditionally appropriate to funerals or weddings, he must have additional qualifications beyond those required for the performance of other rites. All of these qualifications—singing, the playing of certain musical interludes, the performance of techniques specific to dealing with a corpse, and so on—have to be learned orally from an acknowledged expert. Yet, although he must serve an extended apprenticeship, a shaman is considered to inherit his calling, in contradistinction to a ritualist, per se, and thus may not be referred to, strictly speaking, as a ritualist.[69] Furthermore, while both the ritualist and the shaman must be trained by a master, and while both must pay fees for the knowledge they acquire, the activities of the shaman and the ritualist are quite different.[70] The shaman must explore the *Yeeb Ceeb*, or the Otherworld. He must travel to and familiarize himself with the "unseen part of reality in order to chase devils and restore somebody's health."[71] Separating an ordinary person and a shaman is chiefly that a shaman can, and frequently does, move at will into this unseen part of reality and act there.

In order to do so, the shaman will don a veil that covers his head, indicating that he is blind to the living and absent from this side of reality. A lamp is then lit on an altar, which aids the shaman in his travel to and through the unseen.[72] Furthermore, in order to enter the world of the unseen, a shaman must achieve a specific state of consciousness, which is accomplished through trance; a distinctive feature of Hmong shamanism.[73]

So important is this trance to the shaman's profession, that no one may become a shaman who lacks the ability to achieve this altered state of consciousness. In addition, trance is not merely a skill that can be obtained through physical or mental training. It is, on the contrary, an "inherited ability that one cannot have at will,"[74] and spirit helpers must assist in provoking the trance.[75] Still, such aids as finger bells, rattles, and gongs are used to create a tempo which conduces to achieving the trance state, and their use is often called upon to help the shaman to shift his consciousness while he sings along with the music made by these instruments. Despite the employment of such accessories, however, when the trance, as such, begins, it is invariably because, as the shamans themselves assert, the spirit helpers provoke it.[76]

THE SHAMAN'S VOCATION AND SPIRIT HELPERS

As well-versed as he is in the nature and progress of disease, the shaman knows when time is short. When the shaman is very sick and knows he will die, he calls his sons to his bedside and gives them a bowl of magic water from which to drink. This bowl is called "the dragon pond" (*Lub Pas Zaj*) because when the shaman invites or calls, the dragon that controls thunder and lightning comes to rest at this pond. With the ability to kill suddenly which they occasionally exhibit, the Hmong consider thunder and lightning to be the main sources of the magic arts. Thus, if the shaman invites the Thunder Dragon appropriately, it will become a powerful ally; another spirit helper.[77]

Drinking this dragon water (*Dej Zaj*), the shaman's sons will "absorb the essence of magic in their bones and flesh in order to keep it in the descent line."[78] The shaman's sons ingest the water, and, in so doing, ingest the power of their father, with the hope that any shamans in the family line will retain the loyalty and services of the father's spirit helpers. Ultimately, the father's hope is that one of the sons will achieve the status and abilities of a shaman, or, failing that, that he, himself, will be reborn into the family of one of his sons, become a shaman once again, and maintain the profession of shamanism in the family. When, at last, the shaman dies, his altar is destroyed and discarded in the jungle, while his sons keep his tools.[79]

For their part, the deceased shaman's spirit helpers do not actually set themselves up in the bodies of his sons. What will remain with the sons after they drink the magic water is not the spirit helpers themselves, but a token or mark of the former alliance between the elderly shaman and the spirit helpers. After the shaman has passed on and the funerary rites are completed, the spirit helpers will return to their heavenly home, where all Hmong shamans' spirit helpers are considered to live in the presence of *Siv*

Yis, the first shaman, who initiated the vocation, since all the world's shamans are the heirs of *Siv Yis's* talents.[80]

As for the shaman, master of the next world, upon his arrival in the realm wherein he had spent so many extended periods in life, he will join his spirit troops and be their leader (*Thawj Neeb*). When the shaman thinks the time appropriate, he will send two of his troops, the Spirit of the Trance (*Txheej Xeeb*) and the Inspiring Spirit (*Leej Nkaub*) to importune one of his sons. These two spirits are extremely important to any shaman's vocation, and, in this instance, they will prove their worth once again.[81] With the aim in view of bringing the son to the realization of his true calling, these twin spirits will visit upon him an attack of shivering, with pain and fever, until the son is driven to seek out a shaman's diagnosis. This shaman, making note of the obvious, will tell the patient that he must become a shaman and call the spirit helpers on a regular basis. If the patient agrees to do so, his illness will vanish as suddenly as it began, and he will begin to receive instruction from a shaman who will become his master.[82]

The training of a new shaman usually takes two to three years, since the new shaman must learn a great deal—how to summon the spirit helpers; the ways of the world beyond; the identities of the important souls; the various components of the self; the manners in which to restore the souls when they have been captured by other forces; and the identities and character of the different evil and wild spirits with which he will be called upon to contend.[83] He will find plenty of assistance, for the new shaman's "spirit helpers come to him already structured as a task force, with scout spirits, engineer spirits, horsemen and foot soldiers,"[84] while the "Trance Spirit" and the "Inspiring Spirit," who always accompany him, act as liaison and staff officers.[85]

Spirit help is indispensable to the shaman, and among shamans spirits are referred to with descriptive terms denoting creatures in the animal kingdom and insect world which share characteristics of feature and function. For example, the spider is used to describe the spirit vanguard of the engineers, who are able to wind a "copper and iron" thread for the spirit troops to settle upon. Other engineer spirits will help to build "copper and iron" suspension bridges over which spirit cavalry and spirit foot soldiers can cross from one space to another. Such a bridge and such a thread can be seen in the shaman's house on certain occasions, when cotton thread and a ritual cloth are stretched from the altar to the main door to represent these structures. The woodpecker, meanwhile, is used to denote a type of functional spirit helper which is able to pull worms of illness from the "bamboo" soul. The bear and elephant, both of which have great strength, represent other forms of assistance. Often the shaman will send an eagle spirit or a hawk spirit to catch a "shadow" soul that is flying or drifting away.[86]

PRACTICING SHAMAN

When a new shaman has finished his apprenticeship and is ready to practice his art, he installs a two-storied altar in his house.[87] The altar serves the same purpose as a "diploma" in his future vocation, and, like a diploma, can be seen hanging on the wall, showing prospective clients that he has earned his credentials.[88] There are differences, however. Once this altar has been hung, a newly certified shaman's master will call his spirit helpers and invite them to settle within. Nonetheless, although this altar "diploma" is hanging on the wall, training is not yet totally complete, for the master will come every year to help his disciple send his spirits on an annual holiday to *Siv Yis's* cave.[89]

Inevitably, clients soon begin to consult the new shaman at his home, or, when a prospective patient is very sick and unable to move, a family member will come to request a house call diagnosis. Should the shaman visit, he will bring his medical bag, containing a rattle, a gong, a veil, finger bells, and divination blocks, while the patient's family members set up a temporary altar to which the shaman can summon his spirits. When all is in readiness, the shaman sits on a bench and begins his ceremony. Rocking and bending forward and back, he mimes the riding of a horse, sometimes referred to as his "speedy steed." It is also occasionally considered that he has mounted a "dragon charger," or has even boarded a ship of clouds and wind.[90]

The first ceremony on this shaman's agenda explores the illness, in order to ascertain its cause, and the patient will not participate during this first, exploratory, ceremony.[91] Nevertheless, although no medication or other ameliorative measures are prescribed, if the shaman's diagnosis is correct, the patient will feel better in a few days. Such an abatement of symptoms is taken as prima facie evidence that the shaman's diagnosis was accurate, and the shaman will then be called back to perform the second part of his intervention; the healing per se. If, on the other hand, the patient does not feel better within a few days of the diagnosis, he will call another shaman or healer and request intervention.[92]

If the diagnosis has been a good one, however, and the patient begins to improve, the shaman will make promises to the evil or wild spirits, or gods, in order to effect his cure, and, to fulfill these promises, he must, with the patient's participation, perform a healing ceremony. This reprise of his diagnosis is a "dramatic re-enactment of his findings in the unseen," a revelation of the different causes of the sickness.[93] For example, if the diagnosis was that one of the patient's souls has been wandering away from the body, the shaman will call his spirit helpers to go with him to find the soul and bring it back.[94]

In contrast to the first ceremony, though, the patient is invited to sit in the center of the room during the second. The healing ceremony then progresses, and as soon as the shaman has indicated he has brought back the patient's wandering soul, his assistant will sacrifice a young pig. This pig's soul is used to augment, to protect, or to strengthen the patient's soul, and, in recompense to those spirits who assisted, the shaman burns joss money. The shaman then "builds a fence" around the patient's soul by circumambulating the pole to which the pig was bound, and by stamping blood from the pig on the back of the patient. The pig's soul must then be kept in a spirit prison the shaman has assigned it, even as the shaman maintains possession of the pig's lower jaw in a basket near his altar. At the time the shaman sends his spirit helpers on their aforementioned annual holiday, he will burn all the jaws he has thus collected, and the spirits of the sacrificed animals are then relieved of their duties and are set free.[95] In this way, a pig's life is used to replace, support, or repair a human life, for the Hmong believe that human and animal souls are composed of the same essential substance; one reason it is possible for a human to be reincarnated as an animal.[96]

A Hmong shaman is, in sum, responsible for two things. First, he must take over the patient's fight for life; and, second, he is responsible for the restoration of the self, the essential wholeness, of the patient. According to the lore of the Hmong shaman, this self consists of five different souls: the reindeer soul, or *Nyuj Cab Nyuj Kaus*; the protruding shadow, or *Ntsuj Duab Ntsuj Hlauv*; the running bull, or *Nyuj Rag Nyuj Ris*; the growing bamboo soul, or *Ntsuj Xyoob Ntsuj Ntoo*; and the chicken soul, or *Ntsuj Qaib Ntsuj Noog*.[97] This Hmong conception of the self, with its many components, is, in some sense, similar to the Freudian, and both conceptions serve the same purpose, i.e., by bringing back his runaway soul, the shaman helps the patient to restore his psychic balance.[98] Moreover, in taking over the patient's fight for life, the shaman must use his spirit troops to resist the influence of evil spirits on the souls of the patient. This situation bears certain parallels to that in which the Western doctor prescribes antibiotic medication for a patient who has a bacterial infection. There are, of course, significant differences, and exorcism is the most important part of the healing ceremony. The shaman often breaks into sudden, loud chanting, which is meant to scare away evil spirits, but often stuns the patient. Still, this helps prop up the patient's morale,[99] and the shaman will, in addition, use magic water to cleanse and purify, blowing the water over the patient.[100]

These evil spirits are spiritual entities which may be of several varieties. It may be either the spirit of a deceased family member; a spirit of malicious character which has been sent to do harm by someone who bears one ill will; or a nature spirit, such as the spirit of a river or the spirit of a cave, either of which may have become offended by a human's unwanted approach.

HERBAL MEDICINES

In Laos, Thailand, and China, Hmong villages are generally located hundreds of miles from a modern medical facility, and, as a result, the Hmong are generally called upon to use their own medicines to treat illness. These medicines derive from animals, plants, flowers, leaves and other, comparable, sources,[101] and are used along with shamanism to cure illness.[102]

For the most part, Hmong herbalists absorb plant lore from their mothers or other family members; however, it is widely conceded across the board that the effectiveness of any herbal medicine depends largely on the attention given to preparing it,[103] and, while one herb can be used to cure more than one illness, generally at least two or three herbs are used in combination to cure but a single complaint.[104] More Hmong females than males specialize in herbal medicine,[105] but, of course, not all Hmong women have access to the knowledge of herbs, and, unless the expert is a close family member, anyone who wishes to learn this science is expected to pay a fee.

Much like the shaman, the Hmong herbalist is a highly respected individual in society; one who employs herbal medicines to treat both physical and mental ailments. Through centuries of trial and error, Hmong herbalists have gathered knowledge about medicinal and edible plants, and have learned how to prepare them so that any poisons are removed even as the medical efficacy of the resulting product is maximized.[106]

It is unfortunate that the extremely extensive herbal lore resulting from centuries of folk research will be lost as the elderly die, for few young people are interested to learn the healing practices.[107] Every attempt, one is prompted to assert, must be made to save this storehouse of botanical science for future generations, lest information gleaned from literally hundreds of years of wilderness experimentation be lost forever.

The value of this knowledge to modern researchers cannot be doubted. In an attempt to examine the modern relevancy of medicinal properties in Hmong herbal preparations, Spring identified thirty-seven medicinal plants cultivated by the Hmong community in Minnesota.[108] She used "western biomedical criteria of efficacy," to investigate these plants, conducted literature research, and sent plant samples to a laboratory for chemical analysis. The results indicated that ninety-two percent of the plants were found to have medicinal properties—a staggering statistic by any standard—while about eighty-one percent are used frequently by the Hmong in their diet, something which no doubt serves to inhibit illness.[109]

MASSAGE THERAPISTS

In combination with, and as a supplement to, the above mentioned methodologies, the Hmong use massage as a healing technique to alleviate many kinds of bodily aches. A skillful massage therapist can bring relief to muscle pain, nervous discomfort, and stomach ache, and will do so without causing pain or irritation to the skin,[110] despite occasionally rubbing the affected area with juices extracted from herbs, or with oil or other ointments.

TECHNIQUES OF DERMAL ABRASION

Rubbing the skin is a timeless treatment, and the Hmong and many other Southeast Asians practice dermal abrasion techniques such as coining, pinching, cupping and spooning.[111] A reddening of the skin is often the result of these treatments, and this reddening is, unfortunately, occasionally mistaken for a sign of injury. Such is not the case, and the discoloration associated with techniques of dermal abrasion should not be mistaken for a sign of abuse, particularly child abuse.[112] Hmong use other, somewhat more invasive, methods of dermal treatment, as well, such as burning, acupuncture, and bloodletting. Powders and potions are also applied to the skin, and steam treatment and the maintenance of a hot-cold balance are practiced.[113]

All of the Hmong treatments; all the concepts of health, healing, and illness; and all of the Hmong spiritual beliefs discussed heretofore have a tremendous importance in the lives of the Hmong in America. All bear heavily both upon the experiences of the Hmong with Western biomedicine and on the interactions of the Hmong with those who practice it. Not all of these experiences and interactions have been favorable; in fact, there have been significant difficulties. Several Hmong American parents have been wrongly accused of child abuse due to the temporary reddening left on the skin of their children in consequence of the use of the healing techniques of dermal abrasion.[114] Some Hmong families have been accused of the inhumane treatment of animals due to the practice of animal sacrifice in the various shaman's ceremonies.[115] American courts, holding that Hmong traditional healing practices are not sufficiently effective in the treatment of disease, have ordered many Hmong parents to bring their children in for treatment by mainstream health care physicians and facilities.[116]

A classic presentation of the issues raised by such disagreements and difficulties is the very pertinent and well-written book, *The Spirit Catches You and You Fall Down*, by Ann Fadiman.[117] In a very readable literary style, Fadiman documents the health care interactions between Lia Lee, her parents, and American physicians and nurses. When she was three months old, Lia began to experience a progressive and unpredictable form of epilepsy. Her Hmong parents defined her illness as *Qaug Dab Peg*, which translates as "the spirit catches you and you fall down." Lia's mainstream health care providers, however, defined her problem as epilepsy, and the girl's physicians prescribed Depakene and Valium to control her seizures. Lia's parents, believing one of the girl's souls had become lost, commissioned a shaman's ceremony and sacrificed animals to bring the straying soul back. With each faction aware of the other's treatment, some of the girl's care providers tried to understand and sympathize with the parents' beliefs; many others considered those beliefs simple ignorance.

In the course of her very engaging book, Fadiman vividly illustrates many aspects of Hmong culture, and demonstrates the mistakes, misperceptions, and misunderstandings which may ensue when conventional health care providers attempt to serve Hmong patients and their families. In but one notable instance, the Hmong shaman and Hmong elders who had joined forces in the treatment of Lia tied "blessing strings" around the girl's wrist to protect her soul from evil influences. Shortly thereafter, Lia's American nurses, in a demonstration of acute cultural insensitivity, removed what they referred to as the "dirty ties."

The difficulties were not all on one side, however. Even as the nurses removed Lia's blessing strings, Lia's parents were juggling her medication, and often increased or decreased her dosage according to their assessment of her condition. Not infrequently, they withheld the medication altogether. In addition, more often than not the girl's parents interpreted the physicians' caring and careful actions as harmful and uncaring acts, and maintained a suspicious vigilance of the doctors even as they continued to mistrust American medicine. For their part, the treating physicians were dumbfounded as to why Lia's parents would refuse to follow their instructions, and ultimately obtained a court order to remove Lia from her family and have her parents labeled unfit.[118]

Fadiman's book constitutes an excellent representation of the crosscultural difficulties encountered by one Hmong patient and her family as they attempted to come to terms with the conventional American health care system while, at the same time, viewing health care options through the prism of traditional Hmong medical beliefs and making health care decisions based upon traditional Hmong medical lore. The following pages will serve to further illustrate the dilemma faced by Lia Lee's family and others, as Hmong Americans avail themselves of the American mainstream health care system, and cope—or fail to cope—with its shortcomings in dealing with those who hold cultural expectations very different from those of most Americans.

HMONG AMERICANS' EXPERIENCE WITH CONVENTIONAL MEDICINE

In the literature concerning Hmong social adjustment to life in America, there are several documents dealing with Hmong Americans' experiences in attempting to access conventional medical sources and facilities. This literature includes topics such as Hmong Sudden Unexpected Nocturnal Death Syndrome (SUNDS); interactions with conventional health care providers and concomitant attitudes toward conventional medicine; health status, illness and disease; substance abuse; psychological and psychiatric issues; food preparation, nutrition and diet; preventive medicine; and prenatal care, pregnancy, and birth. Some of these topics will be discussed at length in other sections of this book. It may be said in summary, however, that despite a substantial Hmong presence in the United States for two decades, many United States health care providers still know very little about the Hmong, their history, culture, beliefs, and practices.[119] Acknowledging, understanding, and respecting the beliefs and practices of an ethnic group are essential to providing quality health care to that population,[120] and lead to the improvement of patient satisfaction, trust, and compliance. This, in turn, must result in a greatly enhanced health outcome.[121] Frustration, aggravation, and confrontation are avoided, while the increased knowledge of different peoples and cultures can serve as a source of personal and professional enrichment for medical professionals.[122] Physicians should neither stereotype patients nor generalize about a certain patient population, and, in many ways, Southeast Asians are as different from each other as they are from those born and raised in the West. Beyond this, the level of acculturation among Southeast Asians differs from person to person, with the result that health care interactions need to be tailored to the individual.[123]

Waters et al. and Fadiman argue that it takes patience, time, and a continuum of positive interaction for Western health care providers to establish relationships with Hmong patients.[124] Those authors believe that Hmong mistrust of and suspicion regarding health care providers is the result of a dearth of experience with Western medical practice before coming to America. In a similar vein, Gervais argues that a long history of suppression of the Hmong by the dominant culture wherever they found themselves, taken together with their experiences as refugees, have rendered many of them prone to mistrust authority.[125] One result of this unpleasant history, but by no means the only one, is that most Hmong are concerned they may be made the subjects of medical experiments.[126]

Many Hmong, particularly the elderly, are illiterate, and, in addition, the practice of keeping medical records is something that does not exist in their culture. As a corollary, few patients are accustomed to the practice of asking questions regarding a family's health history, or the causes of death of family members. Neither is the usual practice of Hmong healers.[127] In fact, such interactions tend to remind Hmong patients of the interrogations of communist soldiers which so many have been forced to endure, and, not surprisingly, make them extremely uneasy. For this reason, as much as any other, it is important that health care providers explain to Hmong patients the significance of and necessity for assessing a patient's health history.

Waters et al. state that it is difficult to uncover specific information on a Hmong patient's past medical history inasmuch as dates and diagnoses of previous illnesses are usually not recollected, if they were ever known.[128] Furthermore, a Hmong patient's stated age may not be correct because the Hmong, especially those born in Laos before the 1970s, do not celebrate birthdays and keep no record of the date.[129]

Information that can be ascertained regarding a Hmong family history will often be little more than that one or more close family members have died, usually in Laos and at a young age.[130] A Western health care practitioner may assume that those members died from familial or genetic disorders; but when being probed for the cause of death, the patient will ultimately admit that their loved one died in the war, or became ill and died without seeing a doctor or visiting a health care facility.[131]

Another factor that tends to engender mistrust in the Hmong is that Hmong healers traditionally do not charge their patients a set fee, for Hmong patients usually pay healers according to their ability, and only after the malady has been alleviated.[132] Thus, many Hmong have come to feel that Western medicine is priced too high, and, in consequence, will usually wait until they have insurance coverage before seeking health care.[133]

There are, however, other barriers to the utilization of Western health care facilities aside from mistrust. These include a lack of access to providers, a lack of transportation, and an inability to speak English. All of these factors can and do contribute to delays in seeking and receiving health care.[134]

Beyond all this, many Hmong consider it rude or impolite to "get straight to business." In a health care interaction with a Hmong patient, therefore, it is usually more productive to begin with some small talk, such as an inquiry about family members, or other such pleasantries, prior to inquiring about the patient's health.[135] In general, it may be said that Hmong tend to be reserved, modest, and even shy, and demonstrate a passive-obedient manner. Reluctance to express strong emotions, and stoicism, are recognizable cultural traits.[136] It should not be surprising, in light of this, that to undress for a physical examination is extremely embarrassing, and provokes a good deal of anxiety. In such a situation, most Hmong females will be observably uncomfortable with the presence of male translators and health care providers.[137] By tradition, Hmong women talk about their physical problems only with their husbands, not men in general,[138] and, of course, all matters touching on sexuality, pregnancy, family planning, and birth are sensitive topics that likewise may be difficult to discuss.[139] For all the preceding reasons, an awareness of and respect for Hmong patients' inherent modesty is recommended, together with an attempt to provide same-sex translators and care providers.[140]

CULTURAL INFLUENCES IN HEALTH CARE PRACTICE

Biomedical systems in the United States reflect Western values and culture, which emphasize individualism, patient autonomy, and a "rational model of decision-making."[141] Similarly, Hmong health care practices reflect Hmong cultural beliefs and values. These place a heavy emphasis on family, clan, and communal decision-making.[142] To the Hmong, the Western emphasis on individual patient autonomy is seen as isolation and alienation.[143] Thus, these two opposing world views and sets of expectations, Western and Hmong, often clash when a medical crisis occurs and the Hmong seek conventional health care services.[144] It has been the informal observation of the author that many Hmong and their local health care providers often interact with little understanding of each other's worldview with respect to health care treatment.

Hmong society is male dominant and organized into a large, closely-knit community known as the clan. Within this structure, the well-being of the family and of the clan is considered to be more important than that of the individual, and a clan leader's decisions will therefore reflect what he considers to be the best interests of the whole clan.[145] However, since the first generation of Hmong refugees to be educated in this country have grown up in an American environment of "rugged individualism," to use President Herbert Hoover's oft-quoted phrase, many, having become adults and established their own families, are markedly disinclined to consult with or depend upon clan leaders, parents, or elders to make decisions for them. This group frequently use the conventional health care system, and dealing with them is easier for health care providers than dealing with others. However, inasmuch as there is tension between this younger generation and the older clan leaders or parents, a young adult Hmong patient may not only have to deal with the stress induced by illness and the necessity of accommodating the treatment requirements of conventional health care providers, but, in addition, will be forced to manage the tension induced by conflict with the older generation. If he follows his physician's recommendations, he may contravene the wishes of his parents and clan leaders and be caught in the middle of two opposing camps; not a pleasant eventuality at the best of times, and worse when one is sick.

Many Hmong American patients may therefore consult with both the herbalist, the shaman, the clan leader, or with other family members, as well as consulting with conventional health care providers.[146] Health care providers need to realize that several people may be exerting an influence upon or be involved in a patient's care, and, in such a case, welcoming and accepting clan input can be very helpful.[147] It is suggested, then, that providers be aware of clan influence and prepare to accommodate it early on.[148] The issue of family members making health care decisions for the patient is not, of course, unique to the Hmong culture; this health behavior can also be found among other Asian cultures. Ohnuki-Tierney details the manner in which Japanese family members and doctors form teams to make decisions on health treatment for patients.[149] Kleimen describes health care transactions on Taiwan in a similar manner.[150]

In addition to the above, a generalized respect for authority and for the elderly is emphasized in Hmong society.[151] As a result, Hmong may exhibit a desire to please those in authority and may seem to accept the health care provider's recommendations, while, at the same time, intending to take different actions.[152] Such alternative actions on the part of the patient sometimes result in conflict, even to the extent, in the case of children's care, for example, of requiring the intervention of law enforcement personnel. This can serve to create additional confusion and frustration.[153] When Hmong patients occasionally refuse physicians' recommendations, it will be helpful if providers attempt to respect those choices to the extent they can do so.[154] Historically, it has been the case that older doctors, particularly males, tend to exhibit more respect and deference than others when dealing with Hmong in difficult situations.[155]

It is certainly true that, for those born and raised in the West, dealing with other cultures is a multicultural challenge. However, it would seem that, in order to make the benefits of modern medicine available to all people of non-Western cultural backgrounds, it will be necessary for those concerned to respect values other than their own.[156] Conventional health care professionals may wish to "learn to care for people whose views of the self, family, community, time, causality, and spirituality" differ from the "temporally bounded, individualistic, and mechanistic perspectives that prevail in Western culture,"[157] and there can be no doubt that meeting the health care needs of the Hmong population is an excellent means of coming to grips with the differences to be encountered when crossing cultural lines.

FEAR OF SURGERY AND AUTOPSY

Among those things which stimulate feelings of discomfort and unease in the Hmong, the twin notions of surgery and autopsy are prominent. The Hmong are hesitant to have surgery for several reasons; some fear their surgically removed organs and other body parts will be missing when reincarnation takes place; some fear that after surgery their bodies will be weakened and their life expectancy shortened; some are concerned lest incisions open access into the body for evil spirits.[158] Some Hmong believe that if something is removed from the body, the patient may be reborn in a deformed state, his descendants disfigured in a similar manner.[159] Bliatout reports that all of his seventy Hmong informants in Portland, Oregon, believe that surgery is likely to cause some kind of disability, and that surgery conducted on the lower torso area can impair a person's reproductive capacity.[160] Other Hmong have voiced suspicions that American physicians want to surgically experiment on the Hmong.[161] Finally, Waters et al. argue that Hmong are afraid of surgery because in Laos, surgery has often tended to result in disability or death.[162] Payer, who compares the American perspective on medicine with the French, British, and West German views, concludes that the "American system promotes a far more invasive, aggressive kind of medical treatment, which may well serve certain kinds of medical problems, but which may not always be appropriate or even helpful for others."[163] Lonsdorf et al. posit that, when considering the overall health of the patient, this invasive, aggressive, American model of health treatment may lead to situations in which the cure becomes worse than the disease.[164] Surgery rates in the United States are, after all, "two to three times higher than those in Europe."[165] For instance, the rate of breast cancer in the United States is similar to that in Europe in recent decades, but mastectomies were performed in New England three times more often than in England or Sweden. Even the diagnostic tests in the United States seem invasive and aggressive, and there is more drawing of blood and cutting of flesh for such tests than in any other nation.[166] Since the Hmong are newcomers in the United States, they can be expected to notice and react more strongly to what may be an excessive reliance on surgery than do long-term American residents. Unlike most American citizens, who often express a concern with certain parts of the body only—such as, for example, the heart—demand a quick medical fix, and are thus "supporting a quick-fix system," the Hmong are more concerned about the overall health condition after surgery is performed, and about the surgery's long-term consequences.

The nature and conduct of autopsy is a subject with which few human beings, save coroners and career pathologists, are entirely comfortable, and the Hmong are no different. If they differ from others in their unease with the topic, it is because that, as Cheon-Klessig et al. note, the Hmong believe an autopsy is done because American doctors want to eat the organs of the dead.[167] For that reason, and fearing that autopsy will retard reincarnation,[168] the Hmong routinely refuse to allow autopsies on deceased relatives. In the opinion of the author, however, there is more to it than that. Although it may seem paradoxical to non-Hmong, the Hmong continue to love, revere, and respect their departed dear one as much after death as before. If their loved one were still alive, they reason, he would certainly not allow anyone to dissect him; and, therefore, it is incumbent upon them to ensure that such a procedure not take place now, when their loved one is incapable of uttering a protest. It follows that the corpse must be laid to rest as a whole entity.

Yet another aspect of the rationale for refusing autopsy is that it is central to the Hmong ethos to care for family members and relatives. One of the reasons the Hmong have many children and build large families is to ensure they will always have a loved one to care for them when they are ill, disabled due to injury or age, and even dead. This principle does not apply merely when family members and relatives are still living, but even after they have passed on. We have seen that rituals for the spirits of departed ancestors are mandatory to the Hmong from time to time, and the same sense of perpetual concern for the welfare of ancestors which enables these rituals likewise animates the perpetual Hmong concern for family members, friends, and loved ones. Thus, by tradition, most Hmong will feel they have betrayed a deceased family member, relative, or other dear one in allowing an autopsy to be performed.

MEDICATION

Although a majority of Hmong tend to feel most comfortable using Hmong herbal medicines, or medicines prescribed by Western doctors, and will use them first, many Hmong use a variety of Thai and Chinese medicines purchased without prescription from local Thai or Chinese grocery stores.[169] In Laos, medicines are often shared among family members, and this practice is maintained in the United States.[170]

As is the case with many Southeast Asians, most Hmong tend to stop taking medicine immediately they begin to feel better, or when the medicine seems no longer efficacious.[171] The idea that one needs to continue taking the medication for a period of time even after one feels well is a concept foreign to most Hmong.[172] Similarly, Vawter and Babbitt, Cheon-Klessig et al., and Fadiman suggest that Hmong Americans tend not to take prescribed medicines because they find the side effects of many unacceptable.[173] Uba considers that another reason some Southeast Asians do not take prescribed medications is that some believe "Asians have a different physical constitution than Whites, so...Western drugs and drug dosages that are appropriate for white persons may not be appropriate for Asians,"[174] and Lonsdorf et al. concur with this Asian view of the dangers of conventional health care medications.[175]

Besides considering the United States a "surgical nation," Lonsdorf et al. also label the country a "drug-oriented nation."[176] They point out that American physicians prescribe drugs more often, and with higher doses, than physicians in other nations of the world, and, as a consequence, higher rates of side effects are prevalent in the United States. Cited is the tendency of Americans to resort to medication to alleviate mental health problems, asserting that psychiatrists in America usually recommend drug dosages that are "ten times higher. . . . than elsewhere."[177] Gallin suggests that, even with such large dosages of medication, the success rate of psychological health treatment in the West is not high.[178]

PHYSICIAN-PATIENT RELATIONS

Waters et al., O'Connor, Ohnuki-Tierney, Lonsdorf et al., and Fadiman argue that one of the shortcomings of conventional medicine is that it is so egocentric.[179] By this it is meant that many conventional health care providers, believing that biomedicine is the best approach to treatment of illness and disease—in fact, that that biomedicine is the only correct approach—are, in consequence, intolerant of or uninterested in other medical practices, expect their patients to accept their advice without demur, and take it for granted that their patients will obediently follow their prescriptions. A resistant patient is considered either stubborn, ignorant, or non-compliant, and will tend to make the health care provider impatient, even angry.

Nonetheless, inasmuch as the Hmong have historically never responded well to the authoritarian approach, provider-patient relationships involving the Hmong are extremely delicate. The provider's behavior and actions will have major repercussions and consequences.[180] Hmong patients may feel insulted or confused when health care providers are not interested in their opinion of or impression about their condition.[181] Talking to these Hmong patients in a conversational manner, while, at the same time, soliciting their opinion with regard to their condition, can help to develop rapport and improve culturally sensitive health care issues.[182]

On the community level, too, confidence and trust are of great importance, while relationships which have been established gradually can be ruined with a single mistake or negative experience; something which will result in a bad reputation throughout the Hmong community for a clinic, a doctor, or a hospital. Should a single Hmong have such a bad experience, the story will often spread rapidly through an entire clan; even the whole Hmong community. This can and does result in all clan members, or the whole community, joining to boycott a specific hospital or doctor.[183] It is crucial, therefore, that health care providers take time to educate the patient, listen to his opinions, and explain what is happening.[184]

FORECASTING HARM

When Hmong patients fail to comply with the suggestions or instructions of health care providers, especially in serious or life-threatening situations, health care providers will usually attempt to pressure the patient with a demonstration of the gravity of the situation, saying, for example, "If you don't do what I say, then. . ." This weighty-sounding ultimatum is usually followed by the delineation of some variety of terrifying outcome, very often death.[185] It should be noted, however, that there are a great many Hmong who believe that, in making such a statement, the health care provider is actually forecasting the harm of which he speaks, or even causing it to happen much in the nature of a curse. Few Hmong will listen to providers they believe have hexed them,[186] and, should the harmful event warned of subsequently occur, the patient, together with family and friends, may hold the speaker responsible.[187]

A more positive and indirect approach is usually more successful. Speaking in gently persuasive and friendly tones is recommended. For example, the health care provider might say, "If this medicine is taken regularly, you will feel better and live longer."[188] In other words, health care providers should, whenever possible, avoid making negative statements or predictions and "focus on the patient;" on the "here and now."

KINDNESS IS ESSENTIAL

According to Barrett et al. and Fadiman, Hmong patients almost unanimously state that they desire health care providers who show a sense of caring, together with a happy and positive attitude.[189] The Hmong will consider a kind word or a smile an important adjunct to good care, and, in fact, will go so far as to consider basic human kindness the single most essential attribute of good health care providers. Hmong patients appreciate providers who are friendly, kindhearted people, with a pleasant attitude. O'Connor also observes that Hmong patients are more cooperative when health care providers treat them with respect and deal with them as equals.[190]

COMPROMISING AND BARGAINING

Consonant with the above, Waters et al. state that, when providing health care service to the Hmong, it is often advisable, and sometimes necessary, to compromise or bargain.[191] This can help to establish a rapport in non-life-threatening situations, and will certainly serve as an investment in future health care interactions. However, when Hmong patients and their families disagree with health care providers in more serious, or life-threatening, cases, the situation may become more complex. In addition to involving clan and/or community members in the decision-making process, Hmong patients and their families will, in such a case, often want to have a second opinion from another doctor.[192] In the interim, the patient will be growing increasingly ill. It has happened many times, for example, that an obstetric patient's primary health care provider has had to call the patient's clan leaders in the middle of the night to obtain consent for a Cesarean section.[193]

Western society allows a person who is felt to be of sound mind the right to refuse medical intervention for any reason. In contrast, when Hmong parents' beliefs or wishes prevent their sick child from receiving medical care, United States health care providers are legally required to report the case to government authorities. This abstraction of parental authority has been very problematic when dealing with the Hmong.[194] In some such cases, Child Protective Service (CPS) has been reluctant to get involved unless the case is a life-threatening emergency. Leery of any possibility of antagonistic encounter, they proceed with great caution when involving themselves in the Hmong community.[195] Indeed, any involvement on the part of the government which is considered to be inappropriate may bring adverse consequences, and Hmong families who are under pressure from medical authorities or government officials, or both, may move out of town or go underground,[196] which may only worsen an already bad situation. For these reasons, then, health care providers should use good judgment when acting in advocacy for Hmong children's safety and health.[197]

DRAWING BLOOD

Blood tests are another source of cultural dissonance for the Hmong, and most Hmong do not like to have blood drawn, even when they are sick.[198] Hmong women often refuse prenatal care because they are afraid of blood tests.[199] Some Hmong even believe that tubes of blood are drawn from patients on the basis of a variety of specious excuses, only to be sold later to enhance personal finances. It is even thought that such blood samples are transfused into elderly Americans to enhance their longevity.[200]

Like most people, Hmong believe that blood is essential in maintaining a healthy body. There are, however, additional and culturally sensitive issues involved. Blood, it is felt, keeps the body warm and assists in maintaining a balance between the functions of all the bodily systems. Removing too much blood from the body will thus interfere with that balanced state of those same bodily systems which is such a necessity for good health and a feeling of well-being. In the case of one already sick, drawing an excess of blood from a patient may cause him additional harm.[201] It is important, therefore, to explain to a Hmong patient the reason for drawing blood, and to assure him that only a safe amount of blood will be taken.[202]

PATIENT AIDS

It is common practice for Western health care providers to furnish patients with brochures, reading materials, and handouts for explanatory and educational purposes. However, these materials may be of little use to the Hmong, since many Hmong cannot read English or even their own language.[203] This is only partly due to illiteracy in the Western sense of that term, for Hmong traditional culture has not laid great emphasis on written records. In fact, the Hmong did not have a written language until the 1950s, when Christian missionaries developed a romanized alphabet for the Hmong language. Quite frequently, even literate Hmong patients have some degree of difficulty in making sense of aid materials, inasmuch as they cannot grasp the level of abstraction inherent in the concepts discussed therein.[204] This is not to say that such materials are of no use. Models, illustrations, diagrams, and pictures can be helpful in communicating health information to Hmong patients, but health care providers should make the effort to ensure their presentation of health information is fairly concrete and culturally relevant to Hmong patients.[205] Showing the patients their CAT scans or X-rays can help them to better understand their condition, in addition to demonstrating a friendly and helpful attitude.[206]

INTERNAL CONDITIONS

Internal or "invisible" illnesses, especially those with subtle or few physical manifestations, may be difficult for Hmong patients to understand. Blood abnormalities like anemia, electrolyte imbalances, and hypercholesterolemia are perplexing and new concepts. Hmong patients are more reluctant to treat asymptomatic chronic diseases like diabetes, hypertension, and hyperlipidemia than to treat acute, symptomatic illnesses.[207] The details surrounding one not uncommon condition may serve to illustrate. Hmong children experience the same frequency of incidence and degree of severity in lead poisoning as other inner-city children living in the sorts of older housing that retains lead-based paint, and some Hmong children have been screened with high levels of lead poisoning. At the same time, however, and unbeknownst to health care providers, certain of the Hmong traditional medicines actually include lead, and thus it is not impossible that these medicines may actually contribute to the high level of lead found in Hmong children.[208] At the same time, Hmong children with elevated physiological lead levels show few symptoms, so that it is a challenge to explain the dangers of such an invisible substance to Hmong parents. It is even more complicated to explain the treatment for lead intoxication, which ranges from doing nothing other than strip off or otherwise remove old lead based paint to hospitalizing the child. In the latter case, chelating agents will be given intravenously via painful injections, and, having once seen this, Hmong parents will often refuse permission when additional chelating treatments are medically necessary.[209] The real problem is that, whether or not the child receives treatment, he usually seems the same to the parents, which can result in confusion and in additional hazard to the child's health.

THE HOSPITAL EXPERIENCE

Bliatout states that the Hmong fear of hospital stays consists of two different aspects: 1) fear of ghosts, and, 2) fear of hospital personnel.[210] In Laos, from which nation most Hmong have emigrated to the United States, many doctors are poorly trained and medical facilities are neither modern nor well-equipped, so that what hospital experience most Hmong have had prior to their arrival in this country has not been favorable.[211] In consequence, hospitalization is a frightening experience for Hmong patients, to be avoided if possible,[212] and Hmong will go to the hospital only as a last resort, when traditional healing methods have failed.[213] In such a case, often the patient is already in critical condition, and, nearly as often, he does not return home. Thus, many Hmong view the hospital as a place where people go to die, and are afraid of hospitalization, most particularly the elderly.[214]

The Hmong bear a special antipathy for hospitals affiliated with teaching institutions, being concerned that patients may be used as subjects for experimentation.[215] It bewilders these same Hmong even more when many medical personnel, including nurses, students, doctors, residents, and other specialists are invited to deliveries of health information, as well as seemingly informal and certainly impersonal discussions about and examinations of the patient. It is self-evident, therefore, that efforts to identify and assign a single individual as the patient's doctor throughout the course of treatment will be helpful.[216]

In traditional Hmong culture, ancestor worship and animism form the core of the belief system and influence almost every aspect of daily life. According to this belief system, people, animals, plants, natural phenomena, and even many inanimate objects all possess souls, and therefore must be respected.[217] It follows that Hmong relationships with good and evil spirits are important.[218] Hmong also believe in the yin-yang concept of opposing natural forces, popularized by Sinologists, according to which it is important to maintain balance, bodily warmth, and equilibrium.[219] Hmong elderly patients will accordingly not eat cold food or drink cold liquid when they are sick.

On the practical level, one significant corollary of the above is that string bracelets are very frequently worn by Hmong children, tied onto young wrists by elders as a form of blessing. It is believed that these string bracelets connect the children to the spirits of their ancestors and protect their souls from leaving their bodies.[220] Western health care providers should understand the importance of these bracelets, which should not be removed under any circumstances—for example to start an intravenous line or put in place a hospital identification bracelet.[221]

In addition, most Hmong believe in reincarnation and a form of predetermination according to which an individual's fate and life span are set at birth and cannot be changed,[222] while, somewhat paradoxically, actions taken in this life will positively or negatively affect the next.[223] In conjunction, the Hmong believe that when it is time for a person to die, he will die no matter how hard we may try to prevent it.[224] It follows from this that sometimes the Hmong family of a critically ill patient will not seem to demonstrate the same level of anxiety or concern as Westerners. This, of course, is due both to death's inevitability, and to the fact that death for the Hmong is not a final stage in life, but a chance to be joined with ancestors and to be reincarnated. In further contrast to the Western view, most Hmong value living harmoniously and maintaining a good quality of life over the widely-held Western goal of prolonging life at all costs.[225] Therefore, they feel there is no need to make the patient's life miserable by connecting artificial life support systems or equipment when an illness or condition is not curable. On the contrary, most Hmong, especially members of the older generation, prefer that a person be allowed to die naturally at home, rather than in a hospital.[226]

HMONG HEALTH STATUS AND DISEASES

Upon first arriving in the United States, Hmong refugees displayed a high incidence of malaria, tuberculosis, hepatitis, parasitic infestation, syphilis, anemia, malnutrition, and blood dyscrasias.[227] Less common conditions included hypertension, urinary and vaginal infections, preeclampsia, diabetes, and gonorrhea.[228] According to Smith, this high incidence of disease has shifted as the Hmong have settled in America.[229]

Gjerdingen and Lor estimate that the Hmong have the highest rate of hepatitis B infection among all Southeast Asian populations.[230] They state that the Southeast Asian population in Georgia, for example, which includes Vietnamese, Cambodian, and Lao families, show lower rates of hepatitis B infection than the Hmong population in Wisconsin. Among Southeast Asian children aged nine or ten years in Georgia, approximately twenty percent were infected, compared to twenty-five to forty-two percent of the Hmong in Wisconsin. Infection was defined as "HbsAg positive or hepatitis B core antibody [ant-HBc] positive" in both the Georgia and Wisconsin investigations.[231]

Gjerdingen and Lor conducted a study in a family practice residency clinic in St. Paul, Minnesota, at which Hmong accounted for approximately sixty percent of patient visits.[232] The results of this study showed that among the 434 Hmong sampled, 174 patients (forty percent) were found to be susceptible to hepatitis B, and seventy-seven (eighteen percent) had acute or chronic hepatitis B, with Hmong adolescents aged fifteen to nineteen years having the highest rate of infection (twenty-eight percent). Gjerdingen and Lor did not examine the mechanisms for hepatitis B transmission, but they speculated that the high rate of infection among adolescents may be due to "sexual activity and the use of non-sterile acupuncture needles."[233] As a result, they suggest there is a need to vaccinate Hmong children before they become adolescents, and a need for more research on hepatitis B and its transmission among Hmong Americans.

MENTAL HEALTH

Culture shapes the ways in which people perceive and express physical and emotional distress, and people from different cultures express physical and psychological symptoms in different ways. Kleinman states that Chinese patients express psychological problems and depression mostly in a somatic idiom; for example, "I have a headache," rather than, "I am sad."[234] Bliatout explains that the Hmong use a variety of terms associated with the liver to express mental health symptoms.[235] The term "ugly liver" (*Siab Phem*) usually refers to an individual who has suddenly become abusive and destructive. "Difficult liver" (*Nyuaj Siab*) is a term associated with someone who is experiencing excessive worry, and who, as a result, often cries, feels confused, and/or is unable to sleep. "Broken liver" (*Tu Siab*) indicates that the person is suffering from grief or guilt. "Short liver" (*Siab Luv*) refers to an individual who often swings from a normal state of mind to extreme ill temper. "Murmuring liver" (*Kho Siab*) is associated with a person who often exhibits nervous habits, and common symptoms include humming, coughing, shaking, or hearing a whistling sound in the head. People who experience these symptoms usually start to talk about wanting to commit suicide or wishing to die. The term "rotten liver" (*Lwj Siab*) refers to patients who are not happy with their present lives, or are unable to achieve their goals, and such people often experience delusions and loss of memory.[236]

Due to the experience of cultural repression; war; the loss of loved ones, homeland and personal possessions; and years spent in refugee camps, many Hmong suffer from tremendous physical and emotional distress.[237] As a result, a variety of mental difficulties and complaints are prevalent in the Hmong. These include, but are not limited to, post-traumatic stress syndrome, anxiety disorder, depression, somatization, hostility, paranoid ideation, and psychosis.[238]

Mouanoutoua et al. studied 123 Hmong in California with the aid of the Adaptation of the Beck Depression Inventory (HABDI).[239] They identified seventy-eight percent of non-depressed and ninety-four percent of depressed persons in the sample. Their findings reveal that non-depressed subjects tend to have more education, be more fluent in English, be younger, and be less in need of translation assistance than depressed subjects. Jacobson and Crowson studied forty-three Hmong in Minnesota with the Zung Depression Scale.[240] Their findings showed that sixty-five percent of the sample had Zung index scores of equal to or greater than fifty, an indication of some degree of depression. Twenty-five percent scored equal to or greater than sixty-three, which is usually associated with patients hospitalized for depression. Yet, according to Jacobson and Crowson, only one of the sample complained of depression and only five were previously diagnosed as depressed.[241] These authors noted that patients of larger households, Hmong who had lived in America for a longer period of time, and women had higher scores. They suggest, further, that cultural barriers and communication difficulties serve as major obstacles to accurate diagnosis.[242]

Mental health is a highly sensitive issue, since Hmong view mental illness and retardation as "unclean," and an inherited or genetic transmission. A "clean" family or clan is not likely to allow their sons or daughters to marry into a family or clan that has an "unclean" lineage. From this perspective, mental illness and retardation are viewed as sources of shame, and families and patients often attempt to deny or hide evidence of mental problems, so that emotional difficulties are often presented as physical complaints.[243] Moreover, while Hmong may define any dysfunction as a sign of soul loss, and consult a shaman to treat the problem,[244] a clinician trained in the West will generally define the same dysfunction as a form of mental illness, such as post-traumatic stress or depression, and recommend treatment with counseling or psychoactive medications.[245]

According to Westermeyer and Smith, from the very beginnings of Hmong immigration to America, both Hmong and United States government officials have failed to address properly the issue of mental health.[246] The Hmong have contributed to this failure by virtue of the stigma they attach to mental health problems, and the consequent reluctance of the Hmong American citizen to seek help, or even to admit a mental health problem exists. United States refugee resettlement program planners and policy makers have contributed to the failure both through their ignorance of, and through their disinclination to consider, Hmong sociocultural organization; as well as through their lack of financial support for proven psychiatric treatment programs for Hmong and other refugees. This paucity of United States program planning and funding has been a false economy and, as such, has proved counterproductive, in that it has resulted in additional burdens on other service programs; witness prolonged welfare dependency, and the use of primary health care services for those with mental health symptoms.

Westermeyer believes that, unlike many American psychiatric conditions, most of the mental health problems that Hmong refugees have are treatable with early intervention. According to Westermeyer, most of the anxiety, distress, and depression that Hmong refugees experience is due to an inability to support families, live close to extended families, practice traditional religious ceremonies, find jobs, and so on.[247] If these basic needs are addressed when new Hmong immigrants first arrive in this country, much physical and psychological distress can be prevented.

THE HMONG ARE HETEROGENEOUS

Hmong Americans are widely disparate in age, personality, education, and stage of acculturation. Some Hmong speak no English, while others have achieved a diploma from an American four-year college. There are a growing number who have attended graduate school. Some Hmong still believe in and maintain their traditional animist religion, while others have converted to Christianity.[248] Some Hmong prefer shamans to doctors, while others prefer the most highly advanced technology that Western health care providers have to offer. As is the case with all ethnic groups, Hmong wish neither to be stereotyped nor treated as second class citizens.[249] What they do desire is to be treated by conventional health care providers as those providers would treat representatives of their own racial and cultural heritage; that is to say, as individual human beings.[250] Health care providers will achieve more favorable results if they take the small extra increment of time necessary to explore each person's lifestyle and personal attitudes, rather than treat him simply as "a Hmong patient."[251]

Chapter III

Hmong American Health Care in Colorado

SOCIOLOGICAL/DEMOGRAPHIC

MUCH OF THE RESEARCH FOR THIS BOOK WAS CONDUCTED IN THE Hmong community in Colorado, a community principally centered on the following cities: Arvada, Denver, Westminster, Federal Heights, Northglenn, Thorton, Broomfield, Boulder, Lafayette, and Brighton, with primary concentrations in Arvada, Westminster, Broomfield and Lafayette.[1] According to statistics presented in the *Denver Post*, the Hmong population within the delineated area numbers about seven thousand, with ninety-five percent of Hmong adults working.[2] Employment is primarily in low-paying, unskilled, assembly positions, although the few young adults in their twenties and thirties who have been educated in this country have, for the most part, found entry into professional positions such as accountancy, nursing, teaching, business, computer specialties, and so on.

The majority of Hmong in the target area own their own homes, and the preponderance maintain their traditional animist religion. Of those who do not, most have become Christians. There are three Hmong Christian Alliance groups; one in Denver, one in Westminster, and one in Lafayette. There is one Mennonite group in Arvada, and a Catholic group in Denver. There are Methodists who worship in Broomfield and a Christian Evangelical group in Thorton. Only the Christian Alliance groups in Denver and Westminster have their own churches, while the remainder of the listed groups share a church with their American parishioners, but hold separate services in the Hmong language. The number of households allied with these different denominations ranges from ten to a hundred.

Hmong who are senior citizens, those with disabilities, and single Hmong parents with dependent children, are eligible for Medicaid/Medicare in Colorado. Most of these people use public health care facilities, such as the county health clinics in Boulder, Adams, Jefferson, and Denver. The heads of Hmong American families who are working are enrolled in a variety of health insurance programs, ranging from Health Maintenance Organizations (HMOs) to Preferred Provider Organizations (PPOs), which run the gamut from Kaiser Permanente, Pacificare, and CIGNA to Blue Cross/Blue Shield of Colorado. The associated health services are rendered in such hospitals as Boulder Community Hospital in Boulder; Avista Hospital in Louisville; St. Anthony North in Westminster; North Suburban Medical Center in Thorton; St. Anthony Central in Denver; Exempla Lutheran Medical Center in Wheatridge; and the Denver Medical Center and University Health Science Center in Denver.

For the forty health history surveys—one-on-one interviews—taken for this book, the age of the interviewees ranged between twenty to eighty-six years, with a median age of fifty years. The majority of the interviewees were over the age of forty. Thirty-two percent were under age forty (table 3.1).

Table 3.1. Age of Interviewees

Age	Frequency	Percent
20 – 29 yrs.	5	12.5
30 – 39 yrs.	8	20.0
40 – 49 yrs.	5	12.5
50 – 59 yrs.	9	22.5
60 – 69 yrs.	7	17.5
70 – 86 yrs.	6	15.0
Total		100.0
Median 50 yrs.		

In terms of gender representation, forty percent of the interviewees were female and sixty percent were male. Forty percent of the interviewees, a group comprised of eight males and eight females, aged twenty-eight to eighty-six, had no formal education. Twenty-seven percent, a sampling consisting of two females and nine males, aged thirty-one to sixty-five, had attended classes in English As a Second Language for less than two years. Seven percent, broken down into two females and one male, aged twenty-three to thirty-six, had graduated from high school. Fifteen percent, or three females and three males, aged twenty-seven to fifty, had some college education. Seven percent, encompassing one female and two males, aged thirty-one to forty, were college graduates (table 3.2).

Table 3.2. Interviewees' Education by Gender

Education	Gender Male	Female	Total
No Formal Education	8	8	16
ESL Less Than Two Years	2	9	11
High School	2	1	3
Some college	3	3	6
College Graduate	1	2	3
Missing	1	1	1
Total	16	24	40

In terms of employment, six females reported they were working, while ten were unemployed. Half of the male interviewees, or twelve, had jobs, while the other half did not. One female college graduate was professionally employed as a computer programmer. The other five females worked in various manufacturing assembly lines. One male was an insurance agent, one worked as a supervisor, two were technicians, and the other eight males worked in waste water maintenance, as machine operators, landscapers, assemblers, cooks, in cleaning, and in molding (tables 3.3; 3.4).

Table 3.3. Employment Status by Gender

Employed	Gender Female	Male	Total
Yes	6	12	18
No	10	12	22
Total	16	24	40

Table 3.4. Occupation By Gender

Occupations	Gender Female	Male	Total
None/Not Applicable	9	12	21
Waste Water Maintenance		1	1
Machine Operator	3	2	5
Molder		2	2
Insurance Agent		1	1
Technician		2	2
Manufacturing Associate	1		1
Supervisor		1	1
Cooking/Cleaning	1		1
Electronics Assembler	1	2	3
Landscaping		1	1
Computer programmer	1		1
Total	16	24	40

Eighty-seven percent, or thirty-five, of the interviewees were married. Three interviewees were widowed, and two were separated (table 3.5). Twelve percent of the interviewees reported the number of people in the household as less than three. Fifty percent reported household members numbering from four to six. Fifteen percent of the subjects said that the number of people in the home was between seven and ten. One interviewee stated that the number of people in his household was over eleven (table 3.6). The size of these families is, for the most part, modest by Hmong standards, and reflects the impact of the extended family breakup policy mentioned earlier, as well as an adaptation to the American nuclear family structure. The nature of American housing also plays a role, and it is occasionally necessary for large Hmong families to break into smaller units in order to find suitable housing.

Table 3.5. Marital Status

	Frequency	Percent
Married	35	87.5
Widowed	3	7.5
Separated	2	5
Total	40	100

Table 3.6. Number in Household

	Frequency	Percent
1 – 3 Persons	5	12.5
4 – 6 Persons	20	50.0
7 – 10 Persons	14	35.0
Over 11 Persons	1	2.5

Seven percent of the interviewees reported that they had lived in the United States for less than ten years. Forty-seven percent said they had lived in America for ten to twenty years, while forty-five percent said they had lived in the United States for more than twenty years (table 3.7).

Table 3.7. Length of Residence in the United States

	Frequency	Percent
Less Than 10 yrs.	3	7.5
10—20 yrs.	19	47.5
More Than 20 years	18	45.0
Total	40	100.0

Forty-two percent of the interviewees continued to involve themselves in their animist tradition, thirty percent were Catholic, twenty-two percent Protestant, and five percent of the subjects did not worship any particular religion (table 3.8).

Table 3.8. Religion of Interviewees

	Frequency	Percent
Animist	17	42.5
Catholic	12	30.0
Protestant	9	22.5
No Religious Affiliation	2	5.0
Total	40	100.0

Eighty-five percent of the interviewees reported they spoke Hmong at home, while fifteen percent said they spoke both Hmong and English equally at home.

Thirty-two percent of the interviewees considered themselves to be Hmong, twelve percent of them identified themselves as Lao-Hmong, fifty percent considered themselves to be Hmong Americans, and five percent of the interviewees identified themselves as Lao-Hmong Americans (table 3.9).

Table 3.9. Self Identity

Self identity	Label	Percent
Hmong	13	32.5
Lao-Hmong	5	12.5
Hmong-American	20	50.0
Lao-Hmong-American	2	5
Total	40	100.0

Approximately fifty-seven percent of the interviewees thought that they were healthy, while thirty-seven percent said they were not healthy (table 3.10).

Table 3.10. Self Report of Health Status

"How healthy do you think you are?"

	Frequency	Percent
Very Healthy	2	5.0
Healthy	21	52.5
Not Healthy	15	37.5
Don't Know	1	2.5
Half Healthy/Half Not Healthy	1	2.5
Total	40	100.0

HEALTH STATUS OF SUBJECTS

Half of the interviewees reported that they exercise regularly, while the other half said they did not exercise. Thirty-five percent cited walking as their main form of exercise. Eighty-five percent of the subjects said they do not smoke, while fifteen percent reported that they do. Eighty percent said no one in their household had problems with alcohol, twenty percent said someone in the household did have a problem with alcohol.

HEALTH PROBLEMS REPORTED: PHYSICAL HEALTH PROBLEMS

Fifty-two percent of the interviewees reported that someone in their household had been ill in 1998, and fifty-seven percent said someone in their household had been ill in 1999. The significant illnesses reported by subjects of one-on-one interviews as occurring in 1998 are as follows: one person had kidney stones, one had a brain tumor, one had hepatitis C, one had a heart attack and two had anemia. Illnesses reported for 1999 were: two cases of kidney stones, one brain tumor, one incidence of appendicitis, one cerebral hemorrhage, and one instance of hepatitis C. Of those reporting on illness for the year 1998, one person related she had had a heart attack, and three indicated tuberculosis.

Forty-seven percent of the interviewees reported a problem falling asleep which they characterized as "minor," while twenty percent had a sleeplessness problem which ranged from "often" to "extreme." Twenty-five percent reported they had a "little" problem with poor appetite while twenty-two percent said they had the same problem ranging from "frequently" to "an extremely poor appetite." Forty percent of the respondents stated that they had a "little" problem with dizziness and fifteen percent said they had this problem "chronically." Twelve percent reported that they had chest pains "often." Ten percent said they had the same frequency of coughing. Twenty-two percent stated that they had a "severe" problem with arthritis. Thirty-seven percent reported that they had muscle aches (*Mob Laug*). Twenty percent said they had a "serious" problem with abdominal pain (*Mob Plab*) (table 3.11).

Of those aware of health problems in family members, friends, neighbors, and acquaintances, twenty-two percent of the interviewees reported they knew of someone with a brain tumor. Ten percent said they knew someone with breast cancer. Twenty-two percent of the interviewees knew of another who had suffered a heart attack. Thirty-two percent were aware of someone with diabetes. Sixty-five percent of someone who had had a stroke.

One common symptom of which the elderly frequently complained was muscle ache, or *Mob Laug*, a term which is more specifically employed to refer to those sorts of muscle aches specific to old age, and may be trans-

Table 3.11. Self Report of Physical Symptoms

Symptom	Not at All		A Little		Quite a Bit		Extremely		Total
	No.	%	No.	%	No.	%	No.	%	N
Sleeplessness	12	30.0	19	47.5	7	17.5	2	5	40
Poor Appetite	21	52.5	10	25	8	20	1	2.5	40
Dizziness	18	45.0	16	40.0	6	15.0			40
Nausea	27	67.5	9	22.5	3	7.5	1	2.5	40
Chest Pains	26	65.0	9	22.5	5	12.5			40
Coughing	18	45.0	18	45.0	4	10.0			40
Arthritis	26	65.0	5	12.5	9	22.5			40
Muscle Aches	12	30.0	12	30.0	15	37.5	1	2.5	40
Abdominal Pain	19	47.5	12	30.0	8	20.0	1	2.5	40
Headaches	16	40.0	21	52.5	2	5.0	1	2.5	40
High Blood Pressure	32	80.0	4	10.0	3	7.5	1	2.5	40
Shortness of Breath	29	72.5	8	20.0	2	5.0	1	2.5	40
Faintness	35	87.5	2	5.0	2	5.0	1	2.5	40
Low Energy	13	32.5	14	35.0	11	27.5	2	5.0	40

lated as "old age pain." For men who suffer from this condition, *Mob Laug* is believed to be a consequence of performing heavy work at a young age. For women, the etiology is the same, but, in addition, so it is considered, includes not having had sufficient rest during the first thirty days after giving birth, or, alternatively, not following dietary restrictions during the immediate postpartum month. This *Mob Laug* is often manifested all over the body, or it can be localized in the back, chest, arms, or legs. It is usually a "walking pain," i.e. one for which the individual cannot pinpoint a specific area. The elderly tend to assert that the aches become more severe as the weather changes to cold or to rain. When such muscle aches become severe, the elderly will consult their American doctors, who are generally unable to find anything wrong, which often serves to raise suspicions and doubts in the minds of the sufferers as to whether or not the doctors wish to treat them. Often, as well, doctors prescribe medicines for these elderly patients which do not alleviate the problem, with the resulting frequently heard complaint that consulting with a Western doctor is a waste of time and money.

In summary, many Hmong have suffered serious health crises and/or developed chronic conditions such as heart attack, stroke, diabetes, hypertension, kidney dysfunction, bladder infection, gallstones, gout, arthritis, appendicitis, and cancer. Data from both one-on-one and focus group interviews indicate that stroke, diabetes, arthritis, muscle ache, and hypertension are more prevalent in the older Hmong population, but that heart attack, kidney dysfunction, bladder stones, gout, and cancer do not discriminate by age. Hmong men have more problems with gout than Hmong women. A few Hmong of varying ages have died of cancer. The number of older Hmong who have fallen victim to stroke, diabetes, arthritis, and hypertension increases every year, and the Hmong community is concerned, with some members of the community going so far as to believe that many of these conditions are caused by the medications prescribed by mainstream doctors.

HEALTH PROBLEMS REPORTED: MENTAL HEALTH PROBLEMS

Data from one-on-one interviews revealed that twenty percent of subjects reported high levels of anxiety and a problem with restlessness. Forty percent had a significant problem with forgetfulness. Thirty-two percent of respondents said they often experience feelings of worthlessness, while forty-five percent reported they frequently felt they worry too much. Twenty-two percent stated they frequently felt hopeless. Thirty percent reported that they often "feel trapped," and thirty-five percent said they often felt they must "blame themselves." Fifteen percent stated that they frequently experienced feelings of fearfulness without reason. Seventeen

Table 3.12. Self Report of Mental Health Symptoms

Symptom	Not at All		A Little		Quite a Bit		Extremely		Total
	No.	%	No.	%	No.	%	No.	%	N
Lack of Interest	20	50.0	18	45.0	2	5.0			40
Anxiety	20	50.0	16	40.0	4	10.0			40
Restlessness	21	52.5	15	37.5	4	10.0			40
Forgetfulness	5	12.5	18	45.0	16	40.0	1	2.5	40
Nervousness	30	75.0	8	20.0	2	5.0			40
Feelings of Worthlessness	14	35.0	12	30.0	13	32.5	1	2.5	40
Excessive Worry	8	20.0	11	27.5	18	45.0	3	7.5	40
Loneliness	24	60.0	15	37.5	1	2.5			40
Panic	32	80.0	7	17.5	1	2.5			40
Hopelessness	17	42.5	12	30.0	9	22.5	2	5.0	40
Feeling "Blue"	31	77.5	8	20.0	1	2.5			40
Feeling Trapped	15	37.5	12	30.0	12	30.0	1	2.5	40
Blaming Self	11	27.5	14	35.0	14	35.0	1	2.5	40
Fearfulness Without Reason	20	50.0	14	35.0	6	15.0			40
Tension	28	70.0	11	27.5	1	2.5			40
Weeping Without Reason	21	52.5	11	27.5	7	17.5	1	2.5	40
Everything too Difficult	11	27.5	10	25.0	16	40.0	3	7.5	40
Desire to Die	21	52.5	6	15.0	13	32.5	3	7.5	40

percent answered that they find they often cry easily. Forty percent of the respondents reported they frequently felt that everything was difficult, and thirty-two percent said they often felt they would like to die (table 3.12).

Focus group and in-depth interview data indicate that, in general, Hmong do not like the term—and even the concept of—mental health, and even in the face of a relatively serious mental health problem, such as a desire to commit suicide, a Hmong will refuse to acknowledge the situation as relating to mental health, per se. According to one Hmong psychologist, the Hmong seem to have fewer psychological difficulties than their Vietnamese, Lao, and Cambodian counterparts. The Hmong, it was explained, have more control over themselves, and seem to adjust to life in America very quickly. A certain measure of skepticism at these remarks is warranted, however, and it may simply be the case that, for reasons of pride, a Hmong will not admit to being ill until the problem is very serious.

A Hmong mental health therapist states, "Hmong are not getting proper mental health diagnoses and treatment because they do not want to have anything to do with mental health services. I see a lot of schizophrenia, Post-Traumatic Distress Disorder (PTSD), bipolarization, psychotic episodes, dementia, and other such serious conditions—which should be treated with medication. Nevertheless, those who suffer from these symptoms simply go to a shaman to have them 'fixed' spiritually. A lot of them are not being taken care of until they are so far down the road that they have nothing left, and eventually the diseases kill them."

TREATMENT SOURCES AND THEIR USE: HMONG AND WESTERN

Data recorded on the health history survey indicates that twenty-five percent of interviewees considered themselves to be herbalists; twenty-seven percent considered themselves to be massage therapists; five percent of the interviewees stated they are shamans; while one interviewee proclaimed himself to be a fortune teller. Ten percent said they were magic or ritual healers (*Khawv Koob*). One person categorized himself as a soul caller; however, all shamans are capable of performing a soul-calling ceremony, and are considered to be both soul callers and egg readers. One interviewee considered himself a practitioner of *Hno Koob*, or Hmong acupuncture.

Forty-seven percent of the interviewees reported themselves patients of a shaman. Twenty-seven percent said they had consulted a shaman at some point during the preceding three years. Forty-two percent said they were patients of Hmong herbalists, while ninety-five percent considered themselves patients of traditional massage therapists. Half of the subjects said they were patients of Western doctors and nurses.

Fifty-two percent of the interviewees reported they would consult Hmong shamans in the future. Eighty-seven percent said they would consult Hmong herbalists and massage therapists in the future. About twenty-seven percent maintained they would consult fortunetellers; forty-seven percent egg readers; sixty-seven percent the acupuncturist; fifty-two percent would consult soul callers; and forty-seven percent reported that they would consult other traditional Hmong healers (table 3.13).

Table 3.13. Future (Anticipated) Consultations with Hmong Healers

Healer	Yes		No		Total
	No.	%	No.	%	N
Shaman	21	52.5	19	47.5	40
Herbalist	35	87.5	5	12.5	40
Fortune Teller	11	27.5	29	72.5	40
Massage Therapist	35	87.5	5	12.5	40
Egg Reader	19	47.5	21	52.5	40
Needle User	27	67.5	13	32.5	40
Soul Caller	21	52.5	19	47.5	40
Other	19	47.5	21	52.5	40

Sixty-five percent of the respondents reported that they planted Hmong herbs in their gardens or in the house. Fifteen percent of them reported that they used these herbs planted at home for medicinal purposes, while twenty-five percent said they used the herbs for cooking. Another twenty-five percent said they used the herbs both for medicinal and cooking purposes.

Seventy percent of the interviewees reported that they were not knowledgeable in the use of the conventional health care system, while thirty percent said they were (table 3.14).

Table 3.14. Knowledge in the Use of Conventional Health Care System

	No.	%
Very Knowledgeable	1	2.5
Knowledgeable	11	27.5
Not Knowledgeable	16	40.0
Not at all Knowledgeable	12	30.0
Total	40	100.0

Sixty-five percent of the interviewees reported that they needed and got a translator when they used the conventional health care system. Thirty-five percent said they did not need someone to translate for them. Sixty-two percent of the interviewees who needed translation assistance said their family members and friends translated for them when they used mainstream health care services, while only one interviewee said she had used a professional, bilingual translator (table 3.15).

Table 3.15. Translators

	No.	%
Self	14	35.0
Family Member or Friend	25	62.5
Bilingual Professional Translator	1	2.5
Total	40	100.0

Eighty-five percent of the interviewees reported that they had a family doctor. Ninety percent of the interviewees reported that they had health insurance. Thirty-seven percent of the interviewees said they had not seen a doctor in 1998, while forty-five percent said they had not seen a doctor in 1999. Twenty percent met with a doctor once or twice in 1998, while twenty-two percent had seen a doctor once or twice in 1999. Fifteen percent of interviewees had visited a doctor three to five times in both 1998 and 1999. Twenty-seven percent had seen a doctor more than five times in 1998, and seventeen percent of the interviewees had visited doctors with comparable frequency in 1999.

Seven percent of the interviewees reported that they had seen a neurologist. Twelve percent of them had consulted with a psychologist or psychiatrist. Ten percent had seen a physical therapist, seven percent had consulted with a cardiologist, and twenty-two percent of the respondents had seen other specialists.

REASONS FOR SEEING A DOCTOR RATHER THAN A HMONG HEALER

Reasons interviewees gave for seeing doctors rather than Hmong healers are; 1) having a serious illness; 2) being unacquainted with any Hmong healer; 3) skepticism regarding the methods of Hmong healers; 4) having no access to traditional Hmong herbal medicines; 5) reluctance to resort to Hmong herbal medicines due to a lack of scientific analysis of their composition and effects; 6) conversion to Christianity, with associated aversion to or loss of faith in shamanism; 7) concern that some Hmong massage therapists not being sufficiently skillful, damage to the patient's physiology might result. The majority of interviewees expressed the belief that Western doctors have the ability to diagnose illness, and are more successful in treating illnesses such as gout, blurred vision, kidney problems, gall stones, appendicitis, broken bones, and illnesses of the internal organs. Furthermore, what these doctors may lack in their capacity to understand Hmong cultural priorities and to communicate effectively with their

Hmong patients, they can, in many instances make up with visual aids to illustrate their findings, so that, in the case of the maladies listed above and with all factors considered, Western doctors are equal or superior to Hmong healers.

REASONS TO FOLLOW A DOCTOR'S HEALTH TREATMENT PLAN

Hmong interviewees gave a variety of personal reasons for observing such medical recommendations as, e.g., taking medication, having surgery, making follow-up appointments, arranging for additional tests, or seeing specialists. They follow these suggestions because, 1) they believe such suggestions will help them recover; 2) they do not know any Hmong healers from whom they can seek alternative treatment; and, 3) they are sufficiently fluent in English that there is no language barrier to treatment, or, as an alternative, have reliable Hmong interpreters available to translate everything to them when they visit the doctor.

Interviewees who, by contrast, said they would not follow their doctors' health treatment plans cite the following reasons: 1) they tried at some time in the past to follow a doctor's recommendations, but found their condition did not improve; 2) they quite simply do not trust conventional health care providers to treat their illness; 3) while they feel that conventional health care providers have good methods and medicines, these same providers often refuse to treat Hmong patients in a manner consonant with their wishes; 4) the Western health care system is too costly and/or the profit motive seems to be its primary guiding impulse; 5) they are afraid of the side effects of the medications prescribed by their doctors; and, 6) they do not like the invasive procedures (surgeries or biopsies) utilized by their doctors.

TYPES OF ILLNESS A HMONG HEALER TREATS WITH GREATER SUCCESS THAN A CONVENTIONAL DOCTOR

Interviewees reported the feeling that Hmong healers are more knowledgeable about, and can bring quick relief with a greater degree of certainly for, the common cold, flu, broken bones, sprained ankles, chicken pox, back pain, stomach ache, stress or shock (*Ceeb*), miscarriage or difficulties related to child birth, and soul loss. There seemed to be consensus that Hmong herbalists and massage therapists can treat physical ailments quite well, while shamans, soul callers or performers of magic ritual can effectively treat the spiritual aspects of illness.

REASONS FOR FOLLOWING A HMONG HEALER'S HEALTH TREATMENT PLAN

Interviewees who said they follow their Hmong healers' health treatment plans tend to be those who are themselves healers, or who have family members who are healers. In cases in which a family member is a healer and lives in the same house as the patient, it is this family member/healer who will prescribe and prepare all medications. If the family member/healer does not live in the same house as the patient, the former will instruct parents, spouse, or adult children of the latter in the correct method of preparation and administration of all medicines. In this way, the patient whose energies are at low ebb will be required neither to do nor to remember anything; merely being required to take medicine when told to do so by the person assigned to the task. In fact, a traditional Hmong health treatment is considered inefficacious if the patient is forced either to prepare his own medicine or to initiate treatment.

At all events, by custom it is understood that a Hmong patient and his shaman have entered into an unspoken agreement whereby, should the patient's health improve after treatment has begun, the patient will then be obligated to follow the shaman's subsequent health recommendations. This is both a matter of honor and a matter of survival, for, in order to effect a cure, the shaman will incur debts on behalf of the patient to powerful and potentially mischievous assisting spirits. Even if the shaman would countenance a default on the part of the patient, there are few who will test the restraint of such spirits as may become involved in these healings. In the event of a cure, then, the follow-up ceremony is always performed in order to see to it that the spirits who have assisted in the healing process are paid in full. We have already seen above, however, that the patient is not expected to take an active role in his own cure. It is likewise for this follow-up ceremony, for which the patient is only required to be present; it's the shaman and the patient's family members who will attend to everything.

As we have seen, once the shaman demonstrates, via an improvement in the patient's condition, that he has made contact with powerful healing spirits, there are few Hmong who will fail to put themselves fully into the shaman's hands. Of those Hmong who said they did not follow their herbalist's recommended health treatment plan, the reasons given were, 1) an inability to secure a supply of the necessary herbs; and, 2) ignorance regarding the method of their preparation.

NEGATIVE EXPERIENCES IN THE USE OF TRADITIONAL HMONG MEDICINES AND HEALING METHODOLOGIES

Most interviewees who had undergone traditional Hmong healing treatments reported good experiences. A few related they had seen strong reactions to Hmong herbs in some patients. One interviewee said that, while he was still living in Laos, he had sustained a gunshot wound to one of his legs. Wrapping a compress of Hmong herbs around the wounded area, he had developed intense pain. When he removed the herbs and took penicillin, the pain subsided. Some interviewees did state that Hmong herbs may occasionally cause additional pain, swelling, and/or itching, or, if too much is used or the wrong kind selected, may fail to heal, or even worsen, the condition

NEGATIVE EXPERIENCES IN THE USE OF CONVENTIONAL MEDICINES AND HEALING METHODOLOGIES

There are fewer patients who report problems with conventional medicines and healing technologies than is the case with Hmong traditional medicines and healing technologies. Such problems as the interviewees cite are; 1) side effects of prescription medications; 2) a general discomfort with the doctor's "bedside manner;" particularly the feeling that the doctor did not take sufficient time for a careful examination; 3) extended waiting periods before seeing a doctor, despite having an appointment; 4) anxiety inspired by a lack of familiarity with treatment procedures, particularly due to incomplete or confusing explanations prior to treatment; and, 5) inability to schedule a visit with the doctor in a timely manner when ill.

POSITIVE EXPERIENCES IN THE USE OF CONVENTIONAL MEDICINES AND HEALING METHODOLOGIES

The majority of the interviewees asserted good experiences with conventional health care providers. Most of those interviewees who had been hospitalized or had received outpatient treatment felt their doctors had successfully treated their illness. A few interviewees had never utilized any conventional health care services, and, therefore, had no experience to assess.

HMONG-AMERICANS' EXPERIENCES WITH CONVENTIONAL HEALTH CARE SERVICES

When a Hmong American uses the conventional health care system for the first time, there is a tendency to become bewildered over even routine procedures. Hmong patients are generally not aware that, upon arrival in the doctor's office or at the emergency room, there will be forms to fill out and a subsequent wait for attention. The fact that after being summoned to the examining room there is still a wait before seeing the doctor creates an additional sense of cultural dissonance.

In fact, it is a principle of the Hmong culture with regard to the healing professions that when someone is sick he should be treated right away. He should not be required to wait for hours or fill out endless forms in triplicate before he can be attended by a healer. It is in view of this principle that Hmong tend to assess their interactions with conventional health care services, and they do not understand why, in the technologically and medically advanced West, a lengthy and time-consuming health history must be taken prior to treatment, or why many tests must be performed before a doctor can diagnose an illness. They do not understand the complexities of hospital operations, hospital organization, or the nature of or purpose for the many confusing hospital regulations. They do not understand the cultural priorities which come into play in the management of a hospital. Hmong do not understand that any hospital, or, for that matter, any organization, has both its own, unique, system of operation and a cultural affiliation which are different from those traditional to the Hmong.

Conventional health care practice operates upon assumptions of directness, precision, and speed. It provides no time for socializing or building a rapport between total strangers such as, for example, the new patient and his doctor. Many Hmong have not had such apparently brusque individual encounters before their first visit with the conventional health care professional, and the Hmong character does not permit of an open dialogue with a stranger, let alone a stranger who is direct, a mode of behavior considered rude in Hmong culture. This Hmong reserve is even more affronted if the stranger speaks quickly, since this implies that the speaker is impatient and careless. One Hmong American health care professional said, "Hmong health treatment is different from conventional American health treatment...the two are not the same...what you learn in school is the Western philosophy of doing and seeing things...when you work with Hmong patients, you have to throw all of that away and do something totally different. Doing this makes you feel kind of like...sometimes you feel good because you are helping this family. But sometimes you feel like, 'God, you are throwing away everything you learned in school.' This makes you feel like, a bit unprofessional at times, like you're not using your theory."

Above and beyond all the foregoing, most Hmong patients want their doctors to guarantee they will be healed if they follow the doctors' recommendation in prescribing medicine or ordering surgery. If the doctor cannot guarantee this, the patient will not follow the health regimen or agree to the operation. Moreover, the Hmong patient wants this guarantee in writing, something no doctor can give. The standard medical consent form does not provide this guarantee, either. Instead, it explains the risks involved in the surgery or treatment. To many Hmong, the consent form seems to require them to give up their lives, delineating, as it does, all of the many risks involved while, at the same time, demanding that the patient be both aware of and willing to assume all these risks. Many Hmong view the consent form as a way for health care providers to protect themselves in seeking to fulfill only their own selfish best interests; best interests which are of little benefit to the patient, who, rightly or wrongly, assumes the doctor is merely positioning himself and his hospital to avoid tort action should recommended procedures go wrong.

Many times a doctors will, without adequate explanation, instruct his Hmong patient not to eat certain foods, or even to fast. Without such explanation, it is difficult for the patient to understand why he must do so. The unfortunate result is that some patients will complain, "The doctor is starving his patient." A women in labor, for example, is not supposed to eat, leaving the family to argue, "Well, if she doesn't eat, how is she supposed to have strength to push?"

In sum, like most people, the Hmong tend to stick to their beliefs and their familiar ways of doing things. With regard to this, one Hmong health care provider said, "Many Hmong are not willing to accept information unless something affects them directly in some way. Hmong don't want outsiders to get involved with their business. If you are Hmong, and attempt to impart some bit of new information, or if you habitually do something different from the rest of the community, the majority of Hmong won't like you because you represent all of these new ideas that they have to consider... They don't like it, because you bought into it... you sold out... If you are a woman, oh, my God, it's even worse! Because you are woman, what do you know???"

A third reason for Hmong reluctance to seek help from other Hmong, and from non-Hmong professionals, has to do with the issue of "losing face" (*Poob Ntsej Muag*). Most Hmong adults don't want to talk about their problems with people who are not family members. This includes both non-Hmong professionals and other Hmong. When a Hmong adult must see a counselor, mental health therapist, or social service provider, whether the problem is his own or that of a family member, he will be embarrassed and ashamed. If the problem relates to a child, he may feel, "Oh, my God. My child is so bad; that's why we were forced to come here and see you. . . I'm not a good mother/father!" The adult will be afraid that the counselor or social worker or teacher will gossip about him and tell everyone about his problems. The Hmong tend to be shy.

Naturally, working with the Hmong is rendered very difficult by this reticence and this reluctance to consult with mental health or other social workers. The Hmong client may feel even more uncomfortable if the worker is a woman, particularly if the one seeking help is a man. In such a case, the man may think, "I am a man. I'm not going to throw myself down and ask a woman to help me!" If the female therapist, health care, or service provider in such a case is young, while the client is rather mature or even elderly, the situation is further complicated. In most such cases, the client will feel embarrassed, and may, to salvage injured pride, question the service provider's knowledge and ability to assist or treat him. This male client will, more often than not, be stunned upon first finding himself in this situation, because he has never before consulted with or been treated by a young Hmong, or non-Hmong, professional woman. If this young Hmong female is not a culturally conscious individual, she will also find herself at a loss as she perceives his reaction to her. She may believe that she has been well trained, and may be quite confident of her knowledge and her ability to assist him; nevertheless, and for all that, he will not accept her service or suggestions. Astounding as it may be to her, this very client seated before her, who may never have attended a day of school, and who is, in all likelihood, utterly incapable of understanding how she acquired her knowledge or achieved her professional status, now boldly questions her ability. The subtext of this interaction is that he has been rendered massively insecure because in the cultural context in which he was born and raised, it is incomprehensible that a younger female could know something he does not know; that someone who is clearly weaker then he is sits across from him offering to assist him.

The variety of Hmong cultural imperative demonstrated by the male patient discussed above is widespread, especially in the older generation of immigrants from Laos. Not entirely unrelated to this, about two thirds of Hmong interviewees, whether correctly or incorrectly, held an intuitive feeling that conventional health care providers are as hostile toward Hmong traditional techniques of healing as many Hmong feel toward conventional techniques. When one Hmong woman had a difficult labor, for example, her family brought a therapist into the hospital skilled in Hmong birthing massage (*Tig Plab*). However, the conventional health care providers objected forcefully, and refused to allow the Hmong therapist even to touch the woman. A few of the Hmong interviewees, specifically those who believe that conventional health care providers are gradually becoming much more open to Hmong healing practices than previously, argued that such resistance may occur primarily due to language barriers. They believe that if this situation had been fully explained, the doctor in charge would have allowed the therapist to massage the patient. Naturally, they recognize that some doctors are more open to alternative health treatments than others; however, it should be noted that, as a rule, the Hmong are not used to the necessity of consulting with foreign health care providers whose cultural paradigms, and whose method of acquiring skills and knowledge, are unknown. To illustrate this point, it is might be of benefit to consider that few Americans would be willing to consult with or to take the advice of a Hmong healer under any circumstances, and much less so when the American does not know anything about the healer's skills or training. If we, then, apply this proposition in reverse, we may derive a more clear picture of the dilemma faced by Hmong patients and their families in such a situation.

When they are sick, the majority of Hmong have a tendency first to seek treatment from a traditional Hmong healer first, before resorting to the system of health maintenance more characteristic of the West. One Hmong community leader has estimated that as few as five percent of Hmong will consult conventional health care providers before seeking out a traditional Hmong healer, and these five percent of Hmong will consult a traditional Hmong healer as a last resort only, in the event the Western care provider cannot successfully treat their illness.

Most contemporary adult Hmong believe that shots are more potent than oral medications, and, when they are sick, prefer intravenous or intramuscular injections. Such injections are a staple of the Vietnamese doctors who have their offices on Denver's South Federal Boulevard, and it is for this reason that the majority of Denver's Hmong population prefer to consult these physicians. Indeed, most elderly Hmong who are involved in Medicare/Medicaid have selected these Vietnamese doctors as their primary care physicians. It is said, in fact, that these elderly Hmong frequently tell friends who fall ill, "If you're sick, go see the Vietnamese doctors. They'll give you a shot, and you'll be cured. If you go to the American doctors, they'll just give you medicines to take which won't do you any good. It's a waste of time and money."

It should be borne in mind that, to the Hmong, an ill person is someone who actually feels pain. He may feel heat or cold in a particular part of the body; he may be weak and fragile; he may suffer from loss of appetite and be losing weight; or he may experience all of those phenomena. The Hmong do not consider someone ill who simply cannot fall asleep at night, or who worries too much. They do not, in fact, have any of these conditions in their Lao highland villages. In the case of minor afflictions and low level discomforts, stoicism is the rule, and, for this reason, unless someone is quite sick, he will not seek help at all. Unfortunately, this may mean that, by the time assistance is desired, the patient's condition may be grave, a cure problematic.

Hmong beliefs about the nature of fate are also an influence upon the manner and time frame in which assistance is sought. Fatalism is a staple of Hmong traditional culture, and many Hmong believe that it is fate, rather than the consequences of actions taken by human beings in the exercise of free will, which makes certain things happen. It may simply be fate that has made one ill; fate that has made the illness worse. In such a case, if a cure is meant to be, it is fate which will furnish it, not medicine.

HEALTH CARE DECISION MAKING

When someone contemplates making a decision that may permanently affect his life, he will want to reference all aspects of his situation with regard to that which he has previously known. He will want to assess, compare, and contrast his current circumstances in the light of all prior experience, and this is the manner in which Hmong make health care decisions. However, there is another factor; in contrast to Westerners, Hmong make decisions as a group, not as individuals. When it comes to major health care treatments, it is not the individual alone who makes the final determination; it is the whole group: parents, the elderly, husband, wife, and all.

As an example, a pregnant woman in urgent need of Caesarean section may still have to wait for her parents, parents-in-law, and male relatives to meet and decide on the matter before the surgery can be performed. The doctor may want a decision in a few minutes, but the Hmong involved require an entire day or night to reach a final determination, and this determination often contravenes the doctor's recommendation.

When major health care decisions must be made for parents or other family members, even a member of the younger generation of Hmong, who is fluent in English and is intellectually and temperamentally capable to decide for himself, will still have to consult with his relatives and family members. In many instances a young person will ignore this imperative and make his own decisions. If all is well as a result, no one will say anything. However, caution is necessary because, in case things go wrong, everyone will join in condemning the offender. Thus, while it is true that, in conformity with a certain degree of modernization, members of the younger generation of Hmong may make their own decisions, nevertheless they are forced to endure tremendous pressure from the older generation and the rest of the family, and from clan members generally. To play it safe, therefore, if one is making a major decision that will affect one's life, one is well advised to consult with everyone. The voice of the group is more important in Hmong society than the voice of an individual, and ancient Hmong folk wisdom has it that, "An individual is like a drop of water in a bucket. If it crosses the rim and falls out, it is tiny; it is unable to survive by itself and will soon dry out." There are Hmong who can comfortably make independent decisions; however, they are few in number.

Such an emphasis on the group is not without its benefits. In Hmong society, when a family member is sick, it is expected that someone will always be available to care for that person. It is expected that family members, relatives, and friends will rally around to visit him. If they do not do so, both the patient and his family members will feel offended, hurt, and saddened. When a Hmong is hospitalized in this country, therefore, the attending health care workers may expect a great many visitors to crowd the patient's room. Since it is customary in the West that hospital staff usually allow two people to visit a patient at one time, a large group of visitors will be observed in the waiting room, ready to take their turn to visit the patient when the hospital staff allows them to do so. Should the patient be seriously ill, all of his important family members and relatives will gather in the waiting room, not only to visit as a matter of obligation, but, in addition, to prepare themselves for any major decisions they may be forced to make as a result of any and all eventualities.

An informant described his experience as follows: "I live here in Colorado. My mother lives in Fresno, California, with my father, brothers, sisters, and brothers-in-law. My mother was sick. Her upper leg had some cysts. She could not walk. Before they took her anywhere, they called me up and asked which hospital they should take her to. I recommended a hospital for them. After she was admitted, she had trouble eating food. Her doctor wanted to insert a tube into her mouth to feed her. We all had to gather in one place and decide whether or not we would allow her doctor to put the tube in her mouth. During the discussion, some family members agreed to have the tube inserted, while others disagreed. But the majority of the family members agreed to have the tube done. Before we gave permission for the doctor to put the tube in her, we talked to the doctor to determine if he was listening to us, too. If he paid attention to us, took time to talk to us, and listened to our concerns, then we would allow him to put the tube in her mouth. If he did not listen to us, we would not allow him to place the tube in her, since he would just do what he liked. We knew that our mother was raised in another country. She ate rice, meat, and vegetables all her life. But the foods that the doctor would feed her through the tube are only milk and sweet and mixed liquid, which her stomach was not used to. Although the foods were supposed to help my mother, they could also kill her. This was how we viewed it. If the doctor agreed with us to try the tube to see how she reacted, and he would agree to remove the tube if she reacted negatively and we told him to remove it, then we would allow him to place the tube in her mouth. If the doctor insisted that, once the tube was in, he would not remove it, then we would not give permission for him to place the tube in her mouth. This was how we handled my mother's case."

ISSUES OF TRUST

It is a universal of human nature to place one's trust in something that is well understood, in someone with whom one is familiar, and in which or in whom one has confidence. In that way, one may feel reasonably certain that the investment of this trust will not yield negative consequences.

Hmong Americans apply this familiar concept to their dealings with conventional health care professionals. One reason many Hmong do not trust conventional health care providers is that they are not familiar with the diagnosed symptoms, do not understand the seriousness of the health threat, and do not have confidence in the proposed treatment plan. For example, sometimes a Hmong woman will deliver her baby at the hospital. Afterward, her attending physician diagnoses a low fluid level, but the Hmong present do not believe it. "We Hmong have always delivered babies this way," they will respond. "We've never heard of this 'fluid is too low' business in all our lives." They will then decline to follow the doctor's recommendations for treatment. To recapitulate, they disagree to the treatment because, 1) they are not familiar with the symptom(s) being diagnosed; 2) they do not think the problem at hand is life threatening, and; 3) they do not feel the doctor's treatment will be helpful or even necessary.

The often confused and occasionally adversarial nature of interactions between the Hmong and their professional conventional health care providers provokes a raft of complex and often invisible undercurrents that may not always be recognized as barriers. Since the Hmong have long been a minority group wherever they find themselves, they have experienced discrimination in many societies throughout their lives and historically. It is to be expected that they feel vulnerable to discrimination when they are ill, and are quick to become suspicious. Many interviewees cite discrimination as a barrier to placing trust in conventional health care professionals. Some strongly believe they do not receive good treatment due to the fact that they are culturally different and/or non-White. Since their physical appearance is different from those in the mainstream, they often feel they get less attention than they merit, even when loved ones are seriously ill. Some Hmong even believe that doctors or other health care providers will intentionally do them harm because, 1) these health care providers do not care about the Hmong; 2) the Hmong are poor; and, 3) the health care providers do not really want to treat Hmong patients. It is widely felt that some conventional health care professionals treat Hmong patients' bodies as objects which they may with impunity toss, turn, slice, and saw as they please.

In addition, since most Hmong patients do not speak English fluently, health care professionals often appear to be impatient in their communications, either speaking very loudly or even yelling, as if the patients are dumb or have hearing problems. Hmong patients naturally feel humiliated and hurt by such interactions. They feel that, as first generation immigrants, it is not their fault that they cannot yet speak English well, and the sort of unwarranted cruelty of which they are made the butt is merely adding insult to the "injury" of being ill. Hmong who have had, or have heard of, this sort of experience or treatment are very fearful of and reluctant to seek conventional health treatment.

Although it may seem surprising to mainstream Americans, who are used to taking their social institutions in stride, the sort of fear one may feel in what is, for the Hmong, an endless series of new and unfamiliar experiences, is a major issue, and has a tremendous impact on their search for health care and their relations with conventional health care providers. The fear of the unfamiliar is a powerful one for a people who have been subjected to political and military oppression as a matter of course over the span of generations and even centuries. An aspect of this that has been mentioned above is the fear of being used as subjects for experiment by American doctors. Hmong patients normally do not inform their interpreters or health care providers of this, but it is a real concern, nonetheless, and all such anxieties and fears become fodder for conversation at home when chatting with family members or relatives.

At the same time, and not without reason, some Hmong health care providers argue that the Hmong need to develop more faith and trust in the conventional health care system. Still, an abiding fear of the unknown, as has been mentioned, something which is inherent to all human beings, inhibits this trust. This, once again, returns the discussion to communication. If Hmong patients do not speak or understand English, and get interpreters who cannot translate in a clear and comprehensible manner, then patients will not know what is happening to them or what to anticipate. This is especially true when one has no past experience on which to draw; experience which may serve as a basis for comparison in the present instance. The anxiety engendered by uncertainty about what will happen next can create tremendous doubt, suspicion, and a variety of uncomfortable emotions for patients and their families. This uncertainty, moreover, can naturally lead to distrust, and to feelings of vulnerability to abuse, negligence, and experimentation on the part of health care providers. If this distrust persists, it will destroy the impulse to seek future health care.

Since the majority of Hmong Americans still organize themselves according to their traditional social system, whereby they rely heavily on kinsmen, they must, perforce, place great trust in the judgment of their leaders. If these leaders do not or will not put their trust in something, the clan members will follow suit. The contrary is also the case; if the clan leaders do place their trust in, and can clearly explain the details of, various procedures, then the clan members will therein follow suit. The role of the leaders in promoting trust in the conventional health care system thus becomes a central one.

It cannot be overemphasized that the issue of trust is very important to the Hmong, and Hmong Americans will quickly render an overall judgment as to whether a hospital is good or bad by the experiences of friends, relatives, and acquaintances who have been patients there. An interviewee explains: "Even though some hospitals do not have actual records indicating that they are bad, we have the feeling they are, and saw a lot of people hospitalized there who frightened us. We knew a lot of people who went to the hospital that we chose, and we were more pleased with its service than the other hospitals. The things that made us distrust them were the way they talked to us. They did not take time to explain procedures to us. Sometimes they did things without informing us first. Sometimes they did things that we did not like, and we told them so, but they would not listen to us. Many times they did not agree with the decisions a Hmong family made. These are the obstacles that prevent Hmong from returning to those hospitals. A Hmong person may not have been sick, and never used the hospital. But he has friends and relatives who have been sick and used the hospital before. If his friends and relatives have had bad experiences with a particular hospital, he will be scared away and will also avoid that particular hospital."

Broadly speaking, the Hmong take two approaches to a hospital and its staff. The first approach is to scrutinize the way doctors and nurses treat them. Do they take time to listen to the patient and his family members? Sometimes Hmong saw "nurses whose faces are as dark as storming skies and who are very clumsy, unfriendly, and rude." Hmong do not like this kind of attitude, especially when they are sick or have a loved one who is sick. The second approach is to consider the hospital as a whole. Unfortunately, when a Hmong former patient who has had a bad experience with a nurse or doctor does not know the name of the person involved, the former patient will say, simply, "That hospital was bad," thus tarring the entire hospital for what may have been merely a single unhappy episode. This report, that the hospital is not good, will nevertheless spread throughout the Hmong community. This acts as a kind of multiplier, in that if a single Hmong has had a bad experience and has become fearful as a result, many Hmong will become likewise fearful.

HABITS OF TAKING MEDICINE

Many Hmong do not like to take the medicines prescribed by a conventional health care doctor, and, when they do take the medicine, do not always follow the doctor's recommendation. While it may be true that a Hmong patient in hospital has no choice but to take the medicine administered by nurses, if a doctor simply prescribes dosages to be taken at home, most Hmong will not do so. The patient, for example, may be directed to take a particular medicine three times a day until the furnished supply is finished. In the event, however, he will take the medicine inconsistently for a few days, and, if he feels better, stop, reasoning that, since he does feel better, he no longer needs the medicine.

Adding to this problem is the fact that some Hmong have a tendency to doubt the efficacy of the medicines so prescribed. Since competent interpreters are not always available to translate instructions for ingesting dosages, the benefits and risks involved are not fully explained. Without a knowledge of the risks inherent in varying the dosage of the medication in this haphazard manner, the patient may alter the dosage or stop taking the medication altogether. As a corollary, the problem of potential side effects is a concern for many Hmong. One Hmong interpreter said that, in some instances, as soon as she explains these potential side effects to her patients, they immediately decline to use the medicine. For their part, Hmong patients argue that if they do not take the medication, they need contend with only one illness, but if they do take the medication, they run the risk of more than one illness. Thus, they will take the medication as a last resort, but will take only enough to allow them to feel better, then stop in the hope of decreasing the chance of developing side effects. Logically, they feel, medicine is supposed to make one feel better, not worse, and certainly is not supposed to cause one to develop other forms of illness.

Hmong patients also refuse to take medications in the manner directed by their doctors because they hear and believe rumors from other Hmong, who have taken the same or similar medications, that, "I have been taking the medications as directed by the doctors continuously, and now look at what has happened—I have become even worse." Since the person who turns in this sort of negative report believes that it is the medication that has made his illness worse, and since he has talked about his condition openly, this sort of rumor spreads and provokes fear in other Hmong. Sometimes the development of a new and previously unheard of illness will be attributed falsely to medicine. Word of mouth is a powerful force in the Hmong community and, although such rumors are, more often than not, untrue, they are true occasionally enough to provoke many an "I told you so."

It is both the older and the younger Hmong who, in this way, do not follow their doctor's instructions. A Hmong conventional health care provider thinks that, based on his observations and experiences in providing health care to the Hmong, "Hmong seem to listen or pay more attention to things that are not always true.[3] They do not want to listen to or hear things that are true (*Kuv muab xav los ntau tsawv lawm mam peb cov Hmong no ntseeg cov lus dag xwb, cov lus uas luag hais tseeb mas nws tsis tshua ntseeg pes tsawg lawm*)."

USE OF HERBAL AND TABLET MEDICINES SENT FROM ASIA

When they are sick, Hmong Americans use many herbal and tablet medicines sent from Laos, Thailand, and China. In fact, most elderly Hmong will use herbal medicines and other tablets sent from Asia before consulting with American doctors. These import items can be expensive, and sometimes the purchasers will spend over a hundred dollars to obtain mixed results. Although the herbal and tablet medicines are sometimes effective, at other times the illness persists.

For all the mixed results, these herbal and tablet medicines continue to enjoy popularity because the Hmong are familiar with them, or know someone who has used a particular variety of this medicine and has recovered. In other words, the Hmong will tend to follow the advice of a person who has actually used a medicine before they will listen to someone who, while a highly trained expert, has never used the medicine he prescribes. Yet, in many instances, these herbal and tablet medicines have not been systematically examined to determine chemical composition, a fact which, while leaving the older generation unfazed, gives pause to younger and more educated Hmong Americans who tend to be more skeptical regarding the efficacy and potentially harmful side effects of such medications.

HEALTH PROMOTION

Pasick et al. consider that conventional health promotions tend to benefit White, middle-aged, middle class Americans more than other groups.[4] General health promotion campaigns have not been tailored to the needs and concerns of either racial and ethnic subgroups or communities of low economic status. They go on to suggest that the terms of health promotions need to address and incorporate the "unique qualities of different cultures and those common to all humans."[5] That is, effective health promotions should be tailored to appeal to people from different cultural and socioeconomic backgrounds. Examined hereinafter will be ways to promote health education and illness prevention among the Hmong Americans of Colorado, which will inevitably serve to illustrate terms in which appeals might be made to other racial and ethnic minority groups.

Currently, there are many Hmong organizations in Colorado, but all can be categorized into two types: informal and those which are legally incorporated with the State of Colorado and the Internal Revenue Service. Most of the Hmong clan organizations are of the former, informally organized, type. These do not file any legal paperwork with the State of Colorado or the Internal Revenue Service. As a sort of Clan Leader, each clan elects a male representative for a term of one to three years. The duties of this clan representative include calling the other clan members to meetings to discuss an agenda based upon clan problems that arise; attending meetings with the representatives of other clans to discuss such problems as may arise with implications for several or all clans; handling other issues of concern to the entire Hmong community; and organizing the annual

Hmong New Year Festival. By a system of internal arrangement, these clan representatives also serve as a members of the board of directors for The Hmong American Association of Colorado, Inc.

The Hmong American Association of Colorado, Inc., is an example of the legally incorporated Hmong organization. Others are exemplified by the nonprofit mutual assistance association or the church group, and all Hmong belong either to one of the more loosely-knit groups or one of the more formal associations, or both. Approximately ten percent of the Hmong in Colorado belong to a nonprofit organization; thirty percent to a church group; sixty to seventy percent to a clan organization.

Since, as has been discussed, Hmong rely heavily on both kin and clan leaders for support and information, any outreach effort geared to the Hmong community should include a consideration of Hmong social structures as well as perceived authority figures. With such an approach, outreach efforts will be more fruitful. In order for health education information, for example, to reach as many people as possible, it is necessary to work through clan representatives, boards of directors and officers of Hmong non-profit organizations, and church leadership figures, encouraging these various authority figures to organize their members into groups so that health education information can be distributed to them. It has been seen that the Hmong operate on the principle that the group is more important than the individual. What this means on a practical level is that, if an individual health care professional endeavors to come to speak to a Hmong group without going through established channels, the audience may be sparse or nonexistent. It will be most profitable, therefore, in channeling health education information to the Hmong population at large, to "touch base" with all levels of Hmong group leadership in order to reach ensure the widest possible dissemination.

HMONG PROBLEMS WITH WESTERN PREVENTIVE MEDICINE

If one addresses the issue of Hmong health prevention from the Western perspective, one may be led to conclude that the majority of Hmong do not take preventive medicine very seriously. Witness that the majority of Hmong, 1) do not have a physical check up on regular basis; 2) wait too long to consult doctors when they are not well; and, 3) often reject a doctor's recommendations for the amelioration of illness. On the superficial level, these observations, in conformity with Hmong health care-related behavior, would tend to indicate the Hmong have a casual attitude, at best, to preventive medicine. However, Hmong Americans are the product of a traditional culture with autochthonous beliefs for conceptualizing health problems and the means for preventing them. When one, therefore, assesses, in the context of their cultural background, their behavior in seeking, or not seeking, health care, their decisions and approaches are seen as being every bit as logical and valid as those of Westerners. The problem is not so much that the Hmong do not take preventive medicine seriously, but is, rather, that conventional Western and Hmong American health care professionals have sought to impose their perception of preventive medicine on Hmong Americans who still operate within the context of their own cultural beliefs. If the Hmong refuse to comply with these Western medical dicta, it is because such concepts do not make sense in their cultural context, not because they have problems with preventive medicine. Put another way, it is more accurate to state that Hmong Americans have problems accepting Western preventive medicine than to assert that, in their culture, they have no interest in or conception of preventive care.

Hmong Americans' receptivity to preventive medicine is influenced by factors similar to those which affect their behavior in seeking health care from conventional health care services. This receptivity depends largely on an assessment of the benefits, risks, and perceived susceptibility to the health threat or disease being addressed, and this assessment, in turn, is influenced by their degree of Western acculturation. Those who have more exposure to and understanding of the Western viewpoint on various health issues will be more receptive to the Western preventive care methods and techniques presented to them. They will feel more comfortable with the risks involved, and perceive more clearly the ways in which their future lives may be affected by the health issues presented to them.

This acculturation is far from widespread, however, and Hmong may not follow or understand conventional health care providers' recommended health maintenance schedules. As a consequence, children are likely to fall behind with their immunizations, and, when a Hmong child is brought in for an appointment, health care staff may seek to bring the child up-to-date with the administration of a few vaccines at one time. Hmong parents, fearing adverse results, often resist this practice. These parents are hesitant to have their children receive more than one or two vaccines at a time, saying their children are too small, are not strong enough, or are too young to be vaccinated, and request that the shots be delayed until later.[6]

There is no doubt that the inculcation of an appreciation of the need for preventive measures, and general health education, and are needed. A few interviewees showed an interest in learning more about the roles and responsibilities of nurses and doctors, how medicines are approved for use, why it is that following the instructions governing the use of medication is important, and how the conventional health care system works. They felt it would be easier for everyone—Hmong patients and family members, Hmong interpreters, Hmong community leaders, and Hmong and mainstream health care providers—if more Hmong understood such issues. After learning more about the various aspects of managing conventional health care facilities and providing conventional health care, the Hmong may gain more trust in and become less fearful of hospitals and hospital staff. Hmong will also benefit from health education regarding major illnesses, health threats, and chronic diseases such as stroke, diabetes, heart attack, hypertension, and cancer, together with the role played by nutrition and diet. Hmong need to know that if they eat certain foods to excess, such as oily or salty foods, or meat, they may develop certain kinds of infirmities and diseases in later life.

Some Hmong health care professionals observe that, in general, Hmong are not proactive in the sense of taking preventive measures with their health. They tend to wait until they are in crisis or under assault by a serious health condition, then go to see the health care provider. Unless an illness affects them directly and immediately, they do not want to know about it. This attitude is not entirely the result of a stubborn nature or of a "life lived in denial," to employ a currently fashionable idiom. Traditionally, in Hmong society one does not learn about a particular remedy for a particular illness until one has experienced that illness and had need of that remedy. It is, in fact, considered bad luck to discuss something one has not experienced, and, in the past, Hmong have preferred to take information only as and when needed. In some cases, unfortunately, by then it is too late.

Many young Hmong professionals are quite frustrated with this attitude of those Hmong who do not want to learn anything in advance, most particularly to take preventive health measures. Some Hmong professionals feel that these people "just do not want to know, and choose to stay in the dark." In consequence, these professionals deprecate and choose to avoid them. It is nonetheless frustrating for the professional Hmong to "just stand by and watch things happen," and, as young professionals, they can be relied upon for some degree of community engagement, such as adhering to the mandate to report child abuse. The division created between the younger generation and the older, however, is exacerbated by this feature of modern Hmong life, i.e., "the ones who are knowledgeable pulling away from the ones who are not knowledgeable."

In general, the Hmong have a way of establishing awareness of the key aspects of their surroundings. They usually know the important people in the community and have access to them when needed. They often say things like, "Oh, there is Mr. X., the Hmong policeman, who helps our people a lot." Everyone knows Mr. X, and knows that if he gets get into trouble and/or wants information, Mr. X is available. However, if Mr. X were to take the lead in dispensing valuable information, no one would listen. It is for much the same reason that many Hmong interpreters, health care workers, and service providers receive telephone calls at midnight after putting in long hours at the office.

HMONG CONCEPTIONS OF PREVENTIVE MEDICINE

Along with the many differences between the cultures, Hmong and Western, already touched upon, Hmong have a different concept of preventive medicine compared to that held in the Western world. Waters et al. assert that the concepts and practices of preventive medicine are something quite new for the Hmong.[7] However, the Hmong are familiar with the concept of prevention, but do not perceive it in the same way it is seen in the West. The Hmong concept of prevention is inclusive and holistic, but less formal and explicit. For example, Hmong values emphasize hard physical work, eating appropriate food, and taking "appropriate measures," broadly speaking, to prevent sickness, and this sort of folk wisdom with regard to the prevention of illness is embedded in daily life.

The Hmong may not have vaccines, but they do, for example, have folk remedies to assist in safeguarding their children from chicken pox and other such childhood illnesses. In fact, the concept of preventive medicine in the Hmong culture includes attention both to a person's physical and spiritual well-being. As an example, in traditional Hmong society the annual soul calling ceremony performed during the Hmong New Year Festival serves much the same purpose as does an annual health checkup in Western societies. During the New Year Festival, this soul calling is performed to summon all souls of all household members and enjoin them to stay intact within the individuals concerned and the family as a whole. This ceremony is executed to prevent human souls from wandering away and becoming lost. The Hmong believe that if no soul calling ceremony is done, a person's souls may not have a sense of belonging and, in consequence, may stray. If this happens, the individual will fall ill. If the soul calling is delayed, the person's health condition will deteriorate, and, if nothing is done to rescue the souls, eventually he will die. Thus, the soul calling ceremony performed at the New Year Festival is one very dramatic and important feature of Hmong preventive health care.

If omens at the soul calling ceremony indicate that the coming new year may bring illness to family members, then more of the shaman's ceremonies may be commissioned as a further preventative. This procedure is a parallel to the tests and inoculations accepted by the Westerner as he participates in his annual health checkup. If, at that time, abnormalities are found, the individual may be sent to see a specialist who, it is hoped, will help him to ward off any impending problems.

In addition to this, Hmong herbalists and massage therapists take preventive measures in their treatment. For example, Hmong herbalists have prophylactics for chicken pox, common cold and flu, digestive problems, and so on. Instead of administering flu shots or giving oral immunizations,

Hmong herbalists simply boil herbs as insurance for family members against chicken pox, common cold, or flu.

Some Hmong massage therapists also specialize in preventive care. They believe that the human body is similar to a car or other, comparable, machine, in that it that needs to be tuned on regular basis. As people move about executing their daily responsibilities, they use certain parts of the body more than others, stretch certain tissues more than others. Angers and frustrations may etch lines in nerves, or affect the internal organs, which, as a result, may malfunction and even develop illness. It is felt that, on occasion, a person should consult a Hmong massage therapist to alleviate such irregularities before trouble occurs.

Waters et al. go on to mention that the Hmong do not understand the need for cholesterol screening, for vaccines, or for other such measures.[8] Vaccination and cholesterol screening are new concepts, only introduced to most Hmong in the last two or three decades; enhanced efforts will be required to familiarize them with these and similar Western prevention programs.

Nevertheless, ultimately most Hmong consider illness a physical imbalance resulting from a spiritual causality such as soul loss, and often do not see the value of medical care until the onset of illness. That is, they usually delay seeking health care until they are very sick,[9] and will exhaust all traditional healing methods before consulting a Western health care provider.[10]

When Hmong patients finally do visit conventional health care providers, they want medicines to treat their illness. They do not necessarily want diagnosis, a fact which will seem paradoxical to the average Westerner. Nonetheless, the patient expects to receive medication to relieve symptoms, and, if he does not receive medication, may become upset or critical of his care.[11] This is not, however, a paradox to the Hmong, for it is a commonplace in Hmong society that traditional Hmong healers can determine the nature and identity of an individual's illness without touching or questioning the patient directly. Hmong patients may thus be suspicious of conventional health care providers, or doubt the provider's ability, when confronted with an extensive interview, a physical examination, or laboratory tests.[12]

MENTAL HEALTH

A Hmong Christian minister says he addresses the issue of mental health in his congregation every week. Many Hmong have family problems, and he knows that, as a result, various members of Hmong families may develop mental health problems. However, most of these people do not know what constitutes the modern definition of mental health, and will not recognize that they have developed some form of mental infirmity. Although family members develop many mental health symptoms, they continue to believe, and will adamantly maintain, that they are healthy. Certainly, a mental health problem is a health event that the Hmong know very little about. Nor do the Hmong have the slightest inkling about the nature and course of successful mental health treatment. The Hmong Christian minister alluded to above estimates that at least ninety percent of the Hmong population do not know what constitutes mental health or mental illness. If they did, he considers that most would seek treatment.

Yet, the nature of modern mental health counseling is such that when a white, middle class therapist works with a Hmong mental health patient, virtually insuperable difficulties ensue. First, the client will not understand the conversation, and, second, the therapist, for the most part, just sits there, listens, and, if he says anything at all, merely asks questions. This situation is uncomfortable, confusing, and difficult for the Hmong patient, and he will usually consider it a waste of time. Such parameters of interaction are not unique to mental health counselors; many younger Hmong ministers, service professionals, and health workers also experience difficulties in working with Hmong clients and patients. The problem is that these young professionals have been trained in Western schools animated by Western philosophy and ideology. Naturally, when they work with the Hmong, they seek to apply what they have learned in these schools. However, this may not necessarily jibe with the Hmong worldview, Hmong cultural values, or Hmong beliefs, and, when such professionals and their Hmong clients present such contrasting points of view, they will fail to understand one another and fail to achieve the desired end.

Another Hmong Christian minister states, "Whether I am a therapist, a pastor, a shaman, or a doctor, I must have the ability to diagnose and confirm the patient's illness with him. If I have this skill, I am able to treat the patients like humans, and am able to make comparisons of the current symptoms to those of previous patients who had similar problems. This is something that I should continue to do, because it helps me to make sense of everything. The most important point is that, when I must apply the theories I have learned from working with white patients to other ethnic peoples, such as the Khmu, Chinese, and Hmong—when I work with ethnic people—I must be able to apply the same theories to explain symptoms in such a way that the ethnic people can relate to it. If I use the same explanations for both the Hmong and the white person, then it won't work. I cannot apply the same approach for a white individual to a Hmong patient, because the two patients have different conceptions of health and illness."

A Hmong mental health therapist states, "You can't do therapy right away with Hmong people. When you first meet them, you talk about family. They may ask about your age, marital status or parents' names. You are taught in school not to tell any of this stuff. . . . But, with Hmong people, if you don't reveal this stuff, then they are not going to trust you." A health care professional should thus reveal himself to his Hmong client to the extent with which he feels comfortable; after that, he may, if he chooses, say it is policy not to talk about such matters. This the Hmong client will understand.

At the outset of the therapeutic relationship, the therapist will often find he cannot commence the therapy, proper, until he helps the client with some sort of case management, such as, for example, finding a place to live, or obtaining food to eat and clothes to wear. After such basic needs are secured, the therapist can begin to inquire about worries, sleepless nights, or other such symptoms of mental health difficulties.

Most Hmong mental health patients will not take medication. In a prior section, this recalcitrance regarding medication has been seen in questions of physiological ill health; however, the reasons for what appears to be identical behavior in cases of mental health are somewhat different. The Hmong believe that mental health medications are only for the seriously delusional, or "crazy people." Since they are not crazy, they should therefore not be required to take the medicine. Hmong also believe that, even if one is not insane, the ingestion over a prolonged period of time of medications targeted at mental health problems will eventually provoke insanity. This inference has been drawn after observing a few Hmong patients subjected to an intensive mental health regimen, and is congruent with the views expressed in Sue E. Estroff's 1981 book, *Making it Crazy: An Ethnography of Psychiatric Clients in an American Community.* This volume presents substantial evidence to advance the argument that mental health patients rarely recover through treatment. Rather, they tend to become addicted to and dependent upon their mental health medications for the remainder of their lives. This certainly does nothing to persuade the Hmong that a course of mental health medications is salutary or even necessary.

With regard to communication in a mental health setting, most Hmong interpreters report it is very difficult to translate for Hmong mental health patients. For reasons which have been touched on above, if the interpreter explains that the medicines being given are for mental health problems, Hmong patients will reject them all out of hand. If the interpreter employs an alternative strategy, and explains that the medicines are intended to address other, physical, symptoms such as sleeplessness and stress, the patients will take the medicines, but only until they feel better. Then they will stop. Moreover, such an indirect stratagem raises an ethical issue. If the doctor or interpreter does not explain exactly what the medicine is for, he is not telling the truth. If the doctor or interpreter does tell the truth—the whole truth—the patient will not take the medicine. He will also, in all likelihood, not return for future treatment. This "Catch-22" quandary often leads to the Hmong mental health patient to continue endlessly searching for better health treatment, or, worse, abandoning the search for treatment and surrendering to his illness. In that case, if traditional Hmong mechanisms for treating mental health conditions are either unavailable or unsuccessful, the patient is left to suffer on his own without treatment or assistance of any kind.

LANGUAGE PROBLEMS

Patients who lack proficiency in English often experience difficulty in expressing their problems, limited, as they are, to the use of simple English words to explain complex feelings, thoughts, and experiences.[13] This language barrier between patient and health care professional has affected "diagnosis, frequency of misinterpretations, and treatment effectiveness."[14] Those patients who have acquired a limited facility in English understand that, if they attempt to say much beyond the essentials, the English speaking health care provider will not, in any case, understand them, and, therefore, they may as well not talk much at all. Ironically, this reticence can render them more vulnerable to misunderstandings due to misinterpretations and verbal miscues than if they had said nothing at all.[15]

Health care transactions that require translation from Hmong to English and from English to Hmong are difficult and frustrating for all concerned. It is hard for the patient, in that he is not able to express his symptoms directly to the provider.[16] It is complicated for the translator, because there are not always equivalent words or concepts in both languages.[17] It is frustrating for a physician to conduct a medical interview through a translator, and the use of translators presents many other problems, as well.[18] Such medical interviews and other transactions involving interpreters take "two to three times longer than usual."[19] Untrained translators, moreover, often cannot grasp subtle nuances in the conversation, usually altering what is said by adding words or changing the patient's expression to improve images or smooth feelings, and may even replace what the patients has said with their own opinions, for example to accommodate feelings of squeamishness which arise when patients discuss painful illnesses or intimate emotions.[20] Adding fuel to the conversational fire, patients may become resentful if they realize the translator is making changes to their statements and increasingly frustrated and even angry as they attempt inarticulate protests to perceived interpreter transgressions. Finally, the patient may develop an acute sense of embarrassment in observing the interpreter's strong reaction to what he has disclosed. In light of all this, all parties to health care transactions must resolve to maintain sensitivity to what each of the others may be feeling.[21]

TRAINING OF HMONG INTERPRETERS/TRANSLATORS

In interviews conducted with interpreters and translators, only four out of twelve said they had received any formal training. Three of those individuals who had been trained reported that the agency for which they worked had required them to attend the training, while one attended on her own initiative. All four said that the training had been very helpful, and that they would not have been aware of many of the proper methodologies for translation had they not attended such training.

The rest of the interpreters acquired what abilities they have in a haphazard manner. One said she ordered translation training manuals from Minnesota and trained herself. Three are health care professionals who have been called upon to interpret as needed. All of these agreed that translating for Hmong patients is difficult, even with a good grasp of the appropriate medical jargon, because they have never been trained to translate and their Hmong is not up to par. Some of the younger interpreters, although raised with the language, feel they do not know enough Hmong to translate effectively, and often struggle to find the right words. Five of the interpreters interviewed are considered to be Hmong community leaders who frequently interpret for their own family, clan, and community members. These leaders were able to improve their ability through experience, despite the lack of any formal training. Most of the interpreters interviewed felt it would be of value to acquire training—or more training—and a few suggested that local hospitals should train their own interpreters. A Hmong community leader suggested that unless an interpreter has been trained in many fields, he should not attempt to translate in all sectors of service, primarily because each field of specialization has its own jargon.

There was wide agreement that having a family member or friend to translate is not sufficient, and, once again, this is due primarily to a lack of familiarity with the medical terminology or jargon of the specific field involved, as well as having had none of the training which, although admittedly rare, is nevertheless quite apparently needed.

In the typical Hmong family, it is the children and young adults who are usually the most proficient in English, and it is they who will be called upon to translate for elders or parents. However, children usually are incapable of understanding at the requisite level of abstraction, and have a limited ability to translate complex medical problems and treatments. It is, then, in the end best to use bicultural, fully bilingual, trained medical translators.[22] Children will do their best, but will, for instance, often translate words or concepts literally. To cite certain common examples, children will often translate the Hmong *Daj Ntseg* as "yellow ears," instead of as jaundice; or will refer to a *Mob Taub Hau* as a "pain pumpkin cook," rather than a headache. They may refer to the only son of the family, *Tub Twm*

Zeej, as the "buffalo son;" a literal translation. Post traumatic stress disorder symptoms are translated as pains in the liver or heart, leading the doctor to think something must be wrong with the patient's heart, arteries or liver. This sort of miscommunication frustrates both patient and doctor; the former struggling to obtain a cure while the latter struggles to make a diagnosis and render treatment.

LANGUAGE INCONGRUENCE

Another aspect of the problem with translation is that the Hmong and English languages are vastly different, so that there are terms in English that do not exist in a Hmong equivalent, and vice versa. Sometimes the interpreter must translate one English term with many Hmong words, which takes time and patience. This eventuality demands that both the doctor and his patient refrain from speaking too quickly or too long at a stretch, lest the interpreter be unable to remember what has been said and miss important points.

These difficulties are no less apparent when dealing with mental health concepts. When asked how they translate such terms as depression, anxiety, mental health, and schizophrenia, most translators cannot agree on a specific Hmong word for any of them, and are unable to decide quickly which Hmong words may be most appropriate. Some throw up their hands and assert that the Hmong simply do not have words for such concepts. Two of the interpreters—who had been trained specifically to translate in the mental health sphere—said they do not really know how to translate mental health terms into Hmong. In cases of past necessity, they had simply explained in long sentences, or through the use of many words, the intended concepts. To the extent that the Hmong do not like to be associated with mental health problems, and will often decline to view their problems as those of mental health, such translation is a difficult subject to discuss. One Hmong health care provider and interpreter said, "It's really hard to translate. You can get the words, but the meaning. . . . there is the letter of the words and the spirit of the words, and you cannot translate that spirit or tone. It gets totally lost. The emphasis is not there to some degree."

Patients and their family members, or the interpreters they employ, must be able to explain all symptoms in detail to the attending doctor, and a Hmong nurse emphasized that one of the factors contributing to ineffective health care treatment is the lack of patient ability to do so. Patients must be made to understand that they will need to paint a clear picture of their condition in order to obtain effective diagnosis and treatment of their illness.

A Hmong health care provider pointed out that Hmong Americans need to understand that, "Western health care treatment is really an assessment. It's based all on science assessment of things. If the health care providers do not have anything to assess and go by, then they do not know how to treat it. . . . Hmong are very humble. They do not tell you a lot of things. If they do not ask questions, they never get to know. The doctors cannot offer them anything if they do not ask for it."

When they have patients who are not fluent in English, health care providers should simply assume that the information being given them is just a fraction of the whole, and some extra effort will be needed to fill the interstices. A doctor may, for example, be required to take the extra time necessary to phrase questions in simple terms the patients can understand.

When considering all of these factors, it is understandable that four Hmong interviewees said they had gotten interpreters who could not translate in a comprehensible manner. In fact, these interviewees felt they sometimes got interpreters who knew no more than they, themselves, did. Some of the translators were fluent in English but not in Hmong, or fluent in Hmong but not in English. Some interpreters seemed to understand what the doctors had said, but could not translate that into terms which the Hmong patients could understand, and, when the Hmong cannot understand, "they feel like they have been tricked into procedures they do not know and they feel abused because they do not know."

SOCIAL DYNAMICS OF THE TRANSLATION PROCESS

To be sure, the process of translation is quite complex, and it is the rare interpreter who translates everything that has been said. One of the reasons for incomplete translation is that what has been said has been partially forgotten, especially when the conversation is lengthy and without pause. Another reason is that the interpreter may not fully understand the conversation, and is merely translating whatever he thinks he heard. Often, interpreters, motivated by a desire to protect the individuals involved, will screen out and not translate words, phrases or concepts employed either by the patient or the doctor. Translating everything can occasionally create hostile interactions between patients and health care providers, especially when disagreement on a treatment plan already exists. Sometimes Hmong patients will present viewpoints which are quite foreign, and in opposition, to the conventional health care providers' views, such that the interpreter, because he does not agree with one or the other party, may be embarrassed to translate some statements in their entirety. Occasionally, an interpreter may feel that one cannot translate what the Hmong patient has said without framing certain references in the context of Hmong culture. If the interpreter takes this route, and seeks to explain Hmong cultural concepts as he goes along, he will be required to act not only as a language translator, but also as a culture broker. It will, in addition, take considerable time.

Doctors, however, do not have time. They are, on the contrary, perpetually in a hurry. Yet, health care interactions that involve translation inevitably will demand more time than their lingua franca counterparts, and health care service providers should allot that time to the extent they are able to do so. Hmong patients do not care for physicians who are rushed and do not allow a sufficient span to examine or listen to them (Barrett et al. 1998). Such patients feel flouted and consider they are wasting their money, most especially if they do not feel better afterward.

To add to the difficulty, many older Hmong patients explain the symptoms of their illness in lengthy monologue form, some parts of which may not relate directly to the illness. The translator may have to continue probing the patient in order to obtain the information sought. In such cases, the interpreter may assume that much of what has been said is irrelevant or insignificant, and thus there is no need to translate it. Taking this approach, the translator will sum up with a terse, "He says, 'No,'" or, "Yes." This sort of dialogue will lead to consternation on the part of the doctor, who thinks, "But the patient just said a bunch of things. What did he say?" This type of summation, in reality a form of omission, can lead the doctor to question the interpreter's ability.

INTERPRETER/CLIENT RELATIONSHIPS

There are many underlying and unspoken aspects to the relationships between Hmong interpreters and their clients. Some interpreters are related by blood to their clients, or become friends with them in the course of their professional association, while others try to maintain a distant and reserved professionalism. Interpreters who have relationships with their clients will, as a consequence, become involved with their lives. Eventually, those same clients will depend on them to inquire about aspects of health treatment of which they may not be aware, and, eventually, even to help make decisions. They will call upon the interpreter to assist in translation every time someone is sick or in trouble. While such a relationship is warm, friendly, and respectful, it can also be a burden, and will slowly expand until it sometimes seems to have no boundaries of time, no limitation on service. Hmong clients call their interpreters whenever they need someone to translate, even during weekends or at night, and yet, if these interpreters make even a small error, they will quickly lose their client's trust.

Another type of relationship between interpreter and client is illustrated by the Hmong interpreter who strives hard to maintain a highly professional code of conduct. Such a rare and devoted professional will translate exactly and in its entirety everything said by each party. He will tell his clients up front that consultation and advice with regard to personal matters is impossible. He will neither hide nor elaborate upon anything said.

He will not distribute his telephone number, letting it be known that he does not want clients to call at night or on weekends. He will maintain a professional distance from his client, both before and after the translation service has been rendered, by sitting at some remove from the client and by refusing to discuss anything relative to his service on those occasions when he runs into a client in the pursuit of daily life. Although this may seem like the acme of professionalism, such a highly professional individual may find himself widely disliked. If he is young, clients will call his home to complain to his parents or other family members that he is unfriendly, unapproachable, cold, distant, not helpful, and arrogant.

One difficulty reported by most of the Hmong interpreters, health care workers, and service providers interviewed is that their clients and/or employers/coworkers tend to expect them to have more authority or power than they actually have, so that it is often anticipated that they will not only to translate, but also to act as advocate, winning doctors, judges, or other service providers to their side in the case of disagreements. If they should decline to attempt such advocacy, or, having agreed to attempt it, fail to win disagreements, they are liable to be considered inadequate or remiss. On the other hand, the non-Hmong employers or coworkers in such cases will assume that their Hmong clients will be content that there is a Hmong worker now available to assist with translation and any necessary administrative niceties. Some Hmong will be, of course, but some will not. In addition, the non-Hmong coworkers or supervisors often assume that the Hmong health care providers or translators have a complete grasp of all the subtleties of Hmong culture and traditions, and are fully proficient in the language. As we have seen, this is by no means always the case.

All of this tends to create a quandary for the young interpreter, and all the more so for an interpreter who is also a health care provider. A health care provider on the hospital staff who augments employment skills with language skills might be forgiven for expecting to be reflected in the size of the compensation packet. However, the fact is that most interpreters/health care providers' pay rates are the same as those of peers who do no translation. In other words, their employers recognize, and are only too happy to make use of, their bilingual skill—they just do not wish to pay for it. This is not a situation calculated to enhance the motivation of the health care provider/interpreter, nor one which is likely to lead to any voluntary improvement in translation skills.

Chapter IV

Hmong Cultural Beliefs Related to Health, Healing, and Illness

COOPER,[1] LIVO AND CHA,[2] AND JOHNSON,[3] AMONG OTHERS, HAVE recorded various legends about the Hmong's version of the creation of the world and the great flood of the earth. These legends describe how Hmong survived the great flood and how their clan names were formed. They do not address the manner in which Hmong traditional customs and beliefs originated nor do they describe the significance of those beliefs and customs. Rice describes the *Kab Yeeb* couple as responsible for bringing children to their Hmong parents on earth.[4] Cooper and Rice report that the *Saub* is associated with fertility and reproduction.[5] Bliatout, Thao, Lemoine, Ovesen, Cooper, and Rice have written about the *Xwm Kab* as a household spirit that Hmong worship to protect their families.[6] Cooper briefly describes the Water Dragon, *Zaj Laug*, who controls nature.[7] But the following story about the *Dab Pog* couple and the *Xwm Kab* has not been recorded before in the literature. The author herein presents this tale of the *Dab Pog* and the *Xwm Kab* just as it has been related to her; the details and views expressed in the following pages have been drawn from informants.

THE DAB POG COUPLE AND THE ORIGIN OF THE HMONG CULTURAL TRADITION

According to a Hmong traditional massage therapist, the Hmong people are descended from a creator couple who generated the first Hmong man and woman and taught them all of the cultural beliefs and traditional customs they would be expected to follow in order to live prosperous, healthy, and harmonious lives. Since the Hmong do not have a written language, they did not make any record of the creators' names, but, as the years passed by and the Hmong dispersed all over the world, they came to refer to this creator couple with a variety of titles. Some Hmong call them the great grandparents, *Poj Koob Yawm Txwv* or *Poj Yawm Txwv Koob*. Other Hmong call them the spirit couple, *Nkawm Niam Txiv Dab Pog* or *Nkawm Niam Txiv Kab Yeeb*. This *Dab Pog* couple are responsible for sending newborn children to their earthly parents (Rice 2000; Cooper 1991). Inasmuch as child rearing and family life are so important to the Hmong, the *Dab Pog* has become the most-worshipped spirit, together with the house spirit couple, the *Xwm Kab*, who were sent to earth to watch over Hmong homes and protect them from evil spirits and sickness. This latter house spirit couple also watches over household assets and ensures that those who live within are not only healthy, but prosperous.

Thus, at the very beginning of time, the *Dab Pog* couple, *Nkawm Niam Txiv Dab Pog*, and the *Xwm Kab* couple were sent to live with and among the Hmong to watch over them, their houses, and their children. Then, one day, a Hmong couple gave birth to a daughter. When this daughter had grown to adulthood, she desired to marry and start her own family, but her parents loved her so much that they did not want her to leave their home. These parents, as well as the *Dab Pog* and the *Xwm Kab* couples all joined in watching over her. Nevertheless, undeterred, she made up her mind to get married. Yet, concerned about interference if she told her parents about her plan, she told the *Dab Pog* couple what she wanted to do. The *Dab Pog* couple declined to approve her decision, however, and referred her to the *Xwm Kab* couple, saying, "We brought you down to your parents and we assumed the task of watching over you as you grew up. Please consult with the *Xwm Kab* couple, too, since they are the ones who watch over the whole house."

Accordingly, the daughter went to the *Xwm Kab* couple and told them of her desire to get married. After pondering for a while, the *Xwm Kab* couple said, "If you are sure that you have grown old enough to start your own life, we will help you. Tonight, we will make your parents fall into a deep sleep so that they will not hear anything. At midnight, you may get up, open the front door, and run away to marry. But be warned; if your parents see you leave, they will not allow you to go and you will never be able to get married. If you leave quietly with the man you love and marry him, then you can start a new life."

The daughter was pleased with these words and replied, "Oh, let's do that!"

That night, the *Xwm Kab* couple induced the parents to fall into deep sleep so that they would not hear a sound. The *Dab Pog* couple, who had brought the daughter down to earth, helped her open the front door to sneak away.

The next morning, the parents arose and looked around for their daughter, but she was gone. Furious, they called the *Dab Pog* couple and upbraided them, "You brought our daughter to our lives, and you are supposed to watch over her. We love her very much and we do not want her to get married. Why did you allow her to sneak away? We are not happy with what you have done!"

The *Dab Pog* couple were, in consequence, hurt and saddened. They replied, "From now on, we will bring children to their parents on earth, but we will no longer stay with them to watch over their welfare. We will return home. On the third day after a child is born, Hmong parents can kill a pair of chickens, *Ib Nkawm Qaib*, prepare a pair of cut ceremonial papers, *Ob Ntshua Ntawv*, and burn two sticks of incense, taking all these things outside the house. Then we will come and give a blessing to the child."

In this way, the *Dab Pog* couple thenceforth have brought children to their parents on earth only; they no longer stay to watch over the children. When those children grow very old and are near death, the *Dab Pog* couple return to take them home; they cannot return by themselves. The *Dab Pog* couple are, then, to this extent considered to be the creators and protectors of people throughout the world.

But the story is not yet finished. The parents were also furious at the *Xwm Kab* couple. The mother and father thus called them, as well, and scolded, "*Xwm Kab*, we worship you in our house because you are supposed to watch over our family members and our house. But you failed in your duty. You let our daughter sneak away. You are not worthy of our worship."

The *Xwm Kab* couple, like the *Dab Pog* couple, were hurt and saddened at hearing such words. They replied, "Oh, we have stayed with you, watched over you and protected your house. In this case, we did not do your bidding. Your daughter wanted to get married, and we allowed her to do as she wanted in order to start her own life. You are not happy for what we have done. So be it. We will return home and will not stay with you or watch over your house anymore. When you want us to come back to join you or give blessing or protection to your family, you can create an altar for us by hanging a ceremonial paper, *Daim Ntawv Xwm Kab*, on the main wall, *Hauv Plag*, of your house to designate it as our place in the home. You may call us and we will come back to perform those services for you as in the past; then we will return to our own home. If you do not need our assistance and protection and you do not call us, we will never come back."

This is how the Hmong began to worship, *Teev*, the *Xwm Kab* in their houses. The purpose is to protect personal wealth, family members, and the household proper so that everyone in residence may avoid illness and be prosperous and successful in their lives, and so that the children will grow up happy. This is why Hmong only worship the *Xwm Kab*. If there are no major problems and no illness, the Hmong will perform only one ceremony for the *Xwm Kab* per year, and the *Xwm Kab* are considered to visit Hmong families only once a year.

After the *Dab Pog* and *Xwm Kab* couples left the house, there was a major dispute involving the girl and her elopement. Was she really married? The case was argued among the highest authorities in the world, but no one was able to establish his opinion as definitive, and, since human beings could not resolve it, it was taken all the way to the Dragon's Palace, the *Zaj Zeg Zaj Lag*. The Old Dragon, *Zaj Txwg Zaj Laug*, lived under the water, and he was asked to come out to resolve this case in the world of mortals. Applying himself, therefore, the Old Dragon traced the details of the case in order to render an earthly verdict. In doing so, he found an umbrella hanging on the wall of his palace that the people involved had brought with them. He took hold of this umbrella and brought it with him to this world. Holding it as he spoke, he proclaimed to the Hmong people, "Today and henceforth, I will use this umbrella as a symbol for those Hmong who wish to marry. From this day forward, when the marriage negotiator carries an umbrella with him as he walks fondly along the path, all the people who see him should understand that he is engaged in arranging a wedding for someone."

This is how the old Dragon came to resolve the Hmong dispute in this world. He sang the first wedding song, the *Zaj Tshoob Qhib Rooj Tuam Tsa*, created for marriage negotiators to sing in their marriage rituals, which is now used when setting up the table preparatory to marriage negotiations. He began, "It seems like this year, my parents on the other side have prepared ahead well. They have captured the daughter of my parents on this side to run with their son like a herd, in pairs."

Since it was because of the daughter that this marriage dispute developed, the *Dab Pog* couple came to her at the appropriate time and said to her, and to all the Hmong people, "When you have children, you should watch your daughters. When they are ready to get married, they will know how to begin calling to the sky and the land, and how to express their feelings toward the male gender, thus: *"Txawj seev hu lub ntuj daim av txiv leej tub lub npe!"* As parents, you should give them more freedom when they reach this stage, whether they are big or small."

After that, such expressions as these were made into folk songs for Hmong girls to sing. This is the reason why, today, Hmong girls begin singing traditional folk songs by calling to the sky and the land, to the designated male, and then expressing their feelings: *"Ntuj teb yuas txiv leej tub cas kho siab ua luag no!"* when they begin to engage in courtship.

The *Dab Pog* couple advised further that, when a Hmong girl reaches this stage of development, they will not guard her any more, *Tsis Kav*. They will not control her heart. They will set her free to explore as she wishes. When a girl grows up, begins to show interest in the opposite sex, and begins to sing songs to express her feelings, her parents should not try to stop her, so they ruled. If the parents attempt to intervene, they will not be successful because she is ready and the *Dab Pog* couple is no longer controlling her heart. She will not have peace and happiness until she accomplishes her wishes.

If she has not opened her mouth to express such a feeling of interest in and readiness for the opposite sex, the *Dab Pog* couple will continue to guard her heart and control her life, *Tswj*, so that she will experience happiness and peace—even though they do not come to stay with her, as in the beginning. Should she thus continue to refrain from making the prescribed signs and from singing in the prescribed manner, it will indicate to them that she is not yet ready to get married, and they should continue to protect her. Although she may grow older and be single for many years, if she does not open her mouth to express her feelings and show her interest in the opposite sex, the *Dab Pog* couple will continue to control her. People are warned that they should not worry if she appears to be getting old, *Ua Nkauj Hlaug*, does not seem to dress attractively, or manifest an interest in getting married; her time has not arrived.

In the course of this famous case, the *Dab Pog* couple also said to all Hmong sons that, when they have trouble in their lives or experience sickness, they can call the couple by saying, "*plwg, plwg, plwg. . . . tam sis txheev mas tam sis leej*!" Which means, "This calling should be granted!" Whenever someone calls out in this fashion, the *Dab Pog* couple will come to help him. This is why the Hmong shamans and ritualistic healers, to this day, when undertaking a healing ceremony begin their chanting with these words. The *Dab Pog* couple will come back to attend, to assist, and to protect only those people who call upon them.

In addition, the *Dab Pog* couple advised the Hmong people that there are three major events in a person's life. Two are happy events, one is sad. The first happy event is when the new baby is born. When the baby enters this world, he cries aloud. Everybody is happy that the baby has been born, whether it is a girl or a boy. The *Dab Pog* couple, the new baby, and everyone else are happy that the child now has parents and a home.

The second happy event is when the child has grown up and gets married. The child is now an adult and is embarking upon a new life.

The third, sad, event is death. It is at this point that the *Dab Pog* couple come to bring the deceased back to their home with them, while all those left behind, the living, are left saddened by the departure.

As an additional instruction, the *Dab Pog* couple said to the Hmong, "We bring children to you, and we will guide their intuition as they make their decisions in life, but we will not come to take care of them or stay with them anymore. However, when a boy or a girl has grown and is ready to marry, you should invite us—not to see them from the inside of your house, for, if you do, we will not come to see them—but on the way to the wedding you should call us, and we will come to look at the couple, and to see who is the wife and who is the husband."

Therefore, when Hmong have a wedding,[8] no matter how close or far away, they must always pack a lunch consisting of a pair of cooked chickens, some rice, and beverages. On the way to the home of the bride's parents, the wedding troop will stop for lunch. The marriage negotiator will then proclaim out loud, "Oh, *Dab Pog,* please come to bless us! Today we are traveling to negotiate a wedding. Please bless our trip, that it may be safe and that our mission will be successful."

Since this call is made from outside of the home, the *Dab Pog* will come to see and to bless the couple. When the *Dab Pog* hear the call, they will respond thus, "Oh, today they call us to see a couple getting married. Let's go down to look at who is marrying whom."

When they come to see the young couple, and find them well dressed and well prepared, they will make a picture of the couple, so that they will know who is the wife and who is the husband, being pleased to see these two individuals join their lives in marriage.

When the wedding troop returns from the bride's parents' house, her parents will pack a lunch for them. On the way, they will stop for lunch, and once more the marriage negotiator will call the *Dab Pog,* crying, "Oh, *Dab Pog* couple! Today the wedding is completed. Everything went well. There were no problems. Please come to bless us and make our trip home safe. Please protect us from all dangers, harm, evil, and trouble."

Hearing this last call, the *Dab Pog* couple will come to look at the married pair again and make another picture, desiring ensure that the wedding was real and that the bride and groom and their parents and relatives have completed the wedding negotiations and all have agreed that this couple are married to each other. If the *Dab Pog* couple was properly called to bless, protect, and make a picture of the couple together as husband and wife, their married life will be happy, prosperous, and long lasting, and the pair will love, trust, and respect each other until death.

According to a Hmong healer informant, a long time ago the Hmong maintained these blessings and practiced these wedding rituals as set by the *Dab Pog* couple. Thus, they lived happy and long lives together. Their marriages were stable. There were no divorces. However, as the centuries passed, and since the Hmong did not have a written record of these instructions, some later generations forgot these blessings or began to do things according to their own whims and desires. From pride, it is said, people think they can do whatever they want. At some point in time, the majority of the Hmong forgot, altered, or lost the meanings of these marriage blessings dictated by the *Dab Pog* couple. Since the informant who provided this information strongly believed that the strict observance of these blessings is crucial to the well being of the Hmong people, he stated, "Every parent has sons and/or daughters, and each of them needs to be protected; all parents seek to prevent their children's marriages from being short lived. If parents are ignorant, if they are not careful, if they do not follow tradition, they can ruin their daughter's life. When a daughter gets married, parents should not force their son-in-law to drink so much alcohol that he falls down or becomes unconscious and unable to participate in the whole wedding ritual. Nevertheless, if he becomes so sick that he cannot attend to his duties, a male relative of his, sometimes an older or younger man, will be conscripted to substitute for him."

This informant believed that occasional substitutions made for an intoxicated groom during the return procession play an important role in the failure of a marriage. In the course of a properly managed wedding, the wedding rituals are performed at the home of the bride's parents, after which the wedding troop travels back to the home of the groom's parents. On the way, the entire party will stop for lunch, whereupon the marriage negotiator will call the *Dab Pog* couple to come back to bless the newly wedded couple. In a case wherein a conscript substitutes for the groom, whether because the groom has become drunk or for any other reason, the *Dab Pog* couple will notice that the groom is not the same person as before. The groom may be absent, or he may be present but so drunk and looking so terrible that he is seen to be ill-prepared for a lifetime of marriage commitments. In any case, the *Dab Pog* couple will make a picture and compare it to the first one. They will discover that, in the previous picture, the couple was well dressed and well prepared, and looked serious and happy. In the second picture, however, they will see that the groom is not the same well-dressed and well-prepared man as before, and, taking note of this inconsistency, they will withhold their blessings. As far as they are concerned, this bride and groom have neither found their true marriage partners nor made a lasting commitment to each other. In the eyes of the *Dab Pog* couple, the bride is already as good as a widow or a divorcee.

Without the blessing of the *Dab Pog* couple, the hearts of the two will not settle down as they begin their life together. They will be dissatisfied with each other, or find fault with every little thing in their married life, until they break off the arrangement or one of them dies. They will not be happy, and their marriage will not last long. The informant argued that, "Today, even though the majority of Hmong still practice them, many do not know the meanings and purposes of these traditions. Many times, the people who pass on the knowledge of these traditions make mistakes, so that they pass on the wrong way of doing things. Other times, the proper way has been forgotten or was never well known, so that the rituals must be performed as well as may be. Sometimes, people in authority fool themselves, thinking they can do whatever they want and ignore the traditions, adding to the momentum of cultural loss. Since the Hmong do not have a written language, they do not record their traditions in ritual texts. Many of the performers are actually doing things from which they have been enjoined, continuing blindly to follow the mistakes laid down by previous generations. For example, many, if not the majority of, Hmong today will force the new son-in-law to drink so much alcohol at wedding rituals that he passes out before the wedding is over. These people are more concerned with having fun, enjoying excitements, and making an extravagant display at the wedding, than they are with following proper rituals in order to maximize the blessings bestowed by the spiritual entities upon the living. In the United States, moreover, Hmong Americans seem to be even more abusive of the wedding rituals than others, since they can afford to buy a great quantity and variety of drink. Alcohol has thus come to serve no longer as a symbol employed for ritual procedures, but as a symbol of wealth and a sign of ostentation.

"Many Hmong in the modern world do not care to know, and would not understand, the traditional Hmong wedding rituals, and do not wish to follow them as originally laid out. Often, Hmong marriage negotiators (*Mej Koob*) and parents do not follow all the steps of these rituals."

This informant believes that many Hmong marriages end in divorce, and, occasionally, that married people run away with lovers in consequence of the failure of the Hmong couple to follow proper wedding rituals, and in consequence of the older generation to prepare their children to understand fully both the spiritual and physical aspects of the marriage commitment.

If proper wedding rituals are followed, on the other hand, and the newlyweds have been well prepared for their married life, the marriage will not break up so easily. If the *Dab Pog* couple has blessed the union, the husband may, in his masculine frailty, see a pretty lady and think to himself, "I like her; I want to flirt with her." But should he set out to cheat on his wife, he will meet with failure, foiled by the *Dab Pog* couple, who will control his mind and heart. They will remind, him by forcing him to reflect on his actions, that he is about to create an abundance of trouble and embarrassment for himself and his family, and his marriage will be saved. The same thing holds true in the case of the woman whose marriage has been solemnized according to all the traditional rituals and been blessed by the *Dab Pog* couple. According to the Hmong informant, it is thus highly important that all Hmong respect, understand, and follow their traditional marriage rituals; an important part of Hmong culture from the very beginning of time.

With regard to these marriage rituals, the *Dab Pog* couple have instructed the Hmong male, "You are the man. You go and search for a woman as your bosom companion. You are the one who initiates the relationship. You court her and importune her and persuade her to love, believe in, and trust you. She does not come looking for you. She lives with her parents, while you try everything to win her heart and to make her fall in love with you. Therefore, in the course of your wedding, you must make a vow and you must do it freely and from your heart; no one can help you observe this vow. When you invite another person into your life and bring her to your home, it is different from having a relationship with an animal. Therefore, you must make a vow to the sky and the earth that you will do as you have promised. Even though the sky stays high above, the earth does not. The earth lies beneath your feet. If you do not do as you have vowed, the sky will not punish you because it is so high, but the earth will pull you down until your life ends beneath it. You must make the vow by yourself."

The *Dab Pog* couple told the Hmong marriage negotiators, "You are enjoined from assisting the groom in any way with making his marriage vow; he must do it himself."

When the Hmong wedding begins, a wedding troop—consisting of two marriage negotiators (*Mej Koob*), the bride (*Nkauj Nya*b) and her maid of honor (*Niam Txais Ntsuab*), and the groom (*Tus Vauv*) and his best man (*Tus Phij Laj*)—go to the house of the bride's parents. Upon arrival, the marriage negotiators direct both the groom and his best man to stand in a pair facing the main wall of the house. There, the two pay their respects to the household spirits dwelling in the home of the groom's prospective in-laws.

After this, the marriage negotiators say, "*Nrog niam nrog txiv xyuam lub hlis lauj!*" This translates as, "Pay your respects to the mother and father!"

The groom and his best man must then place their knees on the ground, bend their heads, make fists with thumbs protruding, and impress thumb prints on the ground. This is done quickly, whereupon the groom and best man once again stand up. The Hmong, not having a written language, there is neither paper nor pen to sign a written document of marriage. Thus, the thumb is used to seal the vow, and as a promise to the earth that all vows so made will be honored. If the groom does not thereafter honor his vow, the earth is empowered to punish him. If the bride does not keep her vow, the earth will punish her also. Therefore, in marriage, one has the right to choose his own partner. Whether one marries a pretty or handsome partner or a homely one, it is one's own choice, luck, or fate. When a man has sealed his fingerprint on the ground in this fashion, known as *Tau Pe*, he should understand the commitment he is making in marriage from that day on. It is dishonorable for either partner to do harm to the other in married life. Married people should not rail against, hate, or in any way persecute one another, since they have already, of their own free will, made a vow not to do so.

At the wedding, the *Dab Pog* couple tells the marriage negotiators of the bride's family to give the bride away by saying, "We are representatives of the bride's parents. Today we give our daughter to you, the marriage negotiators of the groom's parents. You take her with you. Your family must promise to protect and love her. As her birth parents, we love her very much. But since she is a female, we can only raise her. Due to the custom of our people, she cannot live with us for the rest of her life. We cannot marry her. We allow her to go with you because our customs allow your son to marry her. Wherever she may go, you must watch over her, protect her, care for her, and love her. If you take her to live with you, but you do not protect and love her, we will not be happy when we hear of it. If our daughter goes with you but does not listen to you, if she does not behave like other people and creates trouble for you, you can bring her back to us. We will talk to her and advise her to improve her life. You must not mistreat her or say bad or untrue things about her. If you do, and we hear about it, we will not be happy."

The bride must then follow the vow that the groom has made by sealing a thumb print on the ground. If she does not, while the sky is very high and may not be able to punish her, the earth is just under her feet and will pull her down and punish her badly. If she cheats on her husband, mistreats him, or divorces him, her life is over. She can remarry and start again, but it will not be as good, and will not last as long, as her first marriage, because, so it is believed, the earth is punishing her severely.

This is why married women do not have the right to date other men or to divorce their husbands who have not mistreated them. If a daughter knows of and understands these traditional marriage customs and commitments, and if she follows these traditions or marriage laws, her marriage will not be ruined. The Hmong have a saying, "The law may be as tiny as a hair, but people cannot cross over it."

If the husband, too, understands the importance of these marriage customs and commitments, he will not create any trouble in his marriage. The couple will not argue over little things, and will not make problems for themselves or each other. Both the husband and wife will be happy, and, thus, they will both find it easy to behave well.

The informant believed that in the Hmong American community today, the majority of Hmong do not teach their children about the meaning of marriage rituals and commitments, and perhaps do not understand such matters themselves. They do not know that violating the rituals, laws, and traditions of marriage can affect the living as well as the spirits. People think, "I love you, and you love me, so let's get married. If things work out and we get along, we'll stay together. If not, we can go our separate ways."

The informant thinks that it is the fault of Hmong adults that they do not take time to carefully teach their children the proper ways to consider and to consecrate marriage, and that is one reason so many Hmong marriages end in divorce. When the meaning of Hmong marriage traditions is carefully explained to all people of all ages, they can fully understand the significance of those traditions, and, understanding them, will behave well and treat each other with respect. They will not disagree over trivia, but enjoy each other's presence. They will learn how to grow and evolve in love and patience, and how to improve themselves over time, so that they will be happy.

According to the informant, since the *Dab Pog* couple has blessed these ageless traditions, it is incumbent upon all Hmong parents to teach their children about them. Moreover, Hmong parents must themselves learn the importance of these traditions, so they will better understand themselves and their own lives. This will, in turn, place them in an enhanced position to teach their children. All Hmong need to preserve their marriages in order to live happy and healthy lives.

The above *Dab Pog* story illustrates the interweaving of Hmong beliefs with some of life's major events. The Hmong informant who related this *Dab Pog* story implied that when Hmong do not understand the significance of their cultural traditions, and, in consequence, do not observe those traditions, they will be misled easily in their decisions and will tend to fail in whatever they set out to accomplish. This is because the *Dab Pog* couple having withheld their blessing on the effort, the chances for success are considerably diminished. This informant further suggested that, by contrast, when Hmong maintain and observe their cultural traditions, their overall condition in life will improve. This cannot but have the effect of enhancing the life of the family, the clan, and the Hmong people as a whole.

THE EIGHT MOST IMPORTANT SPIRITS IN HMONG CULTURAL TRADITION (*Yim Tus Tswv Dab Nyob Hauv Hmoob Kev Cai Dab Qhuas*)

Chindarsi, Cooper, Lemoine, and Thao have recorded some of the following spirits.[9] While Chindarsi and Cooper have described the use of the chicken, funeral drum, and ceremonial papers in Hmong rituals, and Cooper and Lemoine have described the use of the *Txwm Kuam* during the shaman's ceremonies, none of these authors has presented the following spirits in the manner presented here.

According to a traditional Hmong massage healer, there are eight spirits (*Dab*) in the Hmong cultural tradition which may, with justification, be called the "most important." These eight spirits play vital roles in propitiating other spirits. Since the Hmong cannot see, touch or feel spirits, of necessity they must use tools or symbols in communicating with them and in acting among them. The following is central to this consideration:

1. The *Txiv Muam Tai*, or owner of a funeral drum is considered to be the father of the spirits, the *Txiv Dab*, or the most important spirit. At the same time, the *Txiv Muam Tai* is a human being who inherits the drum from his father when he dies; by right, this is the eldest son. If the eldest son refuses to receive, or is not available to maintain, the drum and worship its spirit, then the next oldest son is appointed. There is a spirit of or within this drum that the *Txiv Muam Tai* must worship. He keeps the drum in his house, and this drum will be beaten two times by the spirit within a few days before someone dies. After such a death, family members will come to borrow the drum for the funeral, bringing a bottle of wine with them. They will ask the *Txiv Muam Tai* if they may borrow the drum, and the *Txiv Muam Tai* will pour a cup of wine and inform the spirit of the drum that there has been a request for his services. Before the borrowers remove the drum from the house, they will beat it two times. As they walk to the home of the deceased, they will continue to play the drum on and off. *The Txiv Muam Tai* also performs another ceremony, called *Npuas Tai*, which he can perform in his own house if the person who has asked for the rite lives in the same village; otherwise, he will travel to perform it. Unfortunately, since so many Hmong have been uprooted from their traditional villages, it is very often the case that there is no *Txiv Muam Tai* with a drum available. In such an instance, an improvised drum will be made quickly from a tree or bucket which, however, must be destroyed immediately the funeral is over.

2. The pointing-the-way-stick, or *Txhib Ntawg*, is used only during funerals and related death ceremonies. It is made of a split of wood or a bamboo stick for a specific occasion and thrown away after the funeral or ceremony is over. Its purpose is to facilitate communications between the living and the dead, or spirits, and to point the way to the land of the ancestors for the souls of the deceased person. It is also employed to invite the spirits from their place in the other world to come and participate in certain ceremonies, as well as to guide them back to their home.

3. The Shaman's divine split horns, called the *Txwm Kuam*, are used by the shaman to cure illness and to call home the lost souls of the

living during healing ceremonies. The split horns are used again and again during the lifetime of the shaman as a tool for communication between the healer and the spirits.

4. The drum, or *Lub Nruas*, includes all varieties of drum, from the funeral drum to the shaman's ceremonial drum, and is a vital part of Hmong culture; all Hmong clans use the drum. It is employed in clan rituals without fear of offending any spirits. The funeral drum is used in accompaniment with the mouth organ, the *Qeej* or *Kheng*, during a traditional Hmong funeral, while the shaman's ceremonial drum is used to accompany small finger bells during healing ceremonies.

5. The *Qeej*, or mouth organ, is a musical instrument which has a vital role in Hmong social and funerary rites. Among the Hmong of Laos, only men play this instrument, but among the Hmong of China, both men and women play it. The *Qeej* is played for leisure, as well as to entertain crowds at social events such as the Hmong New Year festival. During funeral ceremonies, the ritualists will first recite the texts of the funeral rites in a manner the living can understand; then the *Qeej* is played to the same texts in order that the spirits may understand. Again, the *Qeej* is always played together with the drum during a funeral. When they are played contrapuntally, the voice of the drum is interpreted as, "Where to go? Where to go? *Mus qhov twg? Mus qhov twg?*" and the music of the *Qeej* replies, "Go this way. Go this way. *Mus qhov nov. Mus qhov nov.*" It is in this fashion that the spirits of the drum and *Qeej* help to direct the souls of the deceased to the land of his ancestors.

6. A real umbrella, or *Lub Kaus*, is used during marriage ceremonies. It symbolizes protection for the newly wedded couple in beginning their life together. A paper umbrella, by contrast, is made and used during a funeral. The paper umbrella is placed in a box or a basket with a slain chicken, and this box or basket is placed next to the corpse's head during the funeral. The deceased is fed in a ritual manner three times a day, and this food is likewise placed in the box. After the corpse is buried, the box holding the paper umbrella, the chicken, and the food that was symbolically fed to the deceased, is placed atop of the grave. It is believed that the deceased will then employ the paper umbrella to protect himself from the elements during his journey to the other world.

7. The ceremonial paper cutter, or *Txheej Txam*, is used to cut ceremonial paper into various designs. All Hmong use a similar ceremonial paper cutter, but each person cuts designs according to his ability and creativity. The end product consists of elaborate forms

attached together in huge branch-like figures, which are displayed around the corpse in the course of funeral observances. The older the deceased person, the bigger and more elaborated the ceremonial papers must be. These papers are burned before the deceased is buried, and will be transformed into money to be used in the other world for the deceased to spend on necessities and luxuries alike. The Hmong shaman also uses ceremonial papers in healing rituals. These papers are burned at a specific time during the ceremony, once again as a form of payment; either for debts the sick person may have incurred while wandering, or for services rendered by spirits in releasing the sick person's souls and other such services.

8. The chicken (*Tus Qaib*) is used in many different ceremonies, running the gamut from naming a new baby to the funeral. Traditionally, three days after a new baby is born, Hmong parents perform a naming ceremony. In this ceremony, a pair of chickens is usually killed to call the souls of the new born to occupy his physical body so that he may join the rest of the family members in the house. When a person dies, a chicken is also killed—in this case to help guide his spirits to the other world. Finally, when a person is sick and has been diagnosed by the shaman as having lost a soul, a pair of chickens will be killed for a soul calling ceremony.

All Hmong know of or are familiar with the above eight spirits, and consider that anyone who claims to be Hmong but has no knowledge of these eight, is, in actuality, non-Hmong. Those Hmong who maintain their traditional animist religion still believe in these eight spirits, although Hmong who have converted to other religious systems may have discarded them.

The single most important reason for Hmong clan names is that they originally served to facilitate kinship organization, better enabling young people to find marriage partners. Yet, with the passage of time, clan names have also come to differentiate those with somewhat divergent ceremonial traditions. Nevertheless, all Hmong will accept the existence of the eight spirits listed above.

These clan names are not meant specifically to differentiate one clan from another, or to set apart one clan from the other. From the earliest time, all Hmong, without distinction, have shared essentially the same cultural background and knowledge. They have considered themselves to be related, in that they all maintain the same traditions and believe in the same spirits. However, without a written language it has been necessary to transmit orally from one generation to the next their cultural institutions and religious rituals. In a manner such as this, mistakes will be made and many errors of transmission have occurred over the centuries. Fortunately, the

Hmong have one tradition that addresses this difficulty. If an individual or a group makes a mistake, especially during the performance of a ritual or ceremony, they may ask the "Sister Aunt," *Muam Phauj*, to come and bless their error, and, from that time forward, the ritual will continue, institutionalized, in the new form. The Hmong believe that, once a mistake occurs, it cannot be corrected. This has resulted in the adoption of new forms with relative ease, so that, down the centuries, different Hmong clans or lineages have come to practice slightly different versions of rituals than formerly, and may recite modified texts in the performance of those rituals..

As an adjunct, the majority of modern Hmong assume that since the rituals of their clans or lineages are different from each other, they must be unrelated. In fact, these differences exist as a consequence of the aforementioned mistakes, changes, and adaptations over an enormously lengthy period of time. Another consequence is that, over generations, the Hmong began to emphasize the importance of clan differences and of differing versions of rituals and their texts. Therefore, even though all still believe in and maintain the above eight spirits, the focus of many individuals and clans has shifted to an emphasis on those things that have changed through time, rather than those that have remained static. As a result, clan identity has assumed a heightened importance in later years, with clans emphasizing, and clinging to, a single version of a particular ritual they share or do not share, rather then emphasizing an overview of the whole system. The impact of this gradual shift in emphasis has had a tremendous influence in creating divisions and competition between, and fragmentation of, Hmong cultural beliefs, customs, and religious rituals.

CEREMONIES RELATED TO THE SOULS (*Kev Ua Plig*)

As has been seen time and again, the Hmong perform many ceremonies related to the souls. They perform soul calling ceremonies to bring back lost souls; they tie a string around the wrist to bless the soul; they perform shaman ceremonies to find souls; and they kill chickens and pigs in sacrifice to spirits so that the soul of a suffering individual may be relieved of its torment.

The *Tswv Tsim Neeg* couple taught a blessing for Hmong people on earth to follow. If people worship, believe in, and observe this blessing, life will be happy and fulfilling, but if they do not, then the blessing will be lost and the *Tswv Tsim Neeg* couple will abandon the unbelievers, with the result that life will be lived in suffering. When people on earth experience difficulties in life, are afflicted with poverty and other difficulties, and when they are in ignorance of the reasons for their bitter fate, they should prepare a meal and call the *Tswv Tsim Neeg* couple to bless the food served and endow the caller with good medicine, love, understanding, and a mind of sufficient power to pursue whatever one may desire in life. Whoever asks the *Tswv Tsim Neeg* couple in this manner for blessings will be granted prosperity, good health, and a sharp mind.

However, although a man may make promises to the spirits, he does not necessarily do as he says he will. For example, a man may have had a newborn baby boy and love the child very much. Feeling so strongly, he kills a pig, prepares a feast, and invites his relatives and friends to celebrate with him. He asks each of the relatives to tie a string on the wrist of the child and say a few words of blessing on the child's behalf, so that the child will grow up strong, healthy, and intelligent, becoming educated and a leader. When a man has a son who graduates from high school or college, he is very happy for his son and may want to kill an animal, prepare a feast, and invite everyone he knows to join in the feast and tie strings on the wrist of his son, happy to share this occasion with everyone. Yet, if the man's actions are thought selfish or ostentatious by the *Tswv Tsim Neeg* couple, or if the form for blessing is distorted, the result will not be favorable.

It is to be appreciated that Hmong parents, as parents do everywhere, wish for their children, 1) a successful completion of their education; 2) a prosperous life; 3) health; and, 4) influence in the community, or *Tau Ua Nom Txwv*. To indicate their happiness for their children's success and accomplishments, and to wish the children a bright future, Hmong parents will kill an animal such as a pig or cow, and prepare a feast to celebrate these and other such successful transitions in life. During the feast, people will tie wrist strings on the designated individual and bless him or her with a long, healthy, prosperous, and successful life. If the individual is male, they will wish even more for him, such as that he become well educated and even a just and influential political leader (*Nom Txwv*).

The *Tswv Tsim Neeg* couple have endowed the Hmong with a creed of blessing to be said on such a string tying occasion, and when the Hmong observe this creed and call upon the *Tswv Tsim Neeg* couple to join with them and grant their wishes, the couple are said to do so. However, there were, in the distant past, those Hmong who did not follow the *Tswv Tsim Neeg* couple's creed of blessing carefully, but rather distorted it for selfish ends. Unfortunately, the majority of Hmong, ignorant of this distortion so long ago, continue to use the distorted version today. Since the Hmong do not practice this string tying ceremony in its original form, it is no longer effective, even to the extent that it has a negative, rather than a positive, effect.

The question arises; why did the Hmong distort the string tying creed? It is said that long ago, the Hmong practiced the string tying ceremony by carefully following the creed of blessing enjoined by the *Tswv Tsim Neeg* couple. However, human jealousy became a critical factor. If, for example, if a man had a new son and prepared a feast for his friends and relatives, so that they might tie the string and to bless the boy, the *Tswv Tsim Neeg* couple, in consequence, were thought disposed to grant the child everything. He might grow to have power, and, when he became a leader, punish others if they did not observe his rule or follow his laws.[10] Fearful of just such an eventuality, some, in the course of the blessing at a string tying, would begin in proper fashion, but then intentionally distort the words so that the *Tswv Tsim Neeg* couple would not bless the child, but instead curse him with failure. Since the Hmong do not believe that a mistake can be undone, even a deliberate one, the child would then be doomed to a life of mediocrity, forced to live with the consequences of this "existential sabotage."

However, turn about, as the apothegm has it, is fair play. When the shoe came to the other foot, and it was the neighbor's turn to celebrate the arrival of a son, revenge could be expected. It might be that the sufferer of the original slight would plan and execute a curse of his own, saying, for example, that, should the child grew up with any of a stipulated list of features, he must go abroad to work as the assistant of a foreigner. A child thus cursed, grown into manhood, would be expected to find himself in exile, and not working for the betterment of the Hmong, assisting or leading his people. In such a scheme the *Tswv Tsim Neeg* couple are unable to intervene for the good. The words they gave the Hmong have their own power, and, spoken in this way, to curse, the couple must, perforce, acquiesce, though they shake their heads in disbelief, powerless to turn their eyes away as this cycle of slights and revenge deteriorated into clan vendettas, often lasting generations.

As the years and generations passed, distortions in the formula for blessing the string have become institutionalized in tradition. This distorted tradition is what the Hmong today practice, even without being cognizant of its harm. Modern, young Hmong think that the creed of blessing must be right, since all the old people say it is, and, as a result, they unknowingly perpetuate the mistakes and deliberate distortions of previous generations.

Thus, in their invocations, they continue to importune, albeit inadvertently, the *Tswv Tsim Neeg* couple to bring ill fortune upon others; as, for example, to send intelligent and educated younger Hmong away from their homes to become foreign workers and assistants. They do not, as they believe, ask the *Tswv Tsim Neeg* couple to bless these young people to lead, help, and work for the Hmong. Therefore, no matter how hard these younger people try to work for their own, they are fated to meet with failure.

There are many young Hmong who have, in recent years, completed higher education and earned Ph.D., M.D. or J.D. degrees. But for reasons that are not entirely clear, these people cannot communicate easily with the majority of Hmong, and, as a result, do not work for the Hmong community. Whatever they may propose, the Hmong disagree. Occasionally they are even greeted with censure or threats of death. However, if they choose to work and share their ideas with mainstream Americans, these medical and professional people are given encouragement and respect.

The above discussion will serve to illustrate the extent to which the Hmong often work against their own best interests. In what way, precisely, have the Hmong been misled about and distorted the old rituals? In order for one to understand this well, it may be informative to examine closely a sample ritual; the string tying.

When a would-be well-wisher begins to tie the string on the wrist of the son for whom the occasion is designated, he will intone the first few words, which call for good fortune and are filled with beautiful meaning. Soon thereafter, however, it has become customary to add, "From now on, you should go to eat outsiders' or foreigners' food, speak outsiders' language, sit on outsiders' chairs, work for outsiders, become outsiders' political leaders, and even a king of outsiders."

If it is the case that the *Tswv Tsim Neeg* couple are present and listening, they are certainly convinced that the Hmong do not want to help each other at all, and it would seem logical to infer that the Hmong as a people do not love each other. They are, after all, telling this son of their race not to lead them. They are telling him they do not want him. If the words are to be believed, the Hmong only want him to lead outsiders or foreigners. Nevertheless, it is necessary that the *Tswv Tsim Neeg* couple do as they promised in ages long past, and honor their word that they will come whenever called upon and grant whatever is asked. They may be disappointed that they must grant such terrible wishes, but they are powerless to resist. The feast thus becomes not only a waste of money, but is utterly counterproductive.

The creed of blessing that the *Tswv Tsim Neeg* couple originally bestowed upon the Hmong was not complex; it was a simple means of obtaining a desired end. The couple, in a gesture of extreme generosity, ordained that, whatever the Hmong wanted, if they followed the instructions they would obtain it. If they did something well, it would turn out well. If they asked for something, they would get it, and good results would proceed from good intentions.

What follows is the correct invocation to be observed on the occasion of a string tying: Holding the string in one hand, one should call out, "Oh! Today is a good day, and tonight is a good night. This is a good time. This good day is your day. . . . so I tie you with this string on your day and your night. . . . They said to pull the mountain and valley together for you. . . . tie the copper trunk to the stone trunk, and the stone to the bronze trunk.

. . . I tie them all together to become you. Now I am calling you to come to live with us, to become our political leader and king whom we respect and honor. It's your day, your time, and your tradition to tie you here. We will not let you go to get lost with foreigners or outsiders. Please come to be our political leader and lead the Hmong people."

This is a good blessing; the blessing that the *Tswv Tsim Neeg* couple originally taught the Hmong. If one invokes the blessing in this way and no other, then the son will be granted good fortune, intelligence, leadership skills, and knowledge to prepare him to become an influential man in the Hmong community. When he is mature, he will be knowledgeable and wise. Whatever he says, other Hmong will understand and agree with him. He can become their leader and they will respect him.

It is unfortunate that, as mentioned earlier, the majority of Hmong have distorted this blessing for many, many years—and still use a distorted version today. The Hmong will have to change this blessing, returning it to its original form, in order for the community to respect, trust, and agree with the intellectual, young Hmong in their midst. If the Hmong want to see their children helping and working for their community and leading them into the future, they, themselves, will have to change; otherwise, their children will continue to fail them. If the Hmong follow their traditional rituals correctly and both understand and believe in the meaning of their traditional way of life, they will accrue greater power to do as they want, and, in a very natural way, find themselves becoming more successful.

The informant continued to emphasize the importance of properly following Hmong cultural tradition. This section explains the Hmong ways of dealing with life's events, whether it is birth, marriage, death, or illness. The Hmong need to practice their traditions as they were meant to be practiced so that they may be blessed accordingly. When such a tradition is neglected, ignored, or altered, the intended results may not be achieved. If observing and maintaining their cultural traditions is an essential part of their lives, then it would be logical to argue the converse; namely that a failure to observe and maintain their cultural traditions will lead to difficulties in life. These difficulties can be construed as encompassing a major negative impact on the lifestyle and health condition of any Hmong.

A HISTORY OF ILLNESSES KNOWN TO THE HMONG AND THEIR HEALERS

According to a Hmong healer, illness or disease exists in a manner similar to the nature of politics. That is, a political party may appear very strong during one period of time, but lose influence at another time. People who are not healers or health care providers may have the impression that new illnesses or diseases emerge all the time, but for healers or health care providers, all illnesses or diseases have always existed. They simply become more wide spread during certain periods and among certain groups of the population, then become dormant for a while before awakening once more. Most of the world's major illnesses are never completely and permanently overcome.

What follows is a description of the major illnesses that the Hmong and their healers have known in recent times. These illnesses are fearful to the Hmong due to their powerful and usually fatal impact, but, according to a Hmong healer, they do not last forever. Rather, they tend to last about seven to ten years, then diminish in virulence or become subject to new medicines or treatment techniques developed by health care providers.

It should be borne in mind that, in the following discussion, the ranges of time given for the appearances of the illnesses discussed are approximate. Owing to the imperfect nature of human memory, some of these may have occurred a little earlier or somewhat later than the years given. Nonetheless, according to this informant, a healer, a major illness called *Mob Qhua Tawm Dub* or *Mob Plab Zawv Tshav* made an appearance in circa 1925. Patients who contracted this illness experienced abdominal pain, followed by severe diarrhea with bloody stools, then died suddenly. This illness continued to afflict the Hmong until approximately 1935, when it largely disappeared.

From 1935 to 1945, a new illness manifested itself. The Hmong called it *Mob Yas Yuam*. Those suffering from this illness evinced severe abdominal pains, as of muscles or nerves torn apart, and wracking pains all over the body which caused them to writhe in agony. The patients usually died quickly after these symptoms were noted.

From 1945 to 1959, an illness called *Tswv Xyas* emerged. The etiology of *Tswv Xyas* is often described in mythological or folkloric terms, consonant with which the condition is attributed to a Hmong man who turned into a tiger and roared throughout the forest. Invisible to human beings, he would communicate with people in their dreams, and would come to Hmong villages in search of residents noted for their beauty or other pleasing physical characteristics; their skill in music, needlework, or the performance of ritual, and so on. When he located such a prospective victim, it was his usual practice to extend a foot to trip the unsuspecting individual, and, in this way, capture his soul and carry it away. The victims usually died momentarily, without any visible signs or other symptoms. Many babies noted for their cute appearance, as well as good-looking and/or talented people died suddenly during this period.[11]

From 1959 to 1964, another illness unique to the Hmong emerged, known as *Mob Aws*. Those stuck by this illness became sick for one or two days, then died suddenly. After this illness appeared, it is said, the Sky, considering there had been entirely too many illnesses, replaced the Dragon

King (*Huab Tais Zaj*) with the Thunder King (*Huab Tais Xob*) as the earth's sovereign.[12] This change of leadership, it is said, took place precisely on December 16, 1964, a date known with such accuracy by the occurrence of an earthquake. After the installation of the Thunder King, moreover, fewer major illnesses occurred among the Hmong for a period of approximately ten years, and, although people continued to experience a range of minor illnesses, they usually recovered within a short period of time.

From 1976 to 1985, yet another new illness afflicted the Hmong, referred to as *Mob Kab Xeb*. This infirmity affected both the Hmong of Laos and of Thailand, and became a major threat to the Hmong living at that time in Thai refugee camps, attacking children more often than adults. The single significant symptom of this illness consisted of uncontrollable shaking of the arms and legs, and, without immediate treatment, the patient could die suddenly.

From 1986 to 1995, there have been several widespread illnesses which, although not entirely unique to the Hmong, have nonetheless created fear in the Hmong community. One of these, *Mob Kas Ceeg*, is a variety of sexually transmitted disease which spread quickly during this period. Its dissemination has now slowed, but it is still occasionally encountered.

From 1995 to the present time, the incidence of common cerebral edema, or stroke, has been rising, and this will, before it slows, in all likelihood become a dominant health problem until at least the year 2005.

The year 1997 witnessed the onset of a strange and horrifying illness which, without other signs or symptoms, causes the muscles of the patient's cheek to flex uncontrollably, tearing the flesh all the way back to the ear. At the same time, speech becomes severely reduced in volume and in clarity. According to a Hmong traditional massage therapist, "This is a disease that causes a person's blood and nervous system to malfunction. The nerves in the body have been stressed, twisted, and pulled to cause the mouth to shift to the ears. Some Hmong would attribute this illness to evil spirits, *Dab*, but it is not the case. A virus causes physiological maladjustment to weather conditions, that [in turn] leads to the development of this illness. We don't know how widespread this illness will become or how long it will last."

This discussion of the major illnesses that have affected the Hmong in this century has excluded such minor illnesses as the common cold/flu, chicken pox, and the like; however, this should not be construed to mean they are unknown to the Hmong population. The Hmong have been as much affected by these as the mainstream population.

If the above illnesses are those with which the Hmong and their healers are familiar, then the majority of the diseases currently extant in the United States are new, and the Hmong will not, as a rule, understand the gravity of most of these "new" diseases until they have, themselves, suffered from them, or have seen relatives or friends do so. More importantly, if they cannot conceptualize these new diseases in the same way their conventional health care professionals do, Hmong patients are less likely to follow the health treatment plan recommended for them.

TRADITIONAL HMONG HEALTH TREATMENT TECHNIQUES: PHYSICAL VS. SPIRITUAL TREATMENT

Hmong healers, by and large, hold that people become ill due either to a condition of the spirits or souls, or to a condition of the physiology. A person who becomes sick due to the action of a virus, or a person who has suffered a wound, i.e. someone with diagnosable physical symptoms, may be treated with herbs or other such medicines. The spiritual healer, such as a shaman or magic healer, on the other hand, can treat an individual who is sick but does not have diagnosable physical symptoms. Whether or not he will be able to do so depends largely on his natural power (*Hwj Huam*), and, although the Hmong almost universally believe that, in the course of such healings, contact is made with the spirit world, it should be emphasized that Hmong spiritual healers freely admit that they do not actually see any ghost, spirit or soul; either of the patient or of helper spirits. Nevertheless, if the shaman's natural power is strong, and the shaman says the patient will get well, the patient should get well.

Sometimes the patient's natural power is stronger than the shaman's, however, with the result that the illness, having more "power" than the shaman's remedy, will not be cured. Most Hmong shamans maintain that they know whether or not they will achieve success even before beginning the rite, simply by looking at the patient, and in cases where such prior analysis is not possible, there are prescribed diagnostic techniques that may be called upon. However, if the shaman should decide that he cannot assist the patient, he will generally tell both the patient and the patient's family to ask another shaman for assistance. Naturally, he will refrain from asserting, either in speech or in manner, that the condition or illness is not treatable. In addition, since it is acknowledged that each healer has a different level of natural power, and thus is able to cure some patients but not others, a patient may ask more than one shaman to treat him.

DIAGNOSTIC TECHNIQUES: EGG BALANCING AND POURING (*Tsawv Qe* and *Nchuav Qe*)

There are two diagnostic techniques which employ an egg. The first of these is known as *Tsawv Qe* (egg balancing), and is performed by a diagnostician prior to the shaman's involvement. It is done, in fact, at the onset of illness to assist in the selection of the shaman who will be consulted. This

Tsawv Qe requires the performer to use a raw egg, a large bowl filled with uncooked rice, and a smaller bowl which is placed sideways on top of the rice. As the diagnostician attempts to balance the small end of an egg on the round surface of the lesser bowl, he will call out the name of a shaman in a chanting tone, using a phrase which can be translated roughly as, "Oh, if shaman X is capable of treating (the prospective patient's name), then may this egg balance on this spot!"

If the first shaman named does not "balance the egg," another name will be called, and so on until the egg is balanced. After the diagnostician has completed this rite, and the name of an appropriate shaman has been decided, a family member will approach the shaman and ask him or her to perform a ceremony of diagnosis to determine what is spiritually wrong. At this point, the shaman may express reluctance to perform the ceremony, or he may even refuse altogether. However, when confronted with the fact that his name was approved in the course of a bona fide egg balancing, he will be left with little choice but to acquiesce in treatment.

The second technique of diagnosis which employs an egg is known as *Nchuav Qe* (egg pouring). The diagnostician will hold an uncooked egg in his hand and chant for a while, then break the shell, pour its contents into a small bowl of water, and read the information provided by the egg's configuration; the identity of the evil spirit is causing the illness. In case the diagnostician finds the signs ambiguous, he will issue a tentative diagnosis, then utter additional chants by pouring additional water over the egg. The new formation thus revealed will either confirm or refute the initial diagnosis.

CALLING THE SHAMAN'S SPIRIT HELPERS (*Txhij Qhua*)

When a person is very sick and several treatments have been explored without recovery, a family member will ask a shaman, if one has not been consulted previously or if other shamans have tried and failed, to assess whether the patient can be cured. It is often the case that there has already been great expenditure of funds and of time and energy, and both the family and the shaman will not wish to expend the additional resources required for a full ceremony. In these circumstances, the shaman will perform what is called the *Txhij Qhua* technique. This involves loudly playing his gongs, chanting, and using his *Txwm Kuam* (divine split horns) to call his spirit helpers to his altar. As the chanting continues, the shaman drops his split horns on the floor; if one of the pair opens face up, while the other opens face down, then the shaman knows the outlook is poor. He will repeat this procedure several times, and, if the same result occurs, then the diagnosis is definite; the patient will get worse and eventually die.

DIAGNOSIS THROUGH THE USE OF THE SHAMAN'S DIVINE SPLIT HORNS (*Khov Kuam*)

In addition to the variety of assessment described above, the family member(s) of a patient may ask a shaman to use his divine split horns to make a diagnosis. This he will do by performing the *Khov Kuam* technique, the purpose of which is to uncover both the nature of the illness and its etiology. As he performs the *Khov Kuam*, the shaman will chant and manipulate the split horns in a manner similar to that employed in the *Txhij Qhua*. He will instruct the horns to turn in a certain way if the person's soul(s) have become lost or have wandered away. There may even have been transmigration, in which case the soul(s) will have assumed another form. The shaman will instruct the horns to turn another way if none of these eventualities is the cause of the infirmity, but, rather, it is the case that the spirits of the ancestors want something; or that inadvertent offense has been given the house spirits, or evil and/or wild spirits. In every case, when information has been garnered from a single toss of the horns, the shaman will repeat his actions to be certain of the facts.

As an example of this *Khov Kuam*, we may posit a case in which the shaman has ascertained that the cause of the difficulty is that the spirit of the patient's deceased father wants his earthbound offspring to perform a cow ceremony (*Nyuj Dab*) performed in his honor. In this situation, the shaman will strike a bargain with the father's spirit; he will speak to the father's son, and insist that he commit himself to arranging the performance of a cow ceremony provided the father allows the sick family member to recover in certain number of days. If this recovery occurs, the son will be obligated to prepare the ceremony.

COUNTING THE DATES (*Xam Hnub Nyoog*), COUNTING THE CARDS (*Saib Phaib*), COUNTING THE NUMBERS (*Xam Lej*), AND THE WRITE AND READ TECHNIQUE (*Sau Ntawv Saib*)

"Counting the Dates," "Counting the Cards," "Counting the Numbers," and "Write and Read," are four techniques used in a manner similar to the technique of the shaman's divine split horns, described above, to establish whether it will be possible for a patient to recover from his illness. These techniques may also be used for diagnosing the potential causes of an illness, and for such other, unrelated, inquiries as locating lost articles or determining the best time to plan a journey or other important event. While these techniques have been practiced by the Hmong for centuries, it is widely acknowledged that they originated with other tribes neighboring the Hmong, or with one of the dominant cultures—Chinese, Lao, or Thai—in a locale in which the Hmong have lived.

DIAGNOSTIC SHAMAN CEREMONY (*Ua Neeb Saib*)

The Diagnostic Shaman Ceremony is yet another Hmong diagnostic technique; in this case performed exclusively by a shaman. There are two distinct methods. The first is employed simply to diagnose a patient's health problems, while the second is employed to diagnose a person while the shaman is simultaneously engaged in performing a recovery ceremony for a third party who has been restored to health. In this latter, one or more members of the currently ill individual's family will brings two sticks of incense to burn at the shaman's altar, asking the shaman to diagnose (*Saib*) the relative who is currently ill as he performs the other rite. This may sound like a tall order, but the versatile shaman can do many things while in trance.

As a general rule, when a shaman has achieved trance and is ready to diagnose a patient, he will call his spirit troops to go with him to the house of that individual. While they are there, he will instruct his spirit troops to make a thorough check of all circumstances which may be having an adverse effect on the patient, both within the house and outside. The spirit troops will then determine if all household spirits are in order, will attempt to locate any negative influence, and will, in addition, ascertain if there is anything present in the immediate environment which may constitute a bad omen. After thus checking, the spirit troops will report any disturbing signs to the shaman, who may require them to check for a second time. Once the shaman is satisfied with their report, however, he will gather together his spirit troops and move on to the next case.

CONSULTING THE MASTER HEALER (*Saib Saub*)

The Hmong word, *Saub*, refers to a master healer, and someone who has earned this title is expected to know more or less everything there is to know regarding Hmong traditional health treatment. Thus, to request a *Saib Saub* is to ask a master healer to call upon the sum total of traditional lore in rendering his judgment on the cause and prognosis of an illness. The master healer will then make use of any or all of the diagnostic tools at his command, including all of those discussed above, in arriving at his opinion. Such masters are at the pinnacle of the shaman's craft, and, as such, are rare; indeed, it is generally agreed that, while there are master healers in Laos and Thailand, in the United States all have passed away.

HEALING OR HEALTH TREATMENT TECHNIQUES: SOUL CALLING (*Hu Plig*)

The soul calling is an oft-performed ceremony with which all Hmong become familiar at an early age; in fact, a soul calling is performed three days after the birth of every new Hmong baby. At the time of the Hmong New Year celebration, a soul calling ceremony is performed for the entire family. When a Hmong is ill, has fallen, or merely become frightened, a soul calling ceremony may be performed. In any instance in which it is felt the individual may have lost one of his souls, a soul calling ceremony invariably will be performed. A soul calling ceremony will be held for a newlywed couple on the third day after their union, and may even be performed for a family member who is about to undertake a long journey; or who has just arrived home from such a journey.

The ceremony is not esoteric, and may be performed by any individual who is not shy and knows the method. It is, however, usually performed by an elderly person, by a shaman, or by another variety of healer.

In normal circumstances, the materials required are a pair of chickens, one egg for each person whose soul is to be called, a bowl of uncooked rice in which to place the egg or eggs, incense, and a shaman's gong. The physical presence of the individual whose soul is to be called, on the other hand, is not a requirement, for the caller can simply mention his name during the ceremony.

The ceremony itself consists of two parts. The first of these takes place before the chickens are killed and the eggs are boiled. Subsequently, the chickens are slaughtered, and the chickens and eggs are cooked. Then the caller repeats the ceremony and, once this second part of the soul calling ceremony has been completed, the caller must read the chickens' feet, the top portions of their skulls, and the curves of their tongue bones to determine how willing the soul will be to come back, or, in case the soul has returned, how happy it may be. If any of these readings shows any unfavorable sign, a second soul calling ceremony may be performed or the individual may be advised to take certain precautions in his daily activities, such as, e.g., to avoid certain journeys or to stay in on certain dates. It should be noted, however, that, although this is certainly one of the most common of Hmong rituals, Hmong who have converted to Christianity eschew its performance as a matter of religious principle.

HEALING SHAMAN CEREMONY (*Ua Neeb Kho*)

If it has been emphasized time and again that, in Hmong society, one of the most important healers is the shaman, it is because this fact cannot be overstated. It will not be surprising, therefore, that the Hmong categorize shamanism according to a plethora of types and forms. In the broadest sense, there are two types of shamanism. The first of these, traditional Hmong shamanism, fills its ranks with those who have been selected by circumstance. In conformity with this tradition, no one may become a shaman simply as a matter of personal will; on the contrary, it is the shaman spirits (*Dab*) who will come to the person whom they have selected and make their selection known. This is generally accomplished by rendering him ill until such time as he may agree to become a shaman. When a shaman so selected and so coerced performs healing ceremonies, he will always go into trance. The second, more contemporary, Hmong view of the shaman's selection holds that one may become a shaman merely by desiring to do so. Such a shaman will not necessarily enter a trance state in order to perform his duties.

Although it would seem that, in some sense, a shaman who has been selected by the spirits for his qualifications of temperament and character might be superior, either of these two types of shaman can be expected to be capable of diagnosing and treating illness.

It is thought likely that the Hmong acquired the traditional view of the shaman's selection from other, neighboring, tribes, or from the several cultures dominant in the areas in which they have, throughout the course of their history, resided. That this is, in all likelihood, so is attested by the fact that other aspects of Hmong shamanism, such as the many diagnostic and treatment techniques, often involve skills for which literacy is presumed. Counting cards, counting numbers, or writing and reading, to cite but a few examples, all assume a certain basic familiarity with systems of writing. In addition, there are those rituals which are performed in a language not identifiably Hmong, which lends credence to those who assert that certain, at least, of the Hmong healing rituals are borrowed. (Please refer to the section on the Magic Healing, or *Khawv Koob*, immediately below.) Despite the fact that the aforementioned tribes' and cultures' forms of writing differ from that of the Hmong, the techniques of Hmong healing for the most part antedate any method of transcribing the Hmong language.

THE MAGIC HEALING (*Khawv Koob*)

The Magic Healing technique is performed to frighten, negotiate with, or trick the spirits into leaving the patient alone, and to relieve pain, swelling, vomiting, and bleeding, and it is, by and large, men who learn and practice this technique. Specific incantations are prescribed to cure specific types of illnesses, and the words of these incantations are not Hmong. While some healers maintain that these words are Chinese, others believe they are words and phrases in the language of the spirits. Depending on the type of illness that the healer is attempting to cure, a variety of tools will be used; a bowl of cold water will be utilized in splashing the patient, or a shaman gong employed to make noise. The healer may resort to a drum, a knife, burning rice husks, or other such implements and accessories, all in an effort to frighten evil spirits.

HERBAL MEDICINES (*Tshuaj Ntsuab*)

Many Hmong families in the United States still plant herbs, either outdoors in their gardens or indoors as houseplants. Such herbs, used in many different ways, have been a part of Hmong healing practice for centuries, and there are Hmong specialists, for the most part female, skillful in utilizing these herbs for their medicinal qualities.

As examples, when a couple is infertile; or a person is losing weight, or appetite, or both, or simply feeling weak, the Hmong believe that something is missing from his body. It is held that there is not enough blood or fat to support the body's effective functioning. In order to enhance strength and energy, therefore, and to regenerate the bodily systems, an herbal remedy is prepared. Because herbs are not normally eaten directly, a chicken is killed and cooked in combination with the requisite herbs. When this is done in the prescribed manner and ingested at least three times within a short span, the regimen is believed to yield the necessary healing power to restore the condition.

When a person has stomach ache, on the other hand, the first therapeutic is generally massage, after which, if necessary, herbal medicines are used. In such a case, dry roots are sometimes minced and soaked in hot water, after which the patient drinks the decoction. At other times, dry roots or plants will be mashed until assuming a granular form, some or all of which the patient may simply swallow. Certain green herbs are known to be good for stomach ache, and, of these, there are those which can be steeped to make a tea, while others must be mashed and warmed, then made into a sticking plaster which is applied to the affected area.

In all of these preparations, herbalists follow systematic procedures, and, should these procedures be ignored, the herbs can be harmful. The correct dosage is also of consequence. For instance, when giving certain herbal roots to a male patient, nine slices of the root are called for, while, in the case of a female, seven slices are given. As is the case with more modern biomedicines, the possibility of an overdose is a hazard which cannot be ignored.

MASSAGE TECHNIQUES (*Zaws*)

There exists a variety of massage therapists, each of whom specializes in a different part of the body. A therapist who concentrates on deep anatomy can alleviate sprained ankles and injured hands or feet. This type of massage therapist can bring quick relief to any type of bodily injury. A therapist who focuses on stomach ache and superficial muscle pain is able to diagnose what has become irregular in the condition of the stomach or the aching muscle. When a person feels pain in the stomach, or becomes sick due to the ingestion of bad food, this massage therapist will attend to the stomach, chest, arms and hands. He may, as well, use very fine needles to gently puncture the patient's fingertips and squeeze a few drops of blood out into a bowl of cold water. If this is done correctly, the sufferer will experience a decrease in pain immediately after treatment. For stomach aches unrelated to food, on the other hand, the massage therapist will massage the area, generally at least three times. If pain persists after the third treatment, the therapist usually recommends the patient take some sort of herbal medicine and consult with a shaman.

Another area of specialization in Hmong massage is that of infertility. The massage therapist will begin by feeling the infertile woman's stomach and reproductive system from the outside. Although such a therapist has, in all likelihood, never taken a formal course in anatomy, she can tell where each part of the internal organ lies and what is its condition. If the therapist finds that the patient's reproductive organs are abnormal, she will prescribe a treatment plan which typically will include several massage sessions and the use of herbal medicines. If the infertile woman's internal status is normal, however, then the patient's partner is considered.

This area of focus inevitably touches upon the care of pregnant women, and in the case of a woman with child who is experiencing pain, the massage therapist can bring relief with the application of healing massage to the woman's stomach. In case such a woman also suffers from a delay of labor, the therapist can, by feeling her stomach, know the size and position of the baby. If the baby is not positioned properly, and a difficult delivery is diagnosed, the therapist can massage the stomach to reposition the child, speeding the delivery process and obviating a cesarean section. In such cases, herbal medicines are occasionally also used.

APPLYING PRESSURE (*Xais Ceeb*)

The Hmong believe that, in response to shock, the human nervous system can be shifted out of its state of balance and into an altered condition in which a variety of symptoms present themselves. These symptoms may be mild or severe, according to the severity of the shock's impact, and this altered and unhealthy status of the nervous system is referred to as *Ceeb*. Although the word may be translated as "shock," it is clear that a good deal more is implied, encompassing both the incident which has created the adverse neural or spiritual effect, and the entire panoply of symptoms which may, as a result, occur.

The symptoms of *Ceeb* usually consist of a sensation of chilling cold, which may be felt all over the body or be localized, depending on the degree and type of shock one has experienced. Some sufferers have mentioned coldness in their hands, arms, feet, and lower legs; others have experienced coldness from the waist up to the head, or down to the feet. As mentioned above, some individuals have described a sensation of cold all over. This experience of cold is occasionally described by Hmong patients as being "similar to having a fever, but without the hotness;" by others as a *sticky* cold. This condition can become worse without treatment, for which the Hmong resort to *Xais Ceeb* (applying pressure).

In the course of *Xais Ceeb*, the hands are employed to apply pressure to the patient's body along lines which run up the arms between the palm and the inside of the elbow, between the ankle and the back of the knee; or at the points at the back of the neck, and a good many other places. It is an effective technique for the condition of *Ceeb*, and when a patient is treated by an expert in *Xais Ceeb*, he will generally recover after two to three treatments. At the same time, although the technique is effective, it is not overly complicated, and does not require a specialist. In fact, it can be learned by almost anyone who is interested and has the time and the patience to do so; both Hmong men and Hmong women, therefore, are often found who are proficient.

PROPOSED SACRIFICE (*Fiv Yeem*)

Fiv Yeem is a technique which involves the performance of a sacrifice, and which is used in circumstances which require either that the ill be healed or the well be safeguarded. For *Fiv Yeem*, a shaman or other type of healer performs a brief ceremony and then proposes to the spirits that, if the person suffering illness or other physical complaint recovers in a specific period of time, a chicken, pig, goat or cow will be slaughtered and offered in sacrifice. Such a rite may also be used in some circumstances to ask ancestors or nature spirits for protection. For example, a Hmong patient awaiting open-heart surgery may offer such a *Fiv Yeem* to entreat his ancestors for protection during the operation. If the patient, after doing so, emerges unscathed from the operating room and recovers on schedule, he will kill a cow or pig as an offering. Moreover, in general, all the patient's relatives will attend this sacrifice, transforming a utilitarian into a social occasion.

As what may not be an entirely surprising corollary to the above, it may be noted here that there are some Hmong Americans who decline to purchase automobile insurance in those states where such insurance is not mandatory. Instead, they hold a *Fiv Yeem* for their ancestors, requesting protection for the year, and, if the year is unmarred by accident, these same drivers will kill a cow in fulfillment of their sacrificial pledge and hold a feast. There are those Hmong, in fact, who will join together to offer a single *Fiv Yeem*, and a few families may unite to spend from three hundred to six hundred dollars for the purchase of a cow as guarantor of their annual safety behind the wheel. This, of course, represents a considerable saving over the usual cost of an annual automobile insurance premium, with the added benefit that, if even one or two members of this automotive consortium have accidents, they can all ethically decline to follow through with the proposed sacrifice.

NEEDLE USING TECHNIQUE (*Hno Koob*)

Hno Koob is a technique used to relieve deep bodily tension through a combination of massage and the application of needles, not unlike those used in Chinese acupuncture, to specific areas of the surface anatomy. This treatment relieves tension and stress, as well as gas and the pain created by digestive problems.

TECHNIQUES OF DERMAL ABRASION (*Kav, Kuam, Nqus*)

The efficacy of dermal abrasion and related techniques, according to traditional Hmong medical lore, is due to the fact that both stress and its resulting tension, and 'internal heat,' can cause illness. Thus, Hmong healers employ the *kav* (wrapping and rubbing) technique by boiling an egg until hard, removing the shell and the hardened yolk while the cooked egg is still very hot, and placing a silver bar or a silver coin inside the egg in the yolk's now vacant place. The egg is then wrapped in cloth, and vigorously rubbed over the patient's arms, back, and forehead. The silver bar or coin will, in consequence, turn black, a result considered to arise from chemical action upon the metal by the internal waste and impurity which have been causing the complaint.

Another technique often employed is known as *kua*m (rubbing), in the practice of which a spoon or a coin is used to rub areas of the body with a simple, commercially available cream or ointment, such as Vick's or Tiger Balm.

A third technique is *nqus* (moxibustion), in the course of which a cup fashioned from glass or horn is heated with burning oil, then placed over the skin. With the extinction of the flame, the air inside the cup cools and contracts, forming a vacuum. This vacuum sucks waste from the skin, after the fashion of a small sauna, with the corresponding purification.

These three techniques are generally used in the treatment of the same spots, such as the forehead, back, arms, shoulders, and the backs of the knees. After rubbing and moxibustion, the affected areas will appear reddened or even slightly bruised.

BELIEF IN AND MANNER OF TRANSMITTING TRADITIONAL HMONG HEALING KNOWLEDGE

Many of the traditional Hmong healing methods and techniques discussed herein are quite efficacious, yet, despite the evident value of the knowledge they represent, the method of transmitting these skills and this knowledge has not been standardized. This can prove frustrating to the individual interested in the acquisition of these skills or the study of these methods. Hmong healers tend to be extremely selective about whom they instruct. While it may not be a cause for much astonishment that most Hmong herbalists and massage therapists, for example, will not train any potential apprentices or share their knowledge with anyone until a fee has been paid, in many instances the herbalist or massage therapist will not accept, under any conditions, an apprentice who is not a member of the immediate family.[13] Some will not even teach their own family members. There are even those who refuse to impart their knowledge to anyone at all, regardless of fee. As an example, one Hmong interviewee said, " I have this aunt who is an expert in birthing massage (*Tig Plab*). Many accredited doctors have approached her and asked if she would teach them, but her response was invariably, 'No.' They asked if she would accept a fee in order to teach them, but still she refused."

Another Hmong interviewee said that her husband's grandmother was an herbalist, and that she had asked this woman to teach her. The elderly woman declined without explanation, and soon after passed away. Her knowledge was buried with her.

In one case in which the knowledge was passed on, an interviewee said a Hmong doctor in California learned a version of traditional Hmong birthing massage (*Tig Plab*) when his parents trained him. He has incorporated this skill into his practice and has done wonderfully. He takes care of both Hmong and American patients who are in need of obstetric care, and none of his patients has ever found it necessary to endure a Cesarean section or other surgery. A Hmong nurse said, "If this kind of knowledge could be disseminated among doctors at large, especially in obstetrics-gynecology, the number of women forced to have Cesarean section or other surgeries could be reduced tremendously, and the costs associated with these procedures would be eliminated. That would, of course, increase the demand for these doctors and decrease the overhead expended on advertisements. It's better than any advertisement."

With regard to Cesarean section as performed in the United States, Lonsdorf et al. report that it is the most common surgical procedure in the nation, with hysterectomy ranked second.[14] Both of these procedures are performed on women only, and are of extremely questionable utility. Lonsdorf et al. cited research by Consumer Reports asserting that half of the Caesarean sections and twenty-seven percent of the hysterectomies performed in the United States were deemed to be unnecessary.[15]

One of the central reasons healers are reluctant to teach others is that the approach made by the prospective student is made in a nontraditional manner. In addition, many of these healers have acquired their skills and knowledge in a cultural context very different from the one in which they are now asked to teach, which puts them in an awkward position. When they learned the healing arts, they learned by observation and extended apprenticeship, without asking questions; their teachers neither demonstrated for their benefit, nor offered explanations for their enlightenment. The absorption by the student of skills and knowledge took place over a highly extended period via a process of what might be called intellectual osmosis. Now these same students, advanced in life and career, find they are asked to teach a new generation through the use of targeted demonstrations and extensive personalized explanation, a request which makes them twice uncomfortable. First, because it simply is "not the way things are done;" and, second, because, in any case, they don't know how to do it. Indeed, they may not be able even to conceive how to demonstrate what they know. Additionally, if the student has never suffered from a particular illness or condition, as the result of youth and inexperience, for example, the teacher will assume the student cannot be taught to treat that illness or condition.

HMONG HEALTH CARE PROVIDERS/INTERPRETERS' KNOWLEDGE OF TRADITIONAL HMONG HEALTH CARE PRACTICES

Moua conducted Master's thesis research in Minnesota with forty-eight Hmong bilingual workers.[16] Both her informants and the Hmong informants in Colorado interviewed for this study expressed similar views and detailed similar experiences regarding Hmong traditional healing practices. Most interpreters feel they have a general knowledge of Hmong shamanism, herbal medicine, and massage therapy. They feel they can explain these concepts in a general way to a non-Hmong who wants to know more. But a few, and especially the younger interpreters, feel that they cannot do so, having a poor grasp of the details of the beliefs and practices associated with these healing traditions, and their purposes.

Nevertheless, all of the Hmong interpreters and health care providers strongly believe in the efficacy of the various Hmong massage techniques, because they have seen these techniques work on many patients. A Hmong nurse said, "Sometimes I discover that Hmong massage therapists, especially *Tig Plab*, know more than Western doctors do. When it comes to massage of the abdomen (*Zaws Plab)*, it sometimes seems Western doctors have no knowledge at all about abdominal pain. If they know certain symptoms, as in the case of appendicitis, they may have a way to treat it, surgically removing that part. That's it. But there are other things about which they do not know, such as minor stomachaches or things like that; they do not know what it is or how to treat it."

Yet, in contradistinction to the case with regard to Hmong massage, most Hmong health care providers and interpreters are more critical of or skeptical about Hmong herbal medicine, and evince concern about the chemical composition of the herbs or plants Hmong use, especially those sent from Thailand and Laos. Often medicinal herbs are sent from an expert abroad to a person in the United States who will use or prepare them incorrectly. Exacerbating this problem is the fact that the instructions for the preparation and ingestion of the herbs are not clearly written.

With regard to Hmong shamanism, those Hmong health providers and interpreters who still maintain the Hmong traditional animist religion strongly believe in the power of the shaman's ceremonies to restore a lost soul or negotiate with and through the unseen world. Most of the interviewees who have converted to Christianity, on the other hand, say that while they respect the shaman's method of healing, they would not seek such treatment for themselves. There are others, albeit few in number, who feel that, inasmuch as the Hmong shaman healing tradition is a legitimate way of healing, to categorize it as a religion by Christian converts serves no useful purpose. Rather, it merely discourages the use of the quite valuable and efficacious associated practices.

HEALING: A HMONG AMERICAN CHRISTIAN PRAYER

Prayer is a healing method that Christian Hmong Americans generally use as an ersatz substitute for traditional Hmong spiritual healing methods. A Hmong Christian pastor makes the following statement about his method of prayer for ill members of Hmong American families: "I have helped many Hmong patients who are sick and ask me to go to their houses to pray for them. When I first arrive, they will say, 'Oh, pastor, this illness must be caused by spirits and souls because we have tried everything, but nothing seems to help.' They will tell me that they have seen Western doctors many times, but their doctors could not diagnose anything wrong with their bodies. Some of them have taken medications prescribed by their doctors, but they didn't get better. Many of them complained that Western doctors have treated their illnesses without success. I ask them if they have family problems (*Kev Nyuaj Siab*) that seem to bother them a lot. They say, 'Yes, my son is doing this or my daughter is doing that, and I worry about all of these things. I have so much headache. I cannot eat or sleep, and I feel sicker each day.' When people tell me about their family problems and their worries and when I begin to pray, I ask God to help them deal with these issues. I pray for them to overcome these obstacles. I emphasize these problems during my prayers, not necessarily their illnesses. When people hear these prayers, they have hope and feel good about themselves. When they feel good and believe it, they get better. I was able to help many people recover this way. In fact, the majority of the people who have asked me to pray for them have recovered. However, there are other Hmong Christian pastors who have been invited to pray for their church members, but they didn't take time to talk to the patients, and even though they pray very hard for God's healing power, the patients don't get better."

HMONG PATIENT CASES

THE CASE OF PA MOUA

Pa Moua is a fifty-seven year-old woman living with her husband and her daughter's family in her daughter's apartment, one unit in a fourplex apartment building in Westminster, Colorado. Pa Moua's son-in-law and his cousins bought the fourplex in 1998.

Around noon on March 9, 1999, a policeman delivered a package from Thailand to the apartment next door, which was occupied by relatives. The policeman insisted that the young Hmong man who opened the door sign for the package. He refused, inasmuch as he did not know the sender, nor was he the addressee. Nevertheless, the policeman continued to insist that he sign, since the package was sent to his address. Thinking the parcel might be from her mother's relatives, his wife also advised him to sign, and so the young man acquiesced.

Immediately he was handcuffed for receiving a controlled substance, and, with a wave of his hand, the policeman summoned agents of the FBI, who surrounded the entire building and began handcuffing everyone on the premises.

While this was happening, Pa Moua was inside her apartment with all her grandchildren except her twenty year-old grandson. Hearing the disturbance, she came out of her apartment and observed that police had already handcuffed her grandson and were walking him to their cruiser.

Running to his assistance, she attempted to wrest him from police control and cried, "Why are they doing this to you?"

Then she fainted from shock and fear. When she regained consciousness, she found herself lying on her bed. While she had been indisposed, it had transpired that a Hmong man, who lived upstairs and spoke fluent English, came out and told the police and FBI that the grandson did not live in the apartment they were searching. Subsequently, the police and FBI thoroughly searched the apartment, and, finding no illegal substances, questioned the tenants regarding the identities of the sender of the package and of the addressee. None of the tenants knew them; a careful check of all ID cards, drivers' licenses, Alien ID cards, and other such documents, revealed no matching names, and the lawmen departed.

A few days after this incident, Pa began to feel weak and cold all over her body, lose her voice and her appetite, suffer from sniffles, and feel a sharp pain in her head. Her condition deteriorated with the passing of each week and month. Because she could not eat or sleep, she lost weight precipitously and eventually her family took her to see her primary care physician. The doctor could not diagnose anything wrong with her, despite the fact that, over the course of several visits, he had sent her to see a cardiologist, neurologist, psychologist, and otorhinolaryngologist. She underwent many urine and blood tests, ultrasounds, X-rays, CAT scans, biopsies, and MRIs. Nonetheless, these specialists, likewise, could not find anything wrong with her, and thus could not treat her.

With all of the above, Pa Moua is married to a shaman. He performed two ceremonies and numerous soul callings for her, but none of these were of any help, either. Before she became ill, she had weighed one hundred forty pounds. By October, 1999, as her condition continued to decline, she weighed only a hundred pounds.

By this time, her family were deeply concerned. They began to explore different kinds of traditional Hmong healing techniques. They invited another Hmong shaman to perform a diagnostic ceremony. This shaman discovered that there was a *Cua* (wind—a euphemism for a death omen, called "horse," or *Nees*) in the house. The horse is the spirit within a wooden or bamboo structure upon which the corpse is placed and then carried to the grave in the course of a Hmong funeral. When the corpse is buried, this is cut in half and placed on top of the grave, in the belief that the deceased person will use this horse to ride to the other world. In Asia, among those Hmong who still maintain the animist religion, the spirit of this horse will arrive when a family member is dying, as an omen of and a precursor to this death.

Discovering this *Cua* in the house, the shaman hammered it down and promised to raise it up and liberate it should Pa recover. In the eventuality that Pa did not recover, the shaman would need do nothing, since the *Cua* would then have fulfilled its mission. Despite this, Pa continued to become worse.

Other Hmong told the family that when a sick person has a chilled sensation all over her body, it means she has experienced a shock of such severity that she has been, quite literally, frightened to death. Therefore, they maintained, it was necessary to look for a Hmong healer who knew how to perform *Xais Ceeb* (the application of pressure to relieve shock). Accordingly, the family searched for and eventually found such a man. After this healer treated Pa a few times, the symptom of chilling cold vanished, although her other symptoms persisted.

By October, 1999, Pa had lost her voice completely, could not eat or drink anything, and was unable to get up. As her condition further deteriorated, her family called an ambulance to take her to the hospital, where she lost consciousness.

While Pa lay in a coma, her family located a rare sort of Hmong shaman called *Ua Neeb Xua Nplej* (shaman of the husk rice). This *Ua Neeb Xua Nplej* is different from the shaman who had diagnosed her and from her husband as well, in that those two, and others of the same variety, use incense, gongs, and finger cymbals to call their spirit helpers. These spirit helpers then lead the shamans to the unseen world, where the shamans perform the necessary healing. However, the *Ua Neeb Xua Nplej* does not require any such paraphernalia. Rather, he places a large ceramic bowl in front of him in which he burns rice chaff or rice husks. The fragrance of these burning rice husks is all he requires to call his spirit helpers to lead him to the unseen world. Upon being requested to help Pa Moua, the *Ua Neeb Xua Nplej* performed a long diagnostic ceremony, taking several hours, to establish what had happen to Pa's soul.

Although Pa was still in hospital, the ceremony was performed at her home with her husband in attendance. In the course of the diagnosis, the new shaman and his spirit troops charged along the path her soul had traversed and, as the *Ua Neeb Xua Nplej* followed this path, he called out what he saw. When he arrived at the first gate of the unseen world, the shaman asked the guards if they had seen Pa's soul come by. They replied that her soul had traveled by such a long time before that her foot prints had already disappeared. When Pa's husband heard this, he wept. The shaman and his spirit helpers attempted to bargain with, mollify, and even bribe the guards in an attempt to gain permission to follow her; perhaps even to receive their assistance in guiding them to her. Although initially the guards refused, the proffered payment was increased until the guards relented.

The shaman and his troops then traveled on to next level and the next gate. Here, they asked the guards the same questions. The guards told the pilgrims they had seen Pa Moua's soul come through, but it had already gone on to yet another level and another gate. Again and again, the shaman and his spirit helpers went through gate after gate in the unseen world, and each gate brought them a step higher toward heaven. As the shaman went through each succeeding gate without finding Pa Moua's soul, her husband continued to weep bitterly.

When, at long last, the shaman and his helpers had reached the highest level of the unseen world and its gate, they still could not locate Pa Moua's soul. It thus became necessary to take yet one more step, and so they went on and eventually arrived at the far side of the sky gate; the very heavenly gate itself (*Rooj Ntug*). Here, at last, they found Pa's soul, sitting in the shade of a huge tree. The shaman and his spirit helpers wasted no time, but immediately commenced their efforts to persuade Pa's soul to return to earth, a proposition to which the soul eventually agreed. As this interchange progressed, and the shaman argued for the soul's return to Pa, the guards of the sky gate were also confronted. They were convinced to postpone her admission inasmuch as it was considered that her time had not yet quite arrived. Accompanied, then, by the soul of Pa Moua, the shaman and his spirit helpers reversed course. Once again it was necessary to secure permission to pass through each succeeding gate from each and all of the guards encountered. Once again, the shaman and his spirit helpers bargained, persuaded, flattered, and bribed their way along their chosen course until all had agreed to allow Pa's soul to return to earth.

These negotiations were conducted largely on credit. As the guardians of each gate were confronted, bargaining commenced, and, after both sides had reached agreement on the sums involved, the shaman promised the guards that, if they allowed her soul to return to earth—and if Pa recovered from her illness within thirty days—then he would deliver their payments to them. In this way, the shaman very cleverly guaranteed the assistance of the guardian entities in Pa's recovery, for, should she not get well, the guards would not be paid. The shaman customarily repeated or paraphrased agreements, then promised a few times, until he was sure everyone understood the terms. Each time he did so, he indicated some small thing to be required of the spirit entities to assure recovery. For example, he might say, "You will help to make Pa be able to eat a little each day, starting within the next three days, huh?" If the spirit entities were smiling at him and his troops, the shaman would add, "That's good, friends. That's great." The shaman communicated with the spirit entities in a manner similar to that in which he spoke to the people of this world; sometimes very firm, demanding or diplomatic, at other times emollient or chatty.

When everything had been agreed upon, the shaman and his spirit helpers brought Pa's soul back to earth. Pa's husband, hearing the shaman assert he had captured her soul and brought it home, was ecstatic. The ceremony then ended, and, within thirty days, Pa Moua had recovered from her coma, sat up in bed, begun to eat and drink again, and regained sufficient strength to move around her house. The pain in her head and her other symptoms vanished.

There remained the debts incurred to the spiritual guardians, due and payable by Pa's family. These debts consisted of four hundred *Lub Yeej Khaum* (joss paper, folded into a boat-like shape, which converts to a bar of silver in the unseen world), four hundred *Ntsua Ntawv* (cut branch-like paper, which converts to money in the spiritual world), and four hundred sticks of incense. All of these things were to be delivered by burning them during a second healing ceremony, held by the same *Ua Neeb Xua Nplej* shaman, after the agreed-upon thirty days. The fee that Pa's family paid to this shaman was one hundred dollars for each of the two ceremonies. His assistant received forty dollars for each.

After the second healing ceremony, there was, however, still unfinished business. Upon Pa's recovery, her family called the previous shaman back to perform the promised rite to raise up the *Cua* and liberate it, sending it on its way. In this ceremony, a miniature "horse" was made, and a hand-made doll dressed in Hmong burial clothes (*Nkauj Nyab*) was placed upon it. The shaman then performed his ceremony to raise the *Cua*, and sent it as far away as possible. This ceremony required two pigs; one to raise the *Cua* and the other to send it away. The family paid this shaman two hundred dollars and his assistant eighty dollars, so that the entire ceremony cost eight hundred dollars. Naturally, after Pa had fully recovered and regained all her lost weight, the family never counted the money they had spent to treat her. It is said that, "One can always earn money, but a mother and wife, or other significant person, one can never be replaced."

Interestingly enough, after Pa had recovered, other relatives very naturally had occasion to speak to her, and, in the course of some of these conversations, occasionally attempted to persuade her to convert to Christianity. But both Pa and her shaman husband adamantly refused, however, countering, with good reason, that without Hmong traditional healing techniques Pa would certainly have died.

THE CASE OF MAI NENG YANG

Mai Neng Yang is a sixty-four year-old Hmong woman who lives in Arvada, Colorado. In August, 1998, she was diagnosed with high blood pressure and given a prescription for medication. In November, 1998, she went to Laos to visit her sister and other relatives, who lived in Vientiane, the capital city, and in outlying areas. Vientiane was quite safe; however Mai Neng Yang's sister lived in a remote village, travel to which required a six-hour bus ride and a two-hour walk. Occasionally, anti-government rebels visited this village, and sometimes they created trouble for the villagers. Since Mai Neng had become an American citizen, she was in some fear of being targeted by these rebels.

Mai Neng did not want to visit the village, but, since she and her sister had not seen each other in over thirty years, Mai Neng's sister insisted that Mai Neng come to visit her home. Both the sister and her family wanted to sacrifice a cow to perform a soul calling ceremony in honor and for the benefit of Mai Neng. Having become a Christian, Mai Neng no longer believed in nor placed any value on the soul calling; however, inasmuch as it was her sister's way of showing love and affection, she adopted a tolerant attitude. In the end, she reluctantly traveled with her sister and brother-in-law to their village, but described the nights she spent at her sister's home as sleepless and fearful, owing to the aforementioned concern that rebels might come down from the mountains to attack.

The day after Mai Neng arrived in her sister's house, a cow was sacrificed and the soul calling ceremony performed. Soon after, an occasion arose for her to accompany her sister to the family's rice paddy to carry home some rice. As the group returned, Mai Neng failed to take note of a weed-covered hole on the path about a foot deep, and fell. She was carrying bundles of rice in a basket on her back, and these rice bundles fell off as she toppled. At the time, she was neither afraid nor shocked. In fact, Mai Neng laughed and said, "Well, it would be so funny to watch if someone could have videotaped this fall."

At last, after spending a few days in the village, Mai Neng returned to Vientiane to visit other relatives. It was on these last few days of her trip to Laos that she started to feel sick. Soon she was coughing, registered a fever, and noted an itching sensation all over her body. This was accompanied by chills and a cold sensation in her limbs, despite her fever. She began to feel tired and weak, and was not able to eat much.

It was in early December, 1998, that Mai Neng arrived home in Arvada. With her return, however, her condition did not improve. Rather, her coughing got worse each day, her limbs continued to feel cold, and she reported that she did not feel well at all. In consequence, she went to see her primary care doctor a few times within a period of three weeks, and saw a pulmonary specialist once, as well. Her doctor prescribed various types of cough suppressant medication for her, but none of them helped reduce her cough. Moreover, she continued to run a fever and demonstrate other symptoms. There were a few occasions when she called her doctor with a request to see him, but the doctor simply asked her to explain her symptoms over the telephone, after which she was directed to call the pharmacy to obtain prescriptions. It was thus with a growing sense of helplessness that Mai Neng and her grown children attempted to cope with her condition.

Doctors continued prescribing medicines for Mai Neng that did not help, while her children bought all brands of over-the-counter medications for her to try. Some of these nostrums would be helpful for a few days, but then her coughing would increase again and she would cough all day and all night long, without any sleep, for periods of up to several days. A relative gave her some dried Hmong herbs for her to use, and, when she first used these herbs, they seemed helpful. However, after a few days she began to cough again and she stopped using them.

Mai Neng Yang's coughing and fever continued to grow worse, until, at last, one morning her children noticed that her voice had changed a little, her mouth looked different, and her left hand was not able to hold a spoon when she tried to eat. Neither Mai Neng nor her children knew anything about the nature of stroke. However, since her physical abnormalities were all too obvious, the children took her to the emergency room of the nearby hospital. Two of her children, who are college-educated and speak English fluently, went with her and explained all her symptoms to the hospital's intake staff. Since Mai Neng was able to walk by herself and did not have acute pain, she was seated for two hours in the emergency room's waiting area before being taken to an examination room. Once there, it took the emergency staff a half day to get her health history faxed from her primary care physician and figure out what might be wrong with her.[17] After this, a nurse gave her some aspirin and some medication for high blood pressure, together with a cough suppressant. This nurse then said Mai Neng might have had a stroke, but no one could be sure.

It took three days, with Mai Neng in residence, for the doctor to confirm that she had, in fact, suffered a stroke. During those three days in hospital, Mai Neng was given aspirin, pills for high blood pressure, and cough syrup. Not surprisingly, her condition deteriorated steadily during each of those days. When she had first arrived, she had been able to walk by herself and was able to move her left arm. After the second day, she was struggling to walk to the bathroom of her hospital room. By the third day, she was unable to walk or move her left leg or left arm at all. At long last, her physician found himself able to confirm she had suffered a stroke. In the interim, her left side had become entirely paralyzed.

During those first three, long days in hospital, Mai Neng's children repeatedly asked her doctor and her nurses, "When are you going to know what is wrong with our mother? She's getting worse; is there anything else you can do? What is your treatment plan?"

The answers they got most of the time were stock hospital evasions, such as, "We're scheduling an x-ray of her skull, but the x-ray machine has been completely booked." "They will see if they can squeeze in a time slot for your mom tonight. If not, we'll probably have to take her to another hospital tomorrow for an x-ray. We're still calling around to check." "We're waiting for her test results." "We're waiting for her x-rays to come back." "Let me call her doctor." "You're going have to wait." "There's nothing else we can do."

During this period, Mai Neng had many visits from friends and relatives. The older visitors encouraged her to see a traditional Hmong needle user. Since Mai Neng sensed that her doctor and nurses were neither able, nor, more pointedly, at all willing to do much to help her, she agreed, and begged her children to ask a traditional Hmong needle user to come to the hospital to treat her. Her children approached her doctor about the idea, and initially the doctor agreed. After some time, however, he returned with a very different decision. Having consulted with "higher authorities" in the hospital, so he said, the Hmong needle user would not be allowed on the premises due to "liability issues." The concern, according to the physician, was that, since Mai Neng had been taking aspirin to thin her blood, if a needle user pierced her, she might begin bleeding uncontrollably. This, despite the fact that nurses were allowed to draw blood from her arms whenever they needed to conduct a test, at which times there was no uncontrolled bleeding; actually, there was very little bleeding at all.

In the mean time, other Hmong visitors told Mai Neng that the symptom of coldness she felt throughout her limbs was due to shock, advising her to request her family, therefore, to ask a Hmong healer who specialized in *Xais Ceeb* (applying pressure) to come and treat her in the hospital. Since this Hmong healing technique was not invasive, and knowing that if they asked her doctor for permission for the healer to come he probably would not allow it, the family simply brought the healer secretly to the hospital, where he discreetly treated her. After a few sessions with the man, her symptom of coldness disappeared.

During this same period, two of the relatives who had accompanied Mai Neng to Laos insisted she had become ill because one of her souls had been dislodged and wandered off when she fell down on her way home from the rice paddy; that is, she had literally "fallen ill." They pressed her family to record a cassette tape explaining the onset and symptoms of her illness to her sister in Laos, and asking the sister to perform a soul calling ceremony for Mai Neng. Mai Neng and her family, however, having become Christians, felt this put them in an awkward position, but, after additional pressure was brought to bear upon them by friends, one of the children was prevailed upon to carry out this task. A month after Mai Neng's initial hospitalization, Mai Neng's sister sent a cassette tape from Laos which constituted an aural record of a soul calling ceremony performed on Mai Neng's behalf.

In approximately the same time frame, one of Mai Neng's daughters, who had married into a Hmong family which still maintained the traditional Hmong animist religion, was told by her in-laws that Mai Neng's illness was caused by her soul either being unhappy or being lost. With this in mind, together they determined that they, also, would perform a soul calling for Mai Neng, and, once they had gathered everything necessary, they invited Mai Neng to attend at their home. At first, Mai Neng asserted she did not believe in such things anymore, and insisted they not go forward. After some discussion, however, it finally emerged that her true motive in attempting to quash the proceedings was fear that her church would hear of it. The ensuing debate and dispute became general. Most of her extended family members had become Christians, and some of these insisted she go ahead with the ceremony, while others adamantly disapproved. The in-laws, for their part, insisted they would move forward with the ceremony at all events. Their motive, so they related to Mai Neng, was twofold; first, they believed wholeheartedly that the ceremony would have a positive impact on her condition, and, second, they sincerely cared about her and wanted to do whatever they could to assist in her recovery. Should the church, or any Christians, dislike or disagree with this, they said, it was just too bad. With this, a second soul calling ceremony was performed.

Mai Neng had been hospitalized for over a week before being transferred to the Rehabilitation Unit in another area hospital. There she stayed for three more weeks, during which time she would often tell her children to ask the doctors and nurses to prescribe the best medicines available for stroke patients. Her children did ask about such medications, but again met with what was becoming a stock evasion. The standard response was, "There is no such a thing as a 'best medicine for stroke patients.'" It was difficult for Mai Neng to comprehend this statement. Over the course of many years, she had come to consider that the Western world, and most especially America, was technologically and medically the most advanced region in the world. It puzzled her when one of her doctors told her, "If I had the medicine to make stroke patients recover their normal lives again, I would be one of the richest men in this country." In fact, Mai Neng was appalled to hear this, and wanted to reply, "Well, if you don't have it, who does?" Occasionally she even developed a suspicion that her attending physicians were holding out on her, and complained to her children that the American doctors must have good medicines but simply did not want to give them up.

Throughout, physical and speech therapists in the Rehabilitation Unit worked with Mai Neng every day. Although they worked long and hard with her, and often attempted to cheer her by referring to her as their "Dream Patient," she was still unable to walk alone at the end of three weeks there, and returned home without the use of her left side. The hospital sent a physical therapist to her home, but, when the woman arrived, she spoke at length on a variety of subjects without rendering a great deal of assistance to Mai Neng in doing her exercises. After two weeks of this, Mai Neng told her not to come again and complained bitterly to her children that the therapist had been a mere time-server whose only interest was in her paycheck. Unlike the dedicated therapists at the Rehabilitation Unit, the woman had shown no interest whatsoever in helping Mai Neng.

In the period following her stroke, hospitalization, and eventual return home, Mai Neng continued to cough, and also developed a problem with constipation. She underwent a standardized tuberculosis test, several pulmonary tests, two chest x-rays, and an MRI, but no cause for her persistent cough was found, and, although doctors continued to prescribe cough syrup, it did not help. Fortuitously, one of her sons discovered and purchased for her a Chinese medicine, called *Sem Xyas*. This was mixed with warm water to form a beverage, after consuming which her coughing stopped for a period of two months. Unfortunately, this *Sem Xyas* proved scarce, and when the supply of this medicine ran out, Mai Neng began to cough again. Despite all efforts to secure additional *Sem Xyas*, the family could not find any. Once more, Mai Neng consulted her doctor. Once more, the doctor prescribed Western medicines. Once more, the medicines failed to solve the problem.

Mai Neng and her family continued to exert themselves to discover an effective medicine for her cough. They tried an enormous variety of Hmong herbs; herbs that had proved efficacious for others. In no case did any such herb help Mai Neng. Finally, a relative in Fresno, California, on a routine outing to a flea market, discovered and secured a supply of a Mexican cough remedy previously unknown to the family. This he sent to Mai Neng, who took the medication to a relative undergoing training as a nurse. The medication, taken under the nurse's supervision, was effective, and, after three doses, Mai Neng's cough disappeared and did not recur.

At some point, another relative in Fresno called with the news that certain of the Hmong who live in Crescent City, California, sell medicinal mushrooms which, so some believed, could effectively treat stroke. A name and a telephone number were given, and one of Mai Neng's children put in a call. The man who answered the telephone said that, contrary to what had been reported, he could not guarantee the mushrooms would help her; however, he went on to aver that he knew a Hmong healer in Crescent City who was considered an expert in massage therapy for stroke patients. This healer, the mushroom dealer related, traveled all over the country to help Hmong who had been hit by stroke. Again, a name and a telephone number were given. This number dialed, the callers were informed the healer was out of the country and would not return for a month.

Three months had now passed, and, almost every day for these three months, Mai Neng's family members bought herbs and plants in endless variety from Hmong herbalists. These herbs were boiled, and the decoctions thus created were used to bathe her, while the steam was administered as an inhalant. Mai Neng's sister in Laos also sent dried herbs, but, withal, Mai Neng still was not able to walk by herself. In consequence, she descended into a severe depression, and, after the passage of an additional month, insisted that her children call the Hmong massage therapist—now returned to his home on Crescent City from abroad—to come and treat her. The healer was contacted, and arrangements were made for him to come and spend three days with the family, treating Mai Neng twice each day. Two weeks after his treatment, Mai Neng was able to walk around the house with a cane.

This Hmong massage therapist is in his late thirties. He learned his healing technique from his father, who is still living in Thailand, while his father learned from his grandmother, now deceased. The man commenced his treatment by thoroughly examining Mai Neng's body, informing her as he did so which of her paralyzed extremities would be treatable and which would not. This diagnosis was absolutely on target; the areas for which he predicted progress did, in fact, register improvement, while the areas he said might not regain strength remained paralyzed.

He treated Mai Neng by gently massaging her stomach, followed by massage of her affected shoulder, arm, and leg. He asserted he could thus feel which nerves were damaged, and could then work on those areas to help blood circulate throughout the body as it should. During each treatment, he would spend one and a half hour to two hours massaging the nerves of her stomach, arm, leg, shoulder and head, and, as he massaged, Mai Neng would feel a shaking and a tingling sensation in the affected areas.

As a fee, Mai Neng's family paid for the man's airline ticket, which cost about six hundred dollars and, as was customary in compensating this healer, a calculation was made of the wages lost from his regular job. These lost wages were all he asked as recompense for his healing efforts, and, in this case, the figure of one thousand dollars was reached. Mai Neng's family happily agreed to such a payment over and above the cost of the airline ticket; however, the therapist would accept no more than one hundred dollars.

Subsequently, Mai Neng traveled to see this man two more times. Each time, she paid him one hundred dollars for each treatment and received from three to six treatments. At the present time, Mai Neng is able to walk with a cane without fear of falling down.

As a complement to his therapy for her stroke, this Hmong masseur mentioned the name of a plant in Laos which is effective in the treatment of constipation. One of Mai Neng's nephews, a shaman in Laos, obtained some of this plant, processed it, and sent it to her. He also recorded a cassette tape for Mai Neng and her family, in which he expressed the feeling, which had come upon him as he gathered the plant, that Mai Neng's real problems were not really of the physical body, per se, but consisted in adverse spiritual influences. He strongly believed, so he said, that her soul was either unhappy or had become lost. The nephew asked Mai Neng's family to send him one of her shirts, which he felt would assist him in the performance for her of a shaman's healing ceremony, coupled with a soul calling. This, Mai Neng and her family at first declined to do.

Nevertheless, Mai Neng did use the plant sent from Laos to treat her constipation, and initially it was very helpful. After some time, however, its efficacy diminished and her constipation and appetite problems returned and increased. Before the stroke, Mai Neng had weighed one hundred thirty pounds. After the stroke, her weight declined to approximately one hundred five pounds. Although true that she could now walk around the house, she nonetheless repeatedly developed new and puzzling symptoms. During this period, she was often visited by Hmong elders, who attributed these new symptoms to a lost or unhappy soul. Although the family had converted to Christianity, the elders encouraged them to consult a shaman, arguing that they saw nothing wrong with any variety of healing or health treatment, provided its purpose was to alleviate suffering and help the patient recover.

Yet, to consult a shaman in her home town would have involved the risk of engendering hostility in fellow church members, even to the extent of alienating the family from the congregation. With all of this, one of Mai Neng's children finally sent one of her shirts to her shaman nephew in Laos in order that he might perform the ceremonies he had proposed. The shirt was sent back to her two months later, with a cassette tape recording the shaman and soul calling ceremonies. On the inside of the back of the shirt, he had sewn, with a fine, vegetable fiber thread, symbols of her souls composed of red fabric. When this shirt arrived at the Office of United States Customs Inspection in San Francisco, however, customs officials tore through it, ripping out half of the emblems in a search for controlled substances. None was concealed within, of course, but the damage was done. Mai Neng's appetite and constipation problems, interestingly enough, which had improved steadily for two months, now reappeared.

In summary, then, Mai Neng's health problems have been treated by many health care providers. Her cold symptoms and the paralysis of her leg were successfully treated by Hmong healers. Her coughing problem was eliminated by Chinese and Mexican medicines. Her constipation and appetite problems were eliminated briefly after her nephew's shaman herbs and soul calling ceremony, but recurred.

Chapter V

Hmong Health Behavior: Summary and Conclusions

SUMMARY OF MAJOR FINDINGS

O'CONNOR STATES THAT VERNACULAR HEALING TRADITIONS CANNOT BE fully understood without describing "the ways in which all manner of beliefs about health, illness, and healing are integrated into broader cultural frameworks and larger systems of belief and values."[1] Certainly, Hmong American concepts of health, healing, and illness cannot be understood in the absence of a certain body of accompanying knowledge regarding the ways in which such concepts are integrated into the Hmong cultural framework and system of values. Leslie and Young note that the majority of scholars of Asian medical systems agree that these systems "are intrinsically dynamic, and, like the cultures and societies in which they are embedded, are continually evolving."[2] This writer has demonstrated with this manuscript that the behaviors of those Hmong seeking health treatment reflect Hmong cultural beliefs, Hmong values, and the Hmong experience, broadly considered. These factors have been influenced and shaped by Christianity, exposure to traditional and modern Western ideologies, the various influences felt in the wake of migratory movements, and government policies. Due to this wide range of cultural adaptations, and sometimes owing to a lack of adaptation, one faction of the Hmong population has tended to become increasingly marginalized from mainstream American society, while another faction has acculturated. This is reflected in the evolving heterogeneity of the Hmong American population and the widely disparate natures of those Hmong who will utilize conventional health care services versus traditional Hmong medicine. The author would highlight the major findings as follows:

- With regard to aspects of cultural change, the cultures called "Hmong" have been influenced by, and are themselves a product of, changes resulting from many past migratory experiences. In other words, we may say that what the Hmong are displaying and preserving is not a fixed, calcified, "traditional culture," as such, but a culture that has evolved over many years or centuries of Hmong migration. On a practical level, we have seen that the current culture is very different from even the pre-Vietnam War period in the ways people make a living, in the gender division of labor, in family structures, in religious beliefs, in politics, and in social life.[3]

- Since the Hmong did not have a written language until the late 1950s, their history and cultural traditions have not been recorded in texts. There are neither mass communication, nor library, nor archival resources upon which people may draw in order to assimilate a shared, communal, body of knowledge with regard to Hmong society and what it means to "be Hmong." As a result, Hmong who live in different areas are found to have different customs and traditions, and, while most Hmong know how things are done in their region, they cannot speak for all Hmong.[4] Furthermore, what knowledge of history and tradition exists is varied, not always in-depth, usually does not reach beyond four or five generations,[5] and, in consequence, the 'pristine culture' that many older Hmong yearn for and some younger Hmong Americans imagine and attempt to absorb is, in reality, composed largely of memories of the recent past.[6] This nostalgic cultural memory, although, in truth, relatively recent, may nonetheless be characterized. It seems to reveal a deep-seated desire for an integrated and well-woven cultural fabric, uniting all Hmong in an independent and self-governing state, even though the Hmong have never had such an independent nation state which was recognized in any region in which they have lived. It is not surprising, therefore, that casual conversation with Hmong informants, literature review, and those inferences which may be drawn from this paper indicate that, to most Hmong, especially men, political power equals prestige and authority. Conversely, the lack of same is equivalent to a status of no prestige and no authority. This status of no prestige and no authority, in turn, results in endemic unhappiness, and if, as is widely believed, happiness is the best medicine for a healthy life, then many Hmong Americans are at heightened risk for illness; especially the older Hmong American population.

- A prominent feature of Hmong culture which has not changed much is the essential fabric of Hmong social organization, woven on a pattern of descent lines rather than locality. Even in contemporary America at this writing, the majority of Hmong still organize their allegiances and many of their activities based on the traditional clan and lineage system.[7] There are, it should be noted, Hmong Americans who use their clan names but have little to do with any clan organization. However, even these Hmong Americans will, with some few exceptions, affiliate themselves with church groups and nonprofit organizations. A corollary of this collectivist core social pattern is that Hmong Americans place heavy emphasis on the interests of their kinsmen as a group, rather than on the interests of individuals or themselves. This allocation of allegiance can be found reflected in an examination of the identities of those whom Hmong trust and in the ways in which Hmong make health care decisions and channel information relative to health care service.

- Part and parcel of the pain associated with a history of cultural repression; war; the loss of loved ones, homeland, and personal possessions; and years spent in refugee camps, is tremendous physical and emotional distress, and, as a result, mental illness, such as post-traumatic stress syndrome, anxiety disorders, depression, somatization, hostility, paranoid ideation, and psychosis are prevalent in the Hmong.

- After long-term residence in the United States, many Hmong have developed chronic diseases such as arteriosclerosis and resulting cardiac infarction, cerebral hemorrhage, diabetes, hypertension, kidney dysfunction, bladder infection, gallstones, gout, arthritis, appendicitis, and cancer. Qualitative data generated from the focus group discussions and in-depth interviews held in the course of researching this book indicate that cerebral hemorrhage, diabetes, arthritis, muscle ache, and hypertension occur more often among the older Hmong population, while cardiac infarction, kidney dysfunction, bladder stones, gout, and cancer do not discriminate by age. Hmong men are found to have problems with gout in greater numbers than Hmong women. A few Hmong, of varying ages, have developed cancer and subsequently died. Some Hmong informants believe that the number of older Hmong individuals who have fallen victim to cerebral hemorrhage, diabetes, arthritis and hypertension increases every year, and the Hmong community is concerned about these various chronic diseases.

- In Colorado, the rate of employment in the Hmong is at least ninety-five percent. To make ends meet, many Hmong work two jobs, or interchange day and night shifts between spouses so that one of the pair can care for the children at all times. Hmong adults who are employed experience more physical distress and anxiety than those who do not work. This seems to be the result of a lack of familiarity with the workplace, of language barriers, and of the low-wage, manual labor atmosphere in which many Hmong find themselves.[8] Those Hmong who are unemployed and dependent on public assistance are either elderly, disabled, or single parents with dependent children.

- Since the majority of Hmong Americans in Colorado are employed, most of them have health insurance and, when ill, resort to conventional medical facilities and practices; yet they still depend heavily on traditional methods of addressing illness and infirmity. Non-Christian Hmong have no reservations about using all types of traditional healing methods, while those Hmong who have embraced Christianity tend to limit themselves in this regard, utilizing mostly herbal medicines and therapeutic massage treatments. The herbal and therapeutic massage techniques employed in such cases are non-invasive, and can thus be used to complement Western health treatments without harm or challenge to church doctrine. Nevertheless, some Hmong informants expressed concerns regarding the herbs employed, inasmuch as they are generally of unknown chemical composition and can provoke negative reactions in the case of allergy, overdose, or use in combination with Western medications.[9] Further research is recommended to analyze the chemical composition of Hmong herbs, and to educate the Hmong American population about the potential for negative impact which these herbs may have. Such research may have the incidental benefit of enhancing our knowledge of and understanding about these centuries-old healing herbs and their efficacy, and this might very well, in turn, contribute to the development of new medications.

- Literature review and the findings detailed in this text indicate a lack of culturally appropriate health promotion to and for the Hmong American population. Hmong Americans in Colorado have limited access to health information, especially in the Hmong language, and it is likely that smaller Hmong American communities across the country have similar problems.

- The health problems Hmong patients have are not necessarily somatization, but, in many instances, may also be culturally defined syndromes which conventional health care providers are unable fully to grasp. Being unfamiliar with Hmong health problems, these health care providers indiscriminately utilize the label "somatization." This confusion is in the minds of these same conventional health care practitioners, and not in the minds of the Hmong. Hmong do not hold beliefs about, view, or interpret their health problems in the same way as do Westerners, so conventional health care treatments are often ineffective when a biological etiology is not detectable. Lonsdorf et al. compare conventional medicine to the traditional East Indian health system called "Ayurveda," now gaining popularity in the West, and state that, in conventional medicine, a disease model is applied rather than a health model and "only known illnesses are considered treatable."[10] In other words, a disease has to be named in order to be treatable, and doctors cannot treat patients who are in distress when there is no objectively identifiable disease found during a physical exam, in the results of a lab test, or on an X-ray. In other words, they cannot recognize subtle changes in the state of a person's well-being, such as those which may be indicated by the onset of fatigue, by head pains, by poor or irregular digestion, by increased emotional upset, or a generalized increase in bodily tension. An unknown, uncharted area, then, is the geography upon which Hmong patients find themselves standing when conventionally trained doctors are unable to diagnose or treat their illnesses; yet, the doctors place the judgment of such "somatic" patients at fault for seeking health care treatments that are not commensurate with symptoms.

- In Hmong traditional society, the state of the souls of a person play a vital role in maintaining his health while he is living and in his transmigration after he has died. By carefully structuring his activities in harmony with his cultural traditions, a Hmong can become successful, live a healthy life, avoid many common illnesses, and properly prepare his souls both for life after death and for eventual reincarnation. In accord with such a system of beliefs, health treatment should include both spiritual and physiological components. When the spiritual aspect of a Hmong patient's nature is ignored, or attention to it discouraged, the patient may not be completely satisfied with his treatment. Unlike conventional health treatments, which tend to focus on a specific area of the body of a sick individual, the Hmong focus is on the treatment of the whole person, including unseen aspects, with a genuine concern for his spiritual well-being, and, in cases of gravity, for life after death and reincarnation.

- The majority of Hmong American adults in Colorado are not proficient in English, have a low level of education, low socioeconomic status, and need the assistance of a cultural broker or translator when interacting with mainstream American service providers such as health care professionals. Hmong adults who are not able to express their feelings or opinions to service providers, and must, in consequence, rely on other people to translate for them or to fill out forms, experience tremendous anxiety, emotional distress, and depression.[11] Unfortunately, Colorado has a very limited cross-cultural resource personnel infrastructure available for the assistance of these people.

- In consequence, Hmong adults in Colorado who are not fluent in English frequently must request family members to translate for them. These family members may not have been trained in the specific language ("jargon") of, or with specific reference to, the subculture of the service, and may, as a result, be unaware of essential legal or medical terms and concepts. Such interactions do not serve to maximize the degree of understanding required in decision-making, particularly in health care service situations. Hmong patients usually do not know what is to take place, and may not discover the nature of the treatment or other service until after it has been rendered. There can be little doubt that this has, in many instances, created distrust toward conventional health care professionals and institutions while fostering tremendous frustration and anxiety in Hmong patients and their families.

- There are many conflicts within the Hmong American community. These conflicts cross generational, gender, and "educated" versus "uneducated" boundaries. The intergenerational gap tends to be most evident between parents and their children, notably teenagers and young adults, all in conflict with the elderly, and is in regard to different perceptions of life, different values, and different beliefs. The conflict between the educated and the uneducated, as well, is becoming widespread as more Hmong Americans attain higher educational levels and greater success in professional training in American schools. Although a Hmong healer may see, in the conflict occurring between the more intellectually oriented Hmong and the general Hmong population, a failure of the Hmong people to follow specific rituals, it is more likely that such conflict arises as a result of the tension between two very different philosophies of life; Hmong and Western. Western schools of thought have a tendency to assume the primacy of their ethnocentric world view, and, as a result, those Hmong who absorb such teachings will hold in low regard their own traditions. They may, in fact, be without any Hmong perspective at all; they will be handicapped in speaking the Hmong language, and will reject or demean Hmong culture and its core values and belief systems. Nevertheless, these same Hmong, as professionals schooled in Western thought, are blindly sent to serve their own people with the assumption that since they are, ethnically, Hmong, they can speak the language, understand the culture, and can quite naturally solve Hmong problems. Even though many Hmong professionals have successfully fulfilled such expectations, others may not be able to achieve satisfactory results. One solution to this problem is to provide an opportunity, via some sort of training for Hmong professionals, to address this issue. More importantly, this issue should be included in most of the academic and professional training curricula. It should not be at all far-fetched to propose that such training in the variety of ethnic belief systems prevalent in an increasingly multicultural United States be provided for all those who must deal on a regular basis with them, for this problem of miscommunication creates difficulties for other non-Western ethnic groups which parallel those experienced by the Hmong.

- Unless alternative approaches to helping the Hmong deal with their changing lifestyle and with their health care concerns are explored, greater social stress and the ensuing social problems, increased incidence of violence—both potential and actual—and rising numbers of health complaints may be anticipated in the Hmong American community.

PRIMARY CONCLUSION

In conclusion, the author would assert that the two most important findings to emerge from the research findings elucidated herein are that, 1) Hmong illness is often a culturally defined syndrome and Hmong health treatment approaches are frequently culturally defined methodologies; and, 2) the central problem leading to inadequate health care delivery to Hmong Americans from conventional health care providers is language incongruence. What follows will serve to further illustrate these two key points.

HMONG ILLNESSES AND HEALTH TREATMENT APPROACHES ARE CULTURALLY DEFINED VIEWS

The author has argued that the "somatic" symptoms of which Hmong patients complain when consulting with conventional health care professionals are more accurately viewed as culturally specific illnesses than as somatization. The Hmong phrases *Poob Plig* (soul loss) and *Mob Laug* (muscle aches), to cite but two examples, denote culturally specific symptoms. To Hmong patients, such illnesses are real, in that they can identify the symptoms, feel the pain, and experience the resultant suffering. Hmong healers who have experienced these symptoms, and thus come to understand these illnesses, take a different approach in treating their patients compared to conventional health care professionals. When Hmong healers are asked to treat the sick, they, 1) rarely question the patients directly about their symptoms; 2) avoid invasive tests and assessments in determining the type of illness from which the patient is suffering; 3) encourage family members to seek both physical and spiritual treatment; and, 4) do not tell the patient of the relative gravity of his illness. In much the same way as that discussed by Ohnuki-Tierney—who describes the manner in which Japanese doctors and their patients' family members enter into a teamwork arrangement to make a health care decision or to maintain the secrecy from the patient of a verdict of cancer—when a family member is sick in traditional Hmong society, other family members will take it upon themselves to make the initial move to seek health treatment.[12] It is they who will make the health care decisions for their loved ones, as they seek to obscure from their loved one any potentially distressing diagnosis or problematic outlook for treatment. In this way, both family members and healers play major, and protective, roles in helping the patient recover. It is a Hmong belief, in contradistinction to what often seems to be the conventional American view, that when a person sick it is not his fault. It is either spirits or viruses that have made him sick. Therefore, it is not the patient's duty, it is not even within his power, to find a cure. His main responsibility is to rest and eat good food until he is fully recovered, as the twin tasks of seeking health care and of curing the illness devolve upon family members and healers.

However, due to many changes in Hmong American society, the roles played by the patient, family members, healer(s), and conventional health care providers have shifted and become muddled. Many conflicts and misunderstandings, resulting in poor patient care, occur because each of those who plays a role in the typical health care interaction has an expectation which differs in large measure from that of every other. For example, lately it is not uncommon that Hmong Americans when they fall ill are expected to seek health treatment for themselves. Many in the younger generation, it would seem, are not rendered uncomfortable by this expectation; however, this is not the case with their elders, who are often unfamiliar with the conventional health care system. In addition, dealing with language barriers, as we have seen, is, for them, an often insurmountable problem. Furthermore, seeking out one's own health care, smacking, as it does, of a sort of self-centered individualism, is alien to the traditional Hmong value system and runs contrary to the cultural expectations of these elders. Indeed, when younger Hmong do not recognize these difficulties faced by the elderly, and fail to take seriously the traditional role of family member in seeking health care for an ailing older member of the family, an older person will, as often as not, feel neglected; even unloved. The disappointment and even anger created by this not uncommon scenario contributes to one of the many growing social gaps, the rift between the generations, which tugs at Hmong American society. At the same time, it is not uncommon for younger Hmong to find that, in taking seriously their traditional responsibilities with regard to their elders as they accompany their ailing loved ones to health care service centers, make health care decisions, and crowd in to hospital rooms to lend moral support, these same young people find themselves the butt of the unspoken censure of conventional health care providers for being in violation of American notions of individualism; and may find themselves reprimanded for being in violation of hospital rules.

To reiterate, then, the conflicts that often arise when Hmong Americans seek conventional health care services are twofold: 1) many Hmong illnesses are culturally defined syndromes; and, 2) the beliefs and values which attach to illness and health treatment are culture specific. When these two factors are ignored, redefined, or altered, then conflicts arise.

LANGUAGE INCONGRUENCE

As discussed throughout this book, the language barrier is a major obstacle in obtaining effective conventional health care services for Hmong Americans in Colorado. On a superficial level, the difficulties can be itemized as follows: 1) there are few readily available, competent, bicultural and bilingual Hmong interpreters available to serve the Hmong American population; 2) many Hmong interpreters have received no formal professional training in the translation of health care concepts and treatments; 3) the complexity of the social dynamics involved in the translation process plays a crucial role in obstructing effective health care delivery; and, 4) language incongruence between Hmong and English makes health care translation an extremely painstaking and lengthy process, which is a challenge if not an ordeal.

These factors have all contributed to the obstruction of effective conventional health care delivery to the Hmong. However, the underlying problem is yet more complex. Currently, there is not a standard medical wordbook or dictionary which cross-lists English medical terms with their Hmong counterparts, and conversely. This constitutes a serious obstacle to the training of Hmong medical translators and interpreters, and, in effect, inhibits such personnel and trainees in any effort to establish a fixed and uniformly shared professional standard to which all may adhere. As a consequence, even Hmong informants who had received formal training still had difficulty finding the appropriate term to describe some symptoms and were forced to improvise. With each translator utilizing any terms which may come to mind, confusion across the profession is the inevitable outcome.

In addition, Hmong express symptoms in a somewhat idiosyncratic manner, often employing many linguistic idioms to describe their health. They often ascribe etiologies to the liver, for example, instead of, as in the West, to the heart; and will even characterize difficulties with the liver as the cause of mental health problems. As an example of this latter, we may cite the use of the term *Nyuaj Siab* (difficult liver) to describe someone who is chronically worried.

We can see, then, that even simple terms are difficult to conceptualize across the two cultures. Certainly this fact that has not at all been simplified as the Hmong have undergone tremendous change in their new homeland, being required to use a foreign language as soon as they step out of the house. It can only aggravate this rash of problems that there is no dictionary or textbook available by which to standardize translation; a benchmark upon which all translators may draw as they slowly establish a common vocabulary for new medical concepts. Some of the Hmong interpreters interviewed for this book stated that Hmong simply has no words which will serve to describe a good many of the health symptoms and Western mental health concepts widely understood and frequently discussed by English speakers.

Unfortunately, it is quite true that Hmong has no words which directly translate certain health concepts both from and to English. In certain cases, too, of course, English has no word or words for certain of the health symptoms or names of illnesses that exist in the Hmong language. This single fact results in the frequent necessity for Hmong interpreters to use many words or sentences to describe symptoms to their patients, an approach which is rife with opportunities for misunderstanding. The unfortunate result is that Hmong patients will not get the services of which they are in such need and to which they are entitled.

In addition to having no standardized text from which to study and no standardized dictionary upon which to draw, there is no standardized training course and no standardized set of professional requirements upon which to rely in setting the bar for the qualification or certification of translators. There is not even a standardized manual to be studied and mastered.

Although many interpreters have acquired their skills through years of experience, and are constantly striving to improve them, they nonetheless may still not be able to translate competently and thus to effectively serve their clients in the best possible way. Findings for this book indicate that over sixty percent of interviewees need Hmong interpreters when using conventional social and health care services. Sixty percent of those use family members and friends, who are not professionally trained, as interpreters. It is abundantly clear, therefore, that there is a very real need to develop a standardized health care translation training course, manual, and qualifying test. The core of this course, and of its course materials, must be that body of Hmong and English words or terms that express Hmong and Western conceptualizations of health symptoms and illnesses, cross-listed, one with the other, in order to train Hmong American interpreters effectively.

IMPLICATIONS FOR HMONG HEALTH PROMOTION

This book documents changes in Hmong health related beliefs and practices after long-term residence in the United States, addresses many of the difficulties that Hmong Americans have in utilizing the services of conventional health care providers, and records original health-related Hmong cultural beliefs, values, and ceremonies that have never before been studied. Inasmuch as the writer is a Hmong, who was born in a Hmong community in the highlands of Laos, who emigrated to the United States with the target group, and who is fluent both in English and in the Hmong language, unique qualifications and abilities have been brought to this project which are not possessed by the majority of Western scholars. In consequence, unique insights have been presented.

With this book, light is shed on Hmong American concepts of health, healing, and illness, and Hmong experiences with conventional medical facilities and staff, even as specific recommendations are made to conventional health care providers that may enable them better to meet the health needs of the Hmong, both in Colorado and across the country, and to improve their interactions with Hmong patients and their families. This is important in and of itself; beyond that, the contents of this volume can serve as paradigmatic in understanding the health needs of other non-Western ethnic groups—increasingly prevalent in a multicultural American society. The book can, with profit, be drawn upon by those in the field of medical anthropology, and the data acquired and presented within its pages will serve as an important cultural resource for younger Hmong Americans. Furthermore, the findings can be used to compare Hmong American views of health and healing with those of other societies, and will both promote cross-cultural understanding and indicate ways in which to build an ethical model for intercultural health care relationships, suggesting new modalities by which health care professionals might tailor their efforts to the health needs of one component of an increasingly heterogeneous population. Finally, this study has the potential to make a contribution toward the understanding of culturally defined syndromes, while leading to a heightened public awareness about this abstract, but nonetheless very real, health concern. This, in turn, must, of necessity, lead to a decrease in conflict arising from differing perceptions of quality health treatment.

Glossary of Hmong and Other Terms Used in this Book

Ceeb – stress or shock. The Hmong have a highly developed belief system centered on the potential effects of shock on the psychology and the nervous system. It is held that such shock can lead to adverse consequences which run the gamut from discomfort through illness to death. In brief, however, it is felt that when a person experiences a shocking situation, it may shift his body, and, in fact, his entire nervous system, out of balance. The Hmong refer to this health condition as *Ceeb* (shock), symptoms of which may consist of a chilling cold felt all over the body, or which may be localized, depending on the degree of shock experienced. Other symptoms may be a coldness in the hands, arms, feet, and/or lower legs; coldness from the waist up to the head, or from the waist down to the feet; or coldness throughout the entire body. Hmong patients describe the symptoms of *Ceeb* as being "similar to having a fever, but without the hotness," and victims of severe *Ceeb* describe feeling sick with a "sticky cold." Such a health condition can become worse without treatment, and the Hmong have evolved over time a methodology called *Xais Ceeb* (which see) for dealing with this condition. This methodology involves the skillful application of pressure to various parts of the body.

Chim Heev – very angry.

Cua – wind. This word is employed as a euphemism for the more dreadful *Nees* (which see); a word which nominally means "horse," but which is, in actuality, a reference to the arrival of an omen of impending death. Among those Hmong who still maintain the animist religion, it is thought that when a family member is dying, a horse will arrive as a prelude to the end. The "horse" here intended is not of the

147

equine variety, but is, rather, the spirit within a wooden or bamboo structure, hung along the main wall of the house, upon which the corpse is placed prior to being carried to the grave. This structure is made by the Hmong in the course of funerary preparations. When the corpse is buried, this "horse" is cut in half and placed on top of the grave, in the belief that the deceased person will use the spirit animal within to ride to the other world.

Dab – spirits.

Dab Nyeg – Tame or household spirits. This term encompasses all spirits residing in the house and the ancestral spirits or spirits of deceased family members. It includes the *Xwm Kab* (which see).

Dab Pog – primeval celestial couple who generated the first Hmong man and woman, teaching them all of the cultural beliefs and traditional customs they would be required to follow in order to live prosperous, healthy, and harmonious lives. Due to the fact that child rearing and family life are of such importance to the Hmong, the *Dab Pog*, who are also referred to as the *Dab Pog* couple—together with the *Xwm Kab* (which see), or the *Xwm Kab* couple—are the most-worshipped spiritual entities in Hmong life. Also known as the *Nkawm Niam Txiv Dab Pog* (which see).

Dab Qhuas – rituals that express the unique identities of patrilineal kin groups, including birth, death, and new year rituals.

Dab Qus – wild or evil spirits.

Dab Tshuaj – the spirits of medicine.

Daim Ntawv Xwm Kab – a ceremonial paper hung on the main wall of a Hmong house to designate the place set aside for the *Xwm Kab* (which see) couple.

Daj Ntseg – literally, "yellow ears;" the term refers to the disease jaundice.

Dej Zaj – literally, "dragon water." Drinking this "dragon-water" at the end of their father's life, the shaman's sons will absorb his inner strength and abilities. The water also enables the sons to retain the assistance of the father's spirit helpers. In the course of selected rites and rituals, the shaman spells "dragon-water" over the patient to frighten away evil spirits.

Fiv Yeem – the proposed or promissory sacrifice. This technique of healing involves the proposal or promise, made by a shaman, or any family member, to those spirits thought to be causing the patient's affliction, that a sacrifice will be made to these spirits if they will cease their mischief and allow the patient to recover. This technique is sometimes also employed to ask ancestors or nature spirits for protection prior to undergoing major surgery or a long journey.

God – while there is only one God in Hmong culture, He is known by many names, viz., *Huab Tais Ntuj* (which see), *Vaj Tswv* (which see), *Tswv Ntuj* (which see), *Saub* (which see), *Ntxwg Yug* (which see), *Tus Tswv Tsim Neeg* (which see), *Pog Yawm Txwv Koob* (which see), *Nkawm Niam Txiv Dab Pog* (which see), or *Nkawm Niam Txiv Kab Yeeb* (which see).

Hauv Plag – the common floor area facing the main wall of a Hmong house.

Hmoob Dawb – the White Hmong.

Hmoob Lees – the Blue or Green Hmong.

Hno Koob – technique employing needles. This technique, which is employed to relieve bodily tension, pain, stress, and digestive difficulties, utilizes massage and the puncture of small needles in a manner not unlike Chinese acupuncture.

Hu Plig – soul calling. The soul calling ceremony, which seeks to reunite an individual with one of his souls, considered to have strayed, is one of the most important healing technologies in Hmong traditional medicine.

Huab Tais Ntuj – according to Hmong refugees in Australia, the creator and ruler of the world. He is the King of Heaven; he can see what human beings are doing on earth, but usually does not interfere. He governs everything in the universe, including people and animals. See also "God."

Huab Tais Xob – the Thunder King; current ruler of earth. This celestial entity was sent by the sky in 1964 to rule the earth as a replacement for the Dragon King, *Huab Tais Zaj* (which see), as a result of an excess of illness affecting the Hmong during the latter's tenure.

Huab Tais Zaj – the Dragon King. During the years 1959—1964, the Hmong suffered from a malady known as *Mob Aws* (which see.) Many believe that, as a result of the appearance of this illness, the sky, considering there had been too much illness apportioned to the Hmong, replaced the Dragon King, *Huab Tais Zaj*, as ruler of earth, with the Thunder King, *Huab Tais Xob* (which see). An earthquake, so it is said, marked this transition, which took place on precisely December 16, 1964. At all events, for a long time after this geologic catastrophe, there was a marked decrease in the incidence of major illness, and, although there continued to be a range of minor illnesses, patients suffered little and recovered quickly.

Hwj Huam – a term which refers to a personal attribute which may be translated as "natural power" or "healing power." The healing power of the shaman is critical in the success of a healing ritual; the balance of natural power of the patient as opposed to the natural power of the shaman also figures strongly in this equation.

Ib Nkawm Qaib – a pair of chickens, especially the pair offered to the *Dab Pog* (which see) couple to induce them to give their blessings to a newborn child. See also "*Ob Ntshua Ntawv*."

Kab Yeeb – the spirit couple; this term, like the term *Nkawm Niam Txiv Dab Pog* (which see), is yet another regional variant, used both to refer to the *Dab Pog* (which see) couple, and to God generally. Most Hmong think this celestial couple to be charged with bringing children to their parents on earth. Also known as the "*Nkawm Niam Txiv Kab Yeeb*" (which see).

Kav – a technique of dermal abrasion. The Hmong believe that both stress and tension, and "internal heat," can cause illness. In accordance with this belief, they will often place a small silver bar, or a coin, inside the yolk of a hard boiled egg, wrap the egg and silver in a piece of cloth, and then rub the pack over the arms, back, and forehead. After rubbing, the silver will have darkened, or even turned black. This blackness is believed to be the externalized impurity inside the body which originally caused the complaint. See also "*Kuam*."

Kev Nyuaj Siab – excessive worry due to family problems.

Kev Ua Plig – ceremonies related to, and for the benefit of, the souls.

Khawv Koob – magic healing. This technique is performed to frighten, cajole, or deceive the spirits into leaving the patient alone, and to relieve pain, swelling, vomiting, and/or bleeding. Interestingly, most chanting words used in performing the *Khawv Koob* healing are not Hmong; in fact, they are in an unknown language, the words of which are said by some to be an ancient form of Chinese; by others to be the actual lingua franca of the spirit world.

Kho Siab – literally, "murmuring liver," this is a nervous condition which is said to exist in a person whose behavior is characterized by openly exhibited and obvious nervous habits such as humming, coughing, or shaking; and/or hearing a whistling sound in the head. Those afflicted with *Kho Siab* are often found to speak unreservedly about wanting to die, or even wishing to commit suicide.

Khov Kuam – a diagnostic technique utilizing the shaman's split horns, *Txwm Kuam* (which see). This technique is either performed as part of the ceremony by which the shaman calls his spirit helpers, *Txhij Qhua* (which see) or as an independent diagnostic.

Kuam – literally, "rub." This is a technique of dermal abrasion. The

Hmong believe that both stress and tension, and "internal heat," can cause illness. In accordance with this belief, they will often apply ointment to a patient, then employ a small silver bar, a large coin, or a spoon to rub over the arms, back and forehead. Afterward, the affected areas will appear slightly reddened, or bruised. This discoloration is believed to be the externalized impurity or pressure inside the body which has been causing the complaint. See also "*Kav.*"

Kwv Tij – partrilineal kin group.

Leej Nkaub – the "inspiring spirit." One of a pair of spirits sent by a shaman, who has died and resides in the next world, to press the shaman's son to become, himself, a shaman. The other member of this pair is *Txheej Xeeb* (which see).

Lub Kaus – the ceremonial umbrella. It is one of the "Eight Most Important Spirits in the Hmong Cultural Tradition," or *Yim Tus Tswv Dab Nyob Hauv Hmoob Kav Cai Dab Qhuas* (which see). The ceremonial umbrellas encompassed by this term are of two kinds; a real umbrella is used primarily in marriage ceremonies, and symbolizes the protection of the spirits extended to the newly wedded couple in beginning their life together. A paper umbrella, on the other hand, is used during Hmong funeral rites. It is believed that the deceased will employ the paper umbrella to good effect in protecting himself from the sun and/or rain during his journey to the spirit world.

Lub Nruas – the drum. This term refers to all manner of ritual drums, from a funeral drum to a shaman's ceremonial drum, which are employed in clan rituals. During funeral rites, the drum is often played to the accompaniment of the *Qeej* (which see), one of the "Eight Most Important Spirits in the Hmong Cultural Tradition," or *Yim Tus Tswv Dab Nyob Hauv Hmoob Kev Cai Dab Qhuas* (which see). During healing ceremonies, on the other hand, the drum is most often sounded in conjunction with a set of finger bells or cymbals.

Lub Pas Zaj – literally, "the dragon pond;" the bowl which contains the magic water from which a shaman's sons must drink when the shaman is ill and near death. So called because, when the shaman invites or calls, the dragon that controls thunder and lightning comes to rest at this pond. See also "*Dej Zaj.*"

Lub Yeej Khaum – joss paper, folded into a boat-like shape, which may be converted into a bar of silver in the spirit world. Such *Lub Yeej Khaum* is sometimes offered by shamans to spirits who have been helpful in effecting a cure. Many *Lub Yeej Khaum* are folded and burned during a funeral to provide funds for the deceased person on his journey to the spirit world. See also *"Ntsua Ntawv."*

Lwj Siab – literally, "rotten liver." This term is generally used to describe patients who are not happy with their present lives, or are unable to achieve important goals. Such people often experience delusions and/or exhibit memory loss.

Mej Koob – Hmong marriage negotiators.

Miao – a term used in China as an alternative to "Hmong," and which is generally considered disparaging by the Hmong.

Mob Aws – an illness unique to the Hmong. During the years 1959—1964, sufferers were afflicted by a strange condition which rendered them ill in the fashion of animals for one or two days, after which they died suddenly.

Mob Kab Xeb – one in a series of illnesses unique to the Hmong, this malady appeared in approximately 1976 and lasted until circa 1985, when it disappeared. During the years of its active period, it posed a particular threat to those of the Hmong living as refugees in the camps of Thailand, striking children more often than adults. The symptoms were relatively simple, and consisted chiefly of an uncontrollable shaking in the arms and legs. Immediate treatment was called for, without which the patient could die.

Mob Kas Ceeg – a variety of sexually transmitted disease which affected the Hmong in the closing years of the Twentieth Century, from 1986—1995, and is still to be found as the new millennium opens, albeit less frequently than during the peak years.

Mob Laug – literally, "old age pain." The term refers to muscle aches generally.

Mob Plab – abdominal pain.

Mob Plab Zawv Tshav – an alternative name for *Mob Qhua Tawm Dub* (which see). This mysterious malady, which struck at the Hmong from approximately 1925—1935, was characterized by intense stomach pains and bloody diarrhea, and often resulted in death.

Mob Qhua Tawm Dub – a mysterious malady which occurred at an epidemic rate among the Hmong in approximately the year 1925. Those struck by this frightening condition developed intense abdominal pain, which was followed in short order by severe diarrhea, often with blood in the stool, then death. This illness was widespread until 1935, when it vanished as mysteriously, and as suddenly, as it had arrived.

Mob Tau Hau – literally translated, the meaning is "pain pumpkin cook;" it means, however, headache.

Mob Yas Yuam – an illness common to the Hmong during the period 1935—1945. Those affected experienced sudden, severe abdominal pains, complaining that they felt as if their "muscles or nerves were being torn apart." This was accompanied by intense, wracking pains all over the body which caused the sufferer to writhe in agony. The patient usually died quickly thereafter.

Muam Phauj – literally, "Sister Aunt." The phenomenon of *Muam Phauj* is a device used primarily to atone for mistakes committed in the execution of ritual. In the event that such a mistake is made, a plea will be entered to the Sister Aunt to apply her imprimatur to the error, after which the alteration in procedure will become established ritual. Secondarily, in the event that a natural disaster or other misfortune befalls an individual or a family, then a plea may be entered to the Sister Aunt in the hope that such may never recur.

Mus qhov nov – literally, "Go this way!" A musical response to the question, "*Mus qhov twg?*" (which see) posed during Hmong funerary rites by the drum, *Lub Nruas* (which see), and which means, "Where to go?" The response is delivered by the *Qeej* (which see), answering, "Go this way!"

Mus qhov twg – a musical question posed by the *Lub Nruas* (which see), or drum, and repeated often during all Hmong funerals. Its meaning is, "Where to go?" The answer is furnished by the Hmong mouth organ/flute, the *Qeej* (which see), replying, so it is considered, in musical tones, "*Mus qhov nov!* (Go this way!)"

Nchuav Qe – pouring the egg. One of two diagnostic techniques utilizing an egg. In this exercise, the identity of the evil spirit causing the illness is determined.

Nees – horse. Although this word nominally means "horse," it refers, in actuality, to an omen of impending death. Among those Hmong who still maintain the animist religion, it is thought that when a family member is dying, a horse will arrive as a prelude to the end. The "horse" here intended is not of the equine variety, but is, rather, the spirit within a wooden or bamboo structure, hung along the main wall of the house, upon which the corpse is placed prior to being carried to the grave. This structure is made by the Hmong in the course of funerary preparations. When the corpse is buried, this "horse" is cut in half and placed on top of the grave, in the belief that the deceased person will use the spirit animal within to ride to the other world. Occasionally, the Hmong word for wind, *Cua* (which see), is used as a less frightening euphemism for *Nees*.

Niam Txais Ntsuab - the maid of honor, or the bride's companion/assistant.

Nkauj Nyab – bride; a newly wedded woman. Alternatively, this term may be used to refer to a daughter-in-law.

Nkawm Niam Txiv Dab Pog – *Dab Pog* (which see).

Nkawm Niam Txiv Kab Yeeb – *Kab Yeeb* (which see).

Nom Tswv – political official or leader.

Npuas Tai – literally "pig." This is a ceremony performed in the patrilineal descent line, and is executed when the spirit of an ancestor demands it. The intent is to appease this spirit, which generally makes his desire known by engendering illness in his descendants.

Nqus – literally "sucking." In the health context, this word refers to moxibustion. The Hmong believe that both stress and tension, and "internal heat," can cause illness. In accordance with this belief, they will often fire the air within a cup or a hollow horn, generating a vacuum which affixes the item to the patient's back, forehead or the area specific to the complaint. After treatment, a slight bruising or reddening, especially in a series of circles, may be seen on the treated area. Moxibustion is widely believed throughout Asia to draw out from within the body that impurity or pressure which is causing discomfort.

Ntsua Ntawv – cut, branch-like paper, burned by the shaman during healing ceremonies. This is done to pay debts to spirits incurred for their assistance either in finding, or in returning to earth, the wandering soul of one who has fallen ill; or both. This paper represents currency in the spirit world, and may be exchanged there for the genuine article. *Ntsua Ntawv* is also burned during Hmong funeral rites to provide funds for the deceased in the spirit world. See also "*Lub Yeej Khuam.*"

Ntsuj Duab Ntsuj Hlauv – the "protruding shadow soul." According to the Hmong shaman, the individual possesses five different souls. These are the reindeer soul, *Nyuj Cab Nyuj Kaus* (which see); the protruding shadow, *Ntsuj Duab Ntsuj Hlauv*; the running bull, *Nyuj Rag Nyug Ris* (which see); the growing bamboo soul, *Ntsuj Xyoob Ntsuj Ntoo* (which see); and the chicken soul, *Ntsuj Qaib Ntsuj Noog* (which see).

Ntsuj Qaib Ntsuj Noog – the "chicken soul." According to the Hmong shaman, the individual possesses five different souls. These are the reindeer soul, *Nyuj Cab Nyuj Kaus* (which see); the protruding shadow, *Ntsuj Duab Ntsuj Hlauv* (which see); the running bull, *Nyuj Rag Nyug Ris* (which see); the growing bamboo soul, *Ntsuj Xyoob Ntsuj Ntoo* (which see); and the chicken soul, *Ntsuj Qaib Ntsuj Noog*.

Ntsuj Xyoob Ntsuj Ntoo – the "growing bamboo soul." According to the Hmong shaman, the individual possesses five different souls. These are the reindeer soul, *Nyuj Cab Nyuj Kaus* (which see); the protruding shadow, *Ntsuj Duab Ntsuj Hlauv* (which see); the running bull, *Nyuj Rag Nyug Ris* (which see); the growing bamboo soul, *Ntsuj Xyoob Ntsuj Ntoo*; and the chicken soul, *Ntsuj Qaib Ntsuj Noog* (which see).

Ntxwj Nyug – this celestial personality, largely via the twin mechanisms of illness and accident, calls in the souls of the living whose "mandate of life" has expired. He is also charged with the determination of the appropriate animal, vegetable, or human form for the individual's reincarnation, based upon how well that individual lived his life. See also "God."

Nyuaj Siab – literally, "difficult liver." This term is used to describe someone oppressed by an excess of worry, exhibiting such signs as weeping, confusion, and insomnia.

Nyuj Cab Nyuj Kaus – the "reindeer soul." According to the Hmong shaman, the individual possesses five different souls. These are the reindeer soul, *Nyuj Cab Nyuj Kaus*; the protruding shadow, *Ntsuj Duab Ntsuj Hlauv* (which see); the running bull, *Nyuj Rag Nyug Ris* (which see); the growing bamboo soul, *Ntsuj Xyoob Ntsuj Ntoo* (which see); and the chicken soul, *Ntsuj Qaib Ntsuj Noog* (which see).

Nyuj Dab – literally, "cow spirit." By tradition, once in his lifetime a son may be called upon by his deceased parents to sacrifice a cow for their benefit. They will draw his attention to their desire either by speaking to him in a dream, or by causing someone in the family illness. In the latter case, it will be the shaman who is called upon to alleviate the illness to whom the message is given that a *Nyuj Dab* is requested.

Nyuj Rag Nyug Ris – the "running bull soul." According to the Hmong shaman, the individual possesses five different souls. These are the reindeer soul, *Nyuj Cab Nyuj Kaus* (which see); the protruding shadow, *Ntsuj Duab Ntsuj Hlauv* (which see); the running bull, *Nyuj Rag Nyug Ris*; the growing bamboo soul, *Ntsuj Xyoob Ntsuj Ntoo* (which see); and the chicken soul, *Ntsuj Qaib Ntsuj Noog* (which see).

Nyuj Vaj Tuam Teem – a lord of the spirit world; this entity issues licenses for rebirth.

Ob Ntshua Ntawv – a pair of cut papers offered to the *Dab Pog* (which see) couple in the hope they will confer their blessings on a newborn child. See also "*Ib Nkawm Qaib.*"

Poj Koob Yawm Txwv – literally, "great grand parents." This is a term used by some Hmong to refer to the *Dab Pog* (which see) couple.

Poj Yawm Txwv Koob – a variant of *Poj Koob Yawm Txwv* (which see).

Poob Ntsej Muag – "losing face;" suffering humiliation, embarrassment, or loss of dignity before friends, family, or colleagues.

Poob Plig – literally "falling soul." This term refers to the Hmong concept of soul loss. According to traditional Hmong esoteric thought, an individual has several souls, all of which must be present and functioning in harmony for that individual to experience a feeling of healthy well-being. Occasionally, one of these souls will wander off or otherwise become detached, and may even ascend to the spirit world. In such a case, there is no choice but to go in pursuit and convince the soul to return. This is the object of a soul-calling ceremony, or *Hu Plig* (which see.)

Poob Siab – literally, "dropped liver;" a term used to denote someone who is frightened.

Qaug Dab Peg – literally, "the spirit catches you and you fall down." This is a Hmong term for epilepsy.

Qeej – musical flute or mouth organ made from bamboo and reeds. The *Qeej* (sometimes transliterated as "*Kheng*") is one of the "Eight Most Important Spirits in the Hmong Cultural Tradition," or *Yim Tus Tswv Dab Nyob Hauv Hmoob Kev Cai Dab Qhuas* (which see). It is used both in leisure activities and in ritual; for the latter of which its main service is rendered in tandem with the drum, *Lub Nruas* (which see), to the accompaniment of which it is invariably played during a funeral. When both are thus played, the voice of the drum is interpreted as saying to the newly deceased, who may be in some confusion, "*Mus qhov twg? Mus qhov twg?*" (which see). The meaning of this phrase is, "Where to go? Where to go?" The music of the *Qeej* replies, "*Mus qhov nov! Mus qhov nov!*" (which see), meaning, "Go this way! Go this way!" It is in this fashion that the spirits of the drum and *Qeej* help to direct the deceased to the land of his ancestors.

Rooj Ntug – literally, "door of the sky." A term for the heavenly gate which is the highest and last of a series of gates through which the shaman and his spirit helpers must occasionally pass if they are to seek out and call back a straying soul.

Saib – diagnose.

Saib Phaib – counting the cards. A diagnostic technique not dissimilar to the techniques of counting the numbers, or *Xam Lej* (which see); counting the dates, or *Xam Hnub Nyoog* (which see); and the read and write technique, or *Sau Ntawv Saib* (which see). All of these concepts except *Xam Hnub Nyoog* were originally acquired from peoples among whom or near to whom the Hmong have lived in past centuries.

Saib Saub – consulting the master healer. The word *Saub* refers to a master, and a *Saib Saub* is a master at the arts of diagnosis and treatment of illness and disease. The healer who has earned this title is expected to know everything there is to know in the Hmong culture regarding health treatment. While it is generally agreed that there are master healers in Laos and Thailand, in the United States all have passed away.

Sau Ntawv Saib – the read and write technique. This diagnostic methodology is, in some measure, comparable to the diagnostic and divination methods known as counting the cards, or *Saib Phaib* (which see); counting the numbers, or *Xam Lej* (which see); and counting the dates, or *Xam Hnub Nyoog* (which see). All of these concepts except the *Xam Hnub Nyoog* originated with, and were adapted from, a variety of indigenous peoples among whom or near to whom the Hmong have, at one time, lived.

Saub – master. The word is generally used in the context of a master healer, or *Saib Saub* (which see). Such a man will have developed a command of all the methodologies and techniques of traditional Hmong medicine. In the celestial realm, *Saub* is classified the lieutenant of God or *Huab Tais Ntuj* (which see), who provided the first seeds and made the first hen to lay eggs. After the great flood receded from earth, *Saub* told the surviving Hmong sister and brother to cut their baby into pieces and spread them over the land, forming the twelve original Hmong clans. See also "God."

Sem Xyas – a Chinese cough remedy. When mixed with warm water, *Sem Xyas* forms a sort of cough syrup.

Siab Dawb – literally, "white liver." This term denotes someone who, according to the Hmong ethos, is possessed of a good heart or is generally kind.

Siab Luv – literally, "short liver." This term refers to an individual who often swings suddenly, and, in many cases, inexplicably, from a normal state of mind to a state of extreme ill temper.

Siab Phem – literally, "ugly liver." This term is often used to describe someone who, according to the Hmong ethos, treats others badly. This is a cruel or mean-spirited person.

Siv Yis – the first shaman, sent to earth long ago by the *Saub*, at a time when there were many illnesses and resulting fatalities.

Somatization – the claim to experience physical symptoms without identifiable organic pathological explanation.

SUNDS – Sudden Unexpected Nocturnal Death Syndrome; a terrifying malady that strikes the Hmong with no warning and no discernible cause. The result is sudden death during sleep.

Tau Pe – at the time of his wedding vows, and in conjunction with them, a Hmong male and his best man together seal the groom's oath. This is done in the following manner; standing side by side, the groom and his best man lower themselves so that their knees touch the ground. Then they bow their heads, each of them making a fist from which the thumb protrudes. Finally, each makes a thumb print in the earth, an act which is recognized as testimonial to a binding oath of marriage. This form of sealing the wedding vows is known as *Tau Pe* or *Pe*. This *Pe* is also executed in several other contexts in which a solemn expression of emotion is expected, such as, for example, to thank someone for donating funds at a funeral, or to thank the shaman for performing a healing ceremony.

Tau Ua Nom Txwv – literally "got political power." Someone in the Hmong community who has achieved political office or other position of responsibility and influence.

Teev – worship.

Thawj Neeb – term for a shaman who has died and passed into the next world. The term characterizes the man in his role of leader at the head of spirit troops.

Tig Plab – literally "turning the stomach." This is a technique of massage specially suited to expectant mothers, and is employed to ease a difficult delivery, or to restore a state of well-being to a pregnant woman who has fallen down or suffered other pain or injury.

Tsawv Qe – egg balancing. This diagnostic tool is one of two utilizing an egg. It is performed at the onset of illness to assist in the selection of the shaman who will be consulted.

Tshuaj Ntsuab – literally "green medicine." The reference is to all varieties of herbal medicine. Hmong specialists, for the most part female, are skillful in utilizing many different types of herbs for their medicinal properties. These herbs, either in raw form or already processed into medicinal form, are often obtained via international air mail from Laos, and the Southeast Asia region generally, by Hmong resident in the United States. Many Hmong families in this country also plant herbs, either outdoors in their gardens or indoors as houseplants.

These herbs, used in many different ways, have been a part of Hmong healing practice for centuries.

Tswv Tsim Neeg – a spirit couple; alternative to *Tus Tswv Tsim Neeg* (which see). When believers are afflicted with difficulties such as poverty, bad luck, or illness, they are enjoined to prepare a meal and call upon the *Tswv Tsim Neeg* couple to reverse this downward trend in fortune. Whoever does so is promised prosperity, good health, and a sharp mind. See also "God."

Tswv Xyas – an illness unique to the Hmong, which occurred during the years 1945—1959. Those who contracted this condition simply fell down and died inexplicably. For this reason, it was said that the victim had been attacked by a Hmong outcaste who had turned into a tiger and lived in the forest, occasionally coming to a Hmong village to prey particularly on the beautiful, the handsome, or the talented.

Tu Siab – literally, "broken liver." This is generally someone suffering from grief or guilt.

Tub Twm Zeej – literally, "single buffalo son." This term refers to an only son.

Tus Phij Laj – the best man, or the groom's companion/assistant.

Tus Qaib – the chicken. In the ceremonial context, the chicken is one of the "Eight Most Important Spirits in the Hmong Cultural Tradition," or *Yim Tus Tswv Dab Nyob Hauv Hmoob Kev Cai Dab Qhuas* (which see), and is used in a great variety of Hmong rituals.

Tus Tswv Tsim Neeg – a Hmong term for God. See also "God."

Tus Txawj Khawv Koob – healing through chanting or magic.

Tus Vauv – this somewhat malleable term may be used to refer to the groom, a son-in-law, or a married man.

Txheej Txam – the ceremonial paper cutter. This item, one of the "Eight Most Important Spirits in the Hmong Cultural Tradition," or *Yim Tus Tswv Dab Nyob Hauv Hmoob Kev Cai Dab Qhuas* (which see), is used by all Hmong during funeral ceremonies to cut paper into various designs, which are then utilized in a ritual manner. It is also used in the course of healing rituals to cut paper money to be burned as offering to the spirits by the Hmong shaman.

Txheej Xeeb – the "spirit of the trance." One of a pair sent by a shaman, who has died and resides in the next world, to press the shaman's son to become, himself, a shaman. The other member of this pair is known as *Leej Nkaub* (which see).

Txhib Ntawg – the "pointing-the-way-stick." Since this stick, fashioned from bamboo or other wood, is considered to house a spirit for the duration of its ceremonially useful life, it is one of the "Eight Most Important Spirits in the Hmong Cultural Tradition," or *Yim Tus Tswv Dab Nyob Hauv Hmoob Kev Cai Dab Qhuas* (which see). This split stick is used once only, during a funeral and the related death ceremonies, and is subsequently discarded. Its purpose is to serve as an implement of communication between the worlds of the living and the dead, and to point the way to the latter, considered to be the land of the ancestors, for the guidance of the soul of the newly departed. It is also employed to invite spirit participation in certain ceremonies, and, following those ceremonies, as an aid to guide the participating spirits back to their world.

Txhij Qhua – calling the shaman's spirit helpers. This technique is employed on behalf of the seriously ill by the shaman, for which he utilizes his divine split horns, or *Txwm Kuam* (which see), to determine the outlook for a cure.

Txiv Dab – a "father of the spirits." This phrase refers to the owner of a Hmong funeral drum.

Txiv Muam Tai – the owner of a funeral drum passed from father to son down the generations. This drum is considered to house an important spirit, which must be worshipped and propitiated. Thus, the drum is considered to be one of the "Eight Most Important Spirits in the Hmong Cultural Tradition," or *Yim Tus Tswv Dab Nyob Hauv Hmoob Kev Cai Dab Qhuas* (which see). Moreover, the owner of this drum is considered to be a "father" to the spirits, or *Txiv Dab* (which see), and, thus, in a sense, is considered to be, himself, a spirit.

Txwm Kuam – the "shaman's divine split horns." These items collectively are counted one of the "Eight Most Important Spirits in the Hmong Cultural Tradition," or *Yim Tus Tswv Dab Nyob Hauv Hmoob Kev Cai Dab Qhuas* (which see), and are used by the shaman as a tool for communication with the spirits or for diagnosing illness. In this manner, they are an invaluable aid in the soul calling ceremony, *Hu Plig* (which see), and serve primarily in efforts to cure illness.

Ua Laib- youth gang.

Ua Neeb Kho – the shaman's healing ceremony.

Ua Neeb Saib – the shaman's diagnostic ceremony. The *Ua Neeb Saib* is a diagnostic ceremony performed by a shaman, and may take one of two forms. The first of these is employed simply to diagnose a patient's health problems, while the second is employed to establish the diagnosis of a third party while the shaman is simultaneously engaged in the performance of an entirely different ceremony on behalf of someone who has already recovered.

Ua Neeb Xua Nplej – shaman of the husk rice. A rare variety of master shaman, who, eschewing the ordinary paraphernalia of other shamans such as gongs and drums, requires only the fragrance of burning rice husks to summon his spirit helpers.

Vij Sub Vij Sw – evil spirits thought to cause illness.

Vwm Ntsuav – literally, "crazy." A person odd in manner, or exhibiting slightly crazy behavior.

Xais Ceeb – a uniquely Hmong technique of applying pressure to relieve the condition of physiological imbalance created by shock, or *Ceeb* (which see).

Xam Hnub Nyoog – counting the dates. This diagnostic technique is employed not only to determine the cause of an illness, but, in addition, can be utilized both to locate lost articles and to decide upon the most favorable date upon which to commence a journey or stage some other variety of important event. It bears certain similarities to the techniques of counting the cards, or *Saib Phab* (which see); counting the numbers, or *Xam Lej* (which see); and the read and write technique, or *Sau Ntawv Saib* (which see). All of these diagnostic techniques or methods of divination except *Xam Hnub Nyoog* were initially acquired from peoples among whom or near to whom the Hmong have lived in past centuries.

Xam Lej – counting the numbers. A diagnostic technique which bears similarities to the techniques of counting the cards, or *Saib Phab* (which see); counting the dates, or *Xam Hnub Nyoog* (which see); and the read and write technique, or *Sau Ntawv Saib* (which see). All of the aforementioned techniques or methods of divination were initially acquired from peoples among whom or near to whom the Hmong have lived in past centuries.

Xeem – the clan system; the main social organization in traditional Hmong society.

Xwm Kab – the house spirits; a celestial couple, like the *Dab Pog* (which see), worshipped by the Hmong. This pair, gratified by such worship, protects the family. The *Xwm Kab* watch over Hmong homes, protecting them from evil spirits and guarding all who live within from sickness. This spirit couple also watch over the household assets to ensures that the people who live within not only healthy, but prosperous.

Yaj Ceeb – according to Hmong cosmology, the world in which people live. See also "*Yeeb Ceeb.*"

Yang – the Chinese world of light, where human beings, material objects, and nature exist.

Yeeb Ceeb – according to Hmong cosmology, the unseen aspect of reality. This is the world of the supernatural spirits and deceased ancestors. See also "*Yaj Ceeb.*"

Yim Tus Tswv Dab Nyob Hauv Hmoob Kev Cai Dab Qhuas – the "Eight Most Important Spirits in the Hmong Cultural Tradition." These are, 1) the *Txiv Muam Tai*, or Owner of the Drum (which see); 2) the *Txhib Ntawg*, or Pointing-the-Way-Stick (which see); 3) the *Txwm Kuam*, or Shaman's Divine Split Horns (which see); 4) the *Lub Nruas*, or Ceremonial Drum (which see); 5) the *Qeej*, or reed musical instrument (which see); 6) the *Lub Kaus*, or Ceremonial Umbrella (which see); 7) the *Txheej Txam*, or Ceremonial Paper Cutter (which see); and, 8) the *Tus Qaib*, or Chicken (which see). It will be noted that none of these items is, strictly speaking, a spirit, and, indeed, with the exception of the *Txiv Muam Tai* (Owner of the Drum) and the *Tus Qaib* (chicken) all are inanimate objects. Nevertheless, in the course of their use in those rituals and ceremonies by which they come into contact with spirits and the spirit world, it is thought that they are themselves, in a sense, transformed into spirits; the "Eight Most Important Spirits in the Hmong Cultural Tradition."

Yin – the Chinese world of darkness, where the spirits thrive.

Zaj Laug – literally, "old dragon." In ancient times, this magical creature was thought to live under the waters of the world, and, from there, to control nature. See also "*Zaj Txwg Zaj Laug.*"

Zaj Txwg Zaj Laug – the "old dragon which lives under the water." See also "*Zaj Laug.*"

Zaj Zeg Zaj Lag – the palace of the water dragon. It is thought that, in ancient times, the water dragon existed as a magical creature, steeped in wisdom and nature lore. It lived beneath the world's waters, and, from there, controlled the forces of nature. It occasionally transformed itself into human form to travel in and investigate the world of the Hmong, and, owing to its knowledge of the universe and its command of the mechanics of nature, as well as its insight, understanding, and compassion, it was sometimes asked to arbitrate disputes for the Hmong.

Zaws – literally "massage." Hmong massage techniques.

Zaws Plab – abdominal massage.

Appendix One

Forms

I. HMONG HEALTH HISTORY SURVEY

ID_____

Date_____

HMONG HEALTH HISTORY SURVEY

Demographic Information

1.   Age _____   2.   Gender _____

3   Marital Status: ___ Single ____Married ___Widowed ___Divorced ____Separated

4.   How long have you been in the United States? _____

5.   How many people are in your household? _____
       Number of children _____ Number of adults _____

6.   Number of bedrooms in your house or apartment? _____

7.   What is your religion? _____

8.   Do you consider yourself a:
       ___ a. Shaman
       ___ b. Herbalist
       ___ c. Massage Therapist
       ___ d. Medical doctor
       ___ e. Nurse
       ___ f. Other healer _____
       ___ g. Patient of the above healers: __a ___b __c __d __e __f (check all that apply to you)

9.   What language do you speak more at home? Hmong:____ English:____

10.   Are you currently working? Yes:___ No:___ If yes, what is your occupation?_____

11.   What is your household annual income? _____

12.   What is your level of education?
       ___ a. No formal education
       ___ b. Enrolled in ESL classes for less than 2 years

___ c. High school
___ d. Some college
___ e. College graduate
___ f. Graduate school
___ g. Other_____

13. Which one of the following do you consider yourself to be?
a) Hmong____ b) Lao-Hmong____ c) Hmong-American____ d) American____

Health Care Information

14. If someone in your household is sick, what is the first thing you do?
_____
_____

15. Has anyone in your household been sick **this year**? Yes:___ No:___
If yes, what type of illness?_____
        Name and number of adult (s) sick? _____
_____
        Name and number of Children sick?_____
_____

16. Has anyone in your household been sick in the **last year**? Yes:___ No:___
If yes, what type of illness?_____
        Name and number of adult (s) sick? _____
_____
        Name and number of Children sick?_____
_____

17. Do you have a family doctor? Yes:____ No:____ If yes, give your doctor's name and phone # _____
_____

18. Do you have health insurance? Yes:____ No:____
If yes, name of your provider? _____

19. How many times have you seen the doctor(s) in 1998 and 1999?
1998:   Reason for visit:
a. None
b. 1 - 2 times   _____
c. 3 - 5 times   _____
d. More than 5 times   _____

1999:   Reason for visit:
a. None
b. 1 - 2 times   _____
c. 3 - 5 times   _____

d. More than 5 times _____

20. Have **YOU** had any major surgery in the last three years?   Yes:___ No:___
     If yes, when and what for?_____

21. Has **ANYONE** in your household had major surgery in the last three years? Yes:___ No:___
     If yes, when and what for?_____

22. Do you have or know someone in your household who has had the following health problems?
     a. Brain tumor   Self: Yes___ No___   Someone else: Yes___ No___
     b. Breast cancer   Self: Yes___ No___   Someone else: Yes___ No___
     c. Heart attack   Self: Yes___ No___   Someone else: Yes___ No___
     d. Diabetes   Self: Yes___ No___   Someone else: Yes___ No___
     e. Tuberculosis   Self: Yes___ No___   Someone else: Yes___ No___
     f. AIDS   Self: Yes___ No___   Someone else: Yes___ No___
     g. Alcoholism   Self: Yes___ No___   Someone else: Yes___ No___
     h. Depression   Self: Yes___ No___   Someone else: Yes___ No___
     i. Mental disturbance   Self: Yes___ No___   Someone else: Yes___ No___
     j. Hypertension   Self: Yes___ No___   Someone else: Yes___ No___
     k. Stroke   Self: Yes___ No___   Someone else: Yes ___No___
     l. Other_____   Self: Yes___ No___   Someone else: Yes___ No___
     m. Somatic symptoms   Self: Yes___ No___   Someone else: Yes___ No___

23. How knowledgeable are you in using the mainstream health care system?
     ___ a. Very knowledgeable
     ___ b. Knowledgeable
     ___ c. Not knowledgeable
     ___ d. Not knowledgeable at all

24. Do you need a translator when you use the mainstream health care system? Yes____   No____
     If yes, who?: ___Family member & Friend   ___Bilingual professional translator   ___Other

25. When you consult with the mainstream health care professionals, you are required to sign a sheet of paper.
     Do you know what it is called? Yes ___ No___ If yes, what? _____
     Do you understand what it is for? Yes ___ No___ If yes, explain: _____

26. Have you seen any of the following health care providers?
     a. Family practice doctor   # of time:_____   Year:_____   For_____
     b. Neurologist   _____   _____   _____
     c. Psychologist/psychiatrist   _____   _____   _____
     d. Physical therapist   _____   _____   _____
     e. Cardiologist   _____   _____   _____
     f. Other _____

27. What made you decide to see a doctor instead of a Hmong traditional healer?
    _____
    _____

28. In the past, when a doctor recommended a health treatment plan for a sickness, did you or a family member go along with the plan? Yes___ No___ Why? _____

29. What type of illness might make you decide to see a Hmong traditional healer instead of a doctor?

30. In the past, when a Hmong healer has recommended a health treatment plan for a sickness, did you or a family member go along with the plan?   Yes___ No___ Why? _____
    _____
    _____

31. Which of the following Hmong healers or diagnosticians have you consulted with in the last three years?

	# of time:	Fee paid? $	Year	For
a. Shaman				
b. Herbalist				
c. Massage Therapist				
d. Fortuneteller				
e. Egg reader				
f. Needle user				
g. Soul Callers				
h. Other healer				

32. How many of the following Hmong healers or diagnosticians do you know in the Hmong community in Colorado?

	Number:
a. Shaman	
b. Herbalist	
c. Massage Therapist	
d. Fortuneteller	
e. Egg reader	
f. Needle user	
g. Soul Callers	
h. Other healer _____	

33. Do you have any herbal plants in your home or garden? Yes:___ No:___ If yes, please write down the name(s)_____
    _____
    _____

34. Have you or anyone in your household ever had an automobile accident? Self: Yes___ No___
    If yes, when? _____ Household members: Yes___ No___ If yes, when?_____

35. How healthy do you think you are?
    ___ a. Very healthy
    ___ b. Healthy

___   c.   Not healthy
___   d.   Don't know

36.   Do you consider yourself overweight? Yes:___ No:___ If yes, what is your weight?___ and height?_____

37.   Do you exercise? Yes:___ No:___ If yes, how often?_____

38.   Do you smoke? Yes___ No____ If yes, how often? _____

39.   Anyone in your household smoke? Yes____ No____ If yes, how often? _____

40.   How often do you drink the following?

	Daily	Weekly	Monthly	Other
a) Coffee				
b) Tea				
c) Wine				
d) Beer				
e) Whiskey				
f) Hmong homemade beer				
g) Herbal broth				
h) Plain Vegetable broth				
i) Other liquids				

41.   Will you consult with the following Hmong healers in the future?

a.   Shaman   Yes _____   No _____
b.   Herbalist   Yes _____   No _____
c. Massage Therapist   Yes _____   No _____
d. Fortuneteller   Yes _____   No _____
e. Egg reader   Yes _____   No _____
f. Needle user   Yes _____   No _____
g. Soul Callers   Yes _____   No _____
h. Other healer _____   Yes _____   No _____

42.   What are some of the obstacles you have experienced in using traditional Hmong medicine? _____
_____
_____
_____

43.   What are some of the obstacles you have experienced in using Biomedicine? _____
_____
_____
_____

44.   Describe some of the positive experience you have had when interacting with mainstream health care
providers? _____
_____

45. Have you had an experience that you were sick but when consulting with mainstream health care providers, they were unable to diagnose or cure your sickness? Yes____ No____
If yes, how long ago? _____ Number of time(s) you have this experience? _____ What was your illness? _____

II. INFORMED CONSENT FORM

Informed Consent Form
Hmong American Concepts of Health, Healing, and Illness
And Their Experience with Conventional Medicine

ID # _____

1. You, _____, have been invited to participate in a research project

   conducted by Dia Cha, a graduate student in the Department of Anthropology, University of

   Colorado-Boulder, conducted under the direction of Professor Robert A. Hackenberg. This

   project will research Hmong American Concepts of Health, Healing, and Illness, as well as

   the experiences of Hmong Americans with Western-oriented biomedicine.

2. The study will involve an interview, in the course of which the researcher will ask you

   questions about Hmong American concepts of health, healing, and illness. Further, you will

   be asked to relate your experiences with biomedicine. Finally, certain demographic

   information will be requested, including, but not limited to, your annual household income,

   family composition, gender, age, and level of education. The interview will be audiotaped and/or videotaped, will last one to two hours, and will be conducted at a convenient location favorable to you, such as home, work, public library study and/or conference room, etc.

3. It may reasonably be expected that the benefits of this project to the Hmong American community shall include:

   a.   A better understanding of Hmong concepts of health, healing, and illness; as well as an enhanced comprehension of the overall Hmong American experience with biomedicine, which should, in turn, result in,

   b.   An improvement in the general health of Hmong Americans.

   c.   It should be noted, however, that your participation in this study may not benefit you directly.

4. Inasmuch as hand-written notes may, on occasion, result in missed information, it should be borne in mind that the use of audiotaping technology, although it may be considered somewhat intrusive by some interviewees, represents the optimal modality for the researcher to conduct interviews.

5. It may be reassuring, however, to point out that all audio and video tapes will be stored in a locked box to which only the researcher will have a key. In addition, all audiotapes will be destroyed after the completion of the study. With your approval and permission, and only with that permission, at the end of the research project certain material from the videotapes of focus group and in-depth interviews may be edited to produce an educational video, should funding become available.

6. The risk of harm to you from participating in this study is minimal. However, certain adverse consequences may ensue, as, for example, as follows:

   a. In sharing your beliefs, perceptions, and experiences with biomedicine and/or Hmong healing practices, you may come to feel a certain discomfort, frustration or emotional negativity.

   b. Although it is emphasized that nowhere will your name be given, since the Hmong community in Colorado is small, other people (i. e. your biomedical providers, Hmong healers or community members) may be able to guess your identity by matching you with the opinions you express in the results of this research.

   c. Other people, such as your biomedical providers, Hmong healers or community members, may disagree with your opinions.

   d. Although your name is not given, some personal information, such as your household composition and annual income, age and gender will become public.

7. Any personal information acquired and/or used in this study will be treated as absolutely confidential. Information which identifies you will not be released. No names will appear in the study. The researcher will try her best not impart, convey or reveal anything about you whatsoever to any others, for any reason, in any way that might lead to your identification without your express permission. This principle of absolute privacy and confidentiality shall extend, as well, to all published and written data resulting from this study.

8. It should be clearly understood that any and all participation in this study is absolutely voluntary. Participation is in no way expected or coerced. It is under no circumstances necessary to participate. You, in addition, having once begun to participate, may cease and desist from participation at any ensuing time, and it will have no adverse effect on the research.

9. Any questions about your rights as a subject, any concerns regarding this study, and/or any dissatisfactions with any aspect of this study that may arise, may be reported in written form, and in confidence, to: The Executive Secretary; Human Research Committee, Graduate School; Campus Box 26, Regent 308; University of Colorado-Boulder; Boulder, CO 80309-0026. The same may be reported verbally, by telephone, to: (30) 492-7401. Copies of the University of Colorado Assurance of Compliance with relation to federal government guidelines regarding human subject research are available upon request from the Graduate School address listed above.

10. I have received a signed copy of this consent form.

11. I have read the above information and/or it has been translated orally to me. I understand the study's aims, scope, and purpose and voluntarily consent to participate in the research project entitled Hmong American Concepts of Health, Healing, and Illness.

Signature of Research Subject   Date

Print Name of Research Subject

12. I agree to be audiotaped and videotaped.

Signature of Research Subject	Date

Print Name of Research Subject

13. I, the undersigned, have witnessed the presentation of the description of the research study,

the details of which are elaborated above, to the above named research subject.

Signature of Witness	Date

Print Name of Witness

Contacts:

Dia Cha
Campus Box 233
University of Colorado-Boulder
Boulder, CO 80309
Telephone: 303-492-8462

Professor Robert A. Hackenberg
Campus Box 233
University of Colorado-Boulder
Boulder, CO 80309
Telephone: 303-492-8022

Department of Anthropology
Campus Box 233
University of Colorado-Boulder
Boulder, CO 80309
Telephone: 303-492-2547

The Executive Secretary
Human Research Committee, Graduate School
Campus Box 26, Regent 308
University of Colorado-Boulder
Boulder, CO 80309-0026

(30) 492-7401

III. PARTICIPANT OBSERVATION FORM

Participant Observation Form

ID # _____

1. I, the undersigned, agree to allow Dia Cha who is conducting a research on Hmong Concepts of health, healing, and illness and Hmong American experience with biomedicine, to observe me as I perform a Hmong shaman ceremony, a Hmong massage technique, a Hmong herbal process or application procedure, other health treatment_____ (circle the one(s) that is/are applicable). Dia Cha agrees to protect my confidentiality and to be a participant observer of the above rituals for the aforementioned research only.

_____   _____

Signature of Research Subject   Date

_____

Print Name of Research Subject

2. I, the undersigned, have witnessed the aforementioned agreement to authorize Dia Cha to be a participant observer for the above research.

_____   _____

Signature of Witness   Date

_____

Print Name of Witness

IV. FOCUS GROUP DISCUSSION FORM

Focus Group Discussions for Hmong subjects*

If someone in your household is sick, what is the first thing you do?

In those instances in which a doctor trained in Western biomedicine rather than a Hmong traditional healer is consulted, what are those considerations which motivate this decision?

What types of illness might make you decide to see a Hmong traditional healer instead of a doctor?

What types of medicinal herbs or other useful plants do you grow in your house or garden?

How healthy do you think you are?

What are some of the obstacles you have experienced in using traditional Hmong medicine?

What are some of the obstacles you have experienced in using Western biomedicine?

Describe some of the positive experience you have had when interacting with mainstream health care providers?

How many of you have had an experience in which you were sick but, when consulting with mainstream health care providers, found they were unable to diagnose or cure your sickness?

What is the most difficult or confusing aspect in the interaction with biomedical health care personnel?

What are some of the Western biomedical procedures or techniques with which you are most familiar?

What are some of your health concerns?

V. IN-DEPTH INTERVIEW FORM

In-depth Interview Questions**

Describe the different types of traditional Hmong healers.

Describe the different types of traditional Hmong diagnosticians.

How many of the above healers and diagnosticians exist in the Colorado Hmong community?

What are some of the aspects of traditional Hmong healing practices that have remained intact?

What aspects have changed?

What are some of the factors that have obstructed biomedical health care delivery to Hmong in Colorado?

What are some of the factors that have enabled health care delivery to the Hmong?

Appendix Two

Informants by Clan

Clan Name	No. of Informants	Type of Interview		
		One-on-One	Focus Group	In-Depth
Chang/Cha	6	6	1	1
Cheng	1	1		
Lee/Ly/Le	6	5	1	
Lor/Lo/Lao	6	3	3	1
Her/Herr/Heu	5	2	2	1
Thao	5	2	3	
Vang	7	6	1	
Vue	3	2	1	1
Xiong	9	6	2	2
Yang	6	4	2	1
Moua	2		2	
Kue	1	1		

Notes

NOTES TO THE FOREWORD

[1] Arax, Mark. *Cancer Case Ignites Culture Clash; Hmong Parents Refuse To Agree To Court Ordered Chemotherapy For Teenage Daughter.* (Case in Fresno, California highlights parents fear that ovarian cancer treatment will render daughter infertile and thus unmarriageable). Los Angeles Times, Nov 21, 1994, v113, pA3, Col 1 (35 col in); Arax, Mark. *Hmong's Sacrifice of Puppy Reopens Cultural Wounds: Immigrant Shaman's Act Stirs Outrage in Fresno, But He Believes It Was Only Way To Cure His Ill Wife.* (Chia Thai Moua's sacrifice incurs racism and dislike of Southeast Asians in Fresno). Los Angeles Times, Dec 16, 1995, v114, pA1, Col 5 (40 col in); Fadiman, Anne. *The Spirit Catches You and You Fall Down: A Hmong Child, Her American Doctors, and the Collision of Two Cultures.* New York: Farrar, Straus and Giroux, 1997; Warner, Miriam E., and Marilyn Mochel. *The Hmong and Health Care in Merced, California.* Hmong Studies Journal, Spring, 1998, 2 (2); Waters, David A., Rama B. Rao, and Helen E. Petracchi. *Providing Health Care for the Hmong.* Wisconsin Medical Journal, 91 (11) 1992: 642–651.

[2] Bliatout, Bruce Thowpaou. *Guidelines for Mental Health Professionals to Help Hmong Clients Seek Traditional Healing Treatment.* In *The Hmong In Transition.* Glenn L. Hendricks et al., eds., 349–363. New York: Center for Migration Studies, 1986; Bliatout, Bruce Thowpaou. *Hmong Attitudes Towards Surgery: How It Affects Patient Prognosis.* Migration World, XVI (1) 1988: 25–27; Cheon-Klessig, Y., D. D. Camilleri, B. J. McElmurry, and V. M. Ohlson. *Folk Medicine in the Health Practice of Hmong Refugees.* Western Journal of Nursing Research, 10 (5) 1988: 647–60; Fadiman, Anne. *The Spirit Catches You and You Fall Down: A Hmong Child, Her American Doctors, and the Collision of Two Cultures.* New York: Farrar, Straus and Giroux, 1997; Thao, Xoua. *Hmong Perception of Illness and Traditional Ways of Healing.* In *The Hmong In Transition.* Glenn L. Hendricks et al., eds. pp. 365–378. New York: Center for

Migration Studies, 1986; Waters, David A., Rama B. Rao, and Helen E. Petracchi. *Providing Health Care for the Hmong.* Wisconsin Medical Journal, 91 (11) 1992: 642–651.

[3] Lin, Elizabeth H. B., William B. Carter; and Arthur M. Kleinman. *An Exploration of Somatization among Asian Refugees and Immigrants in Primary Care.* American Journal of Public Health, 75 (9) 1985: 1080–1084; Nuland, Sherwin B. Review of *A Spirit Catches You and You Fall Down,* by Anne Fadiman. New Republic, 217 (15) 1997: 31–40; Fadiman Anne. *The Spirit Catches You and You Fall Down: A Hmong Child, Her American Doctors, and the Collision of Two Cultures.* New York: Farrar, Straus and Giroux, 1997.

[4] Lin, Elizabeth H. B., William B. Carter; and Arthur M. Kleinman. *An Exploration of Somatization among Asian Refugees and Immigrants in Primary Care.* American Journal of Public Health, 75 (9) 1985: 1080–1084.; Barsky, Arthur J., and Jonathan F. Borus. *Somatization and Medicalization in the Era of Managed Care.* Journal of the American Medical Association, 274 (24) 1995: 1931–1934.

[5] Lin, Elizabeth H. B., William B. Carter; and Arthur M. Kleinman. *An Exploration of Somatization among Asian Refugees and Immigrants in Primary Care.* American Journal of Public Health, 75 (9) 1985: 1080–1084.; O'Connor, Bonnie Blair. *Healing Traditions: Alternative Medicine and the Health Professions.* Philadelphia: University of Pennsylvania Press, 1995.

[6] Lin, Elizabeth H. B., William B. Carter; and Arthur M. Kleinman. *An Exploration of Somatization among Asian Refugees and Immigrants in Primary Care.* American Journal of Public Health, 75 (9) 1985: 1080–1084.; Barsky, Arthur J., and Jonathan F. Borus. *Somatization and Medicalization in the Era of Managed Care.* Journal of the American Medical Association, 274 (24) 1995: 1931–1934.

[7] Lin, Elizabeth H. B., William B. Carter; and Arthur M. Kleinman. *An Exploration of Somatization among Asian Refugees and Immigrants in Primary Care.* American Journal of Public Health, 75 (9) 1985: 1080–1084.

[8] Lin, Elizabeth H. B., William B. Carter; and Arthur M. Kleinman. *An Exploration of Somatization among Asian Refugees and Immigrants in Primary Care.* American Journal of Public Health, 75 (9) 1985: 1080.

NOTES TO CHAPTER I

[1] Tapp, Nicholas. *Sovereignty and Rebellion: The White Hmong of Northern Thailand.* Oxford: Oxford University Press, 1989.

[2] id.

[3] Barney, G. Le. Christianity and Innovation in Meo Culture: A Case Study in Missionization. Unpublished M. A. thesis. Minneapolis: University of Minnesota, 1957; Tapp, Nicholas. Sovereignty and Rebellion: The White Hmong of Northern Thailand. Oxford: Oxford University Press, 1989.

[4] Tapp, Nicholas. *Sovereignty and Rebellion: The White Hmong of Northern Thailand.* Oxford: Oxford University Press, 1989.

[5] Cooper, Robert, ed. Resource Scarcity and the Hmong Response: Patterns of Settlement and Economy in Transition. National University of Singapore: Singapore University Press, 1984; Heimbach, M. At Any Cost: The Story of Graham Ray Orpin. London: Overseas Missionary Fellowship, 1976; Kuhn, I. Ascent to the

Tribes: Pioneering in North Thailand. London: Overseas Missionary Fellowship, 1956; Tapp, Nicholas. Sovereignty and Rebellion: The White Hmong of Northern Thailand. Oxford: Oxford University Press, 1989.

⁶ Cooper, Robert, ed. *Resource Scarcity and the Hmong Response: Patterns of Settlement and Economy in Transition.* National University of Singapore: Singapore University Press, 1984; Tapp, Nicholas. Sovereignty and Rebellion: The White Hmong of Northern Thailand. Oxford: Oxford University Press, 1989.

⁷ Tapp, Nicholas. *Sovereignty and Rebellion: The White Hmong of Northern Thailand.* Oxford: Oxford University Press, 1989.

⁸ id.

⁹ Cooper, Robert, ed., *The Hmong.* Bangkok: Artasia Press Co. Ltd., 1991; Ovesen, Jan. *A Minority Enters The Nation State: A Case Study of a Hmong Community in Vientiane Province, Laos.* Sweden: Uppsala University, 1995; Tapp, Nicholas. *Sovereignty and Rebellion: The White Hmong of Northern Thailand.* Oxford: Oxford University Press, 1989.

¹⁰ Ovesen, Jan. A Minority Enters The Nation State: A Case Study of a Hmong Community in Vientiane Province, Laos. Sweden: Uppsala University, 1995; Tapp, Nicholas. Sovereignty and Rebellion: The White Hmong of Northern Thailand. Oxford: Oxford University Press, 1989.

¹¹ Ovesen, Jan. A Minority Enters The Nation State: A Case Study of a Hmong Community in Vientiane Province, Laos. Sweden: Uppsala University, 1995.

¹² Long, Lynellyn D. *Ban Vinai: The Refugee Camp.* New York: Columbia University Press, 1993; Ovesen, Jan. *A Minority Enters The Nation State: A Case Study of a Hmong Community in Vientiane Province, Laos.* Sweden: Uppsala University, 1995; Tapp, Nicholas. *Sovereignty and Rebellion: The White Hmong of Northern Thailand.* Oxford: Oxford University Press, 1989.

¹³ Ovesen, Jan. A Minority Enters The Nation State: A Case Study of a Hmong Community in Vientiane Province, Laos. Sweden: Uppsala University, 1995; Tapp, Nicholas. Sovereignty and Rebellion: The White Hmong of Northern Thailand. Oxford: Oxford University Press, 1989.

¹⁴ The Hmong words in this paper are written in the White Hmong dialect, and in the format of the Romanized Popular Alphabet (RPA) writing system.

¹⁵ Cooper, Robert, ed., *The Hmong.* Bangkok: Artasia Press Co. Ltd., 1991; Long, Lynellyn D. *Ban Vinai: The Refugee Camp.* New York: Columbia University Press, 1993; Ovesen, Jan. *A Minority Enters The Nation State: A Case Study of a Hmong Community in Vientiane Province, Laos.* Sweden: Uppsala University, 1995; Tapp, Nicholas. *Sovereignty and Rebellion: The White Hmong of Northern Thailand.* Oxford: Oxford University Press, 1989.

¹⁶ Hamilton-Merritt, Jane. *Tragic Mountains: The Hmong, the Americans, and the Secret Wars for Laos, 1942–1992.* Bloomington and Indianapolis: Indiana University Press, 1993; Quincy, Keith. *Hmong: History of A People.* Cheney, WA: Eastern Washington University Press, 1995; Chan, Sucheng. *Hmong Means Free: Life in Laos and America.* Philadelphia: Temple University Press, 1994; Ranard, Donald A. *The Last Bus; The Hmong are Reluctant to Come to America: That is Their Tragedy and Thailand's Trouble.* The Atlantic, 260 (6) 1987: 26; Smalley, William A., Chia Koua Vang, and Gnia Yee Yang. *Mother of Writing: The Origin and Development of a Hmong Messianic Script.* Chicago: The University of

Chicago Press, 1988; Tobin, J. J., and J. Friedman. *Spirits, Shamans, and Nightmare Death: Survivor Stress in a Hmong Refugee.* American Journal of Orthopsychiatry, 53 (3) 1983: 439–48; Warner, Roger. *Back Fire: The CIA's Secret War in Laos and Its Link to the War in Vietnam.* New York: Simon & Schuster, 1995; Warner, Roger. *Shooting at the Moon.* South Royalton, Vermont: Steerforth Press, 1996.

[17] Cha, Dia, and Cathy A. Small. *Policy Lessons from Lao and Hmong Women in Thai Refugee Camps.* World Development, 22 (7) 1994: 1045–1059; Chan, Sucheng. *Hmong Means Free: Life in Laos and America.* Philadelphia: Temple University Press, 1994; Cooper, Robert, ed., *The Hmong.* Bangkok: Artasia Press Co. Ltd., 1991; Hamilton-Merritt, Jane. *Tragic Mountains: The Hmong, the Americans, and the Secret Wars for Laos, 1942–1992.* Bloomington and Indianapolis: Indiana University Press, 1993; Long, Lynellyn D. *Ban Vinai: The Refugee Camp.* New York: Columbia University Press, 1993;

Mottin, Jean. *History of the Hmong.* Bangkok: Odeon Store, 1980; Quincy, Keith. *Hmong: History of A People.* Cheney, WA: Eastern Washington University Press, 1995; Tapp, Nicholas. *Sovereignty and Rebellion: The White Hmong of Northern Thailand.* Oxford: Oxford University Press, 1989; Warner, Roger. *Shooting at the Moon.* South Royalton, Vermont: Steerforth Press, 1996.

[18] Cha, Dia, and Cathy A. Small. *Policy Lessons from Lao and Hmong Women in Thai Refugee Camps.* World Development, 22 (7) 1994: 1045–1059; Chan, Sucheng. *Hmong Means Free: Life in Laos and America.* Philadelphia: Temple University Press, 1994; Cooper, Robert, ed., *The Hmong.* Bangkok: Artasia Press Co. Ltd., 1991; Hamilton-Merritt, Jane. *Tragic Mountains: The Hmong, the Americans, and the Secret Wars for Laos, 1942–1992.* Bloomington and Indianapolis: Indiana University Press, 1993; Long, Lynellyn D. *Ban Vinai: The Refugee Camp.* New York: Columbia University Press, 1993;

Mottin, Jean. *History of the Hmong.* Bangkok: Odeon Store, 1980; Quincy, Keith. *Hmong: History of A People.* Cheney, WA: Eastern Washington University Press, 1995; Ranard, Donald A. *The Last Bus; The Hmong are Reluctant to Come to America: That is Their Tragedy and Thailand's Trouble.* The Atlantic, 260 (6) 1987: 26.

[19] Chan, Sucheng. *Hmong Means Free: Life in Laos and America.* Philadelphia: Temple University Press, 1994; Lee, Gary Yia. *Cultural Identity In Post-Modern Society: Reflections on What is a Hmong?* Hmong Studies Journal, 1 (1) 1996; Long, Lynellyn D. *Ban Vinai: The Refugee Camp.* New York: Columbia University Press, 1993; Mottin, Jean. *History of the Hmong.* Bangkok: Odeon Store, 1980; Quincy, Keith. *Hmong: History of A People.* Cheney, WA: Eastern Washington University Press, 1995.

[20] Hmong National Development, Inc. *Hmong American Population.* Washington, DC: Newsletter (Summer), 2000; Jambunathan, J., and S. Stewart. *Hmong Women in Wisconsin: What Are Their Concerns in Pregnancy and Childbirth?* Birth, 22 (4) 1995: 204–10. Jambunathan and Stewart, 1995, report over 1 million Hmong in the United States. The author disagrees with this figure, and there is no other source to support it.

[21] Pfeifer, Mark. *U.S. Census 2000: Trends in Hmong Population Distribution Across the Regions of the United States.* St. Paul, Minn.: Hmong Cultural Center, 2001.

[22] Hmong National Development, Inc. *Hmong American Population.* Washington, DC: Newsletter (Summer), 2000.

[23] Tapp, Nicholas. *Sovereignty and Rebellion: The White Hmong of Northern Thailand.* Oxford: Oxford University Press, 1989; Cooper, Robert, ed., *The Hmong.* Bangkok: Artasia Press Co. Ltd., 1991; Ovesen, Jan. *A Minority Enters The Nation State: A Case Study of a Hmong Community in Vientiane Province, Laos.* Sweden: Uppsala University, 1995; Rice, Pranee L. *The Hmong Way: Hmong Women and Reproduction.* Westport, CT: Bergin & Garvey, 2000.

[24] Cooper, Robert, ed., *The Hmong.* Bangkok: Artasia Press Co. Ltd., 1991; Tapp, Nicholas. *Sovereignty and Rebellion: The White Hmong of Northern Thailand.* Oxford: Oxford University Press, 1989; Geddes, William Robert. *Migrants of the Mountains: The Cultural Ecology of the Blue Miao (Hmong Njua) of Thailand.* Oxford: Clarendon Press, 1976; Yang, Kaoly. *Problems in the Interpretation of Hmong Clan Surnames (Hais Txog Kev Nrhiav Hmoob Cov Xeem).* Paper presented at the First International Workshop on the Hmong/Miao in Asia at the Centre des Archives d'Outre-Mer, Aix-en-Provence, France, 1998; Ovesen, Jan. *A Minority Enters The Nation State: A Case Study of a Hmong Community in Vientiane Province, Laos.* Sweden: Uppsala University, 1995; Rice, Pranee L., Blia Ly, and J. Lumley. *Childbirth and Soul Loss: the Case of a Hmong Woman.* Medical Journal of Australia, 160 (9) 1994: 577–8.

[25] Ovesen, Jan. *A Minority Enters The Nation State: A Case Study of a Hmong Community in Vientiane Province, Laos.* Sweden: Uppsala University, 1995; Cooper, Robert, ed., *The Hmong.* Bangkok: Artasia Press Co. Ltd., 1991; Tapp, Nicholas. *Sovereignty and Rebellion: The White Hmong of Northern Thailand.* Oxford: Oxford University Press, 1989; Mottin, Jean. *History of the Hmong.* Bangkok: Odeon Store, 1980; Rice, Pranee L. *The Hmong Way: Hmong Women and Reproduction.* Westport, CT: Bergin & Garvey, 2000.

[26] Ovesen, Jan. *A Minority Enters The Nation State: A Case Study of a Hmong Community in Vientiane Province, Laos.* Sweden: Uppsala University, 1995.

[27] Some Hmong believe that the term "Green" Hmong has a negative connotation. Thus, the term Blue Hmong or Hmong Leng (*Hmoob Lees*) is preferred (see Thao 1999 for additional discussion).

[28] Ovesen, Jan. A Minority Enters The Nation State: A Case Study of a Hmong Community in Vientiane Province, Laos. Sweden: Uppsala University, 1995; Rice, Pranee L. The Hmong Way: Hmong Women and Reproduction. Westport, CT: Bergin & Garvey, 2000.

[29] Mottin, Jean. *History of the Hmong.* Bangkok: Odeon Store, 1980; Rice, Pranee L. *The Hmong Way: Hmong Women and Reproduction.* Westport, CT: Bergin & Garvey, 2000.

[30] Cooper, Robert, ed., *The Hmong.* Bangkok: Artasia Press Co. Ltd., 1991; Rice, Pranee L. *The Hmong Way: Hmong Women and Reproduction.* Westport, CT: Bergin & Garvey, 2000.

[31] Rice, Pranee L. *The Hmong Way: Hmong Women and Reproduction.* Westport, CT: Bergin & Garvey, 2000.

[32] Cha, Dia, and Cathy A. Small. Policy Lessons from Lao and Hmong Women in Thai Refugee Camps. World Development, 22 (7) 1994: 1045–1059; Cha, Dia, and Jacquelyn Chagnon. Farmer, War-wife, Refugee, Repatriate: A Needs

Assessment of Women Repatriating to Laos. Washington, DC: Asia Resource Center, 1993; Rice, Pranee L. The Hmong Way: Hmong Women and Reproduction. Westport, CT: Bergin & Garvey, 2000.

[33] Cha, Dia, and Jacquelyn Chagnon. Farmer, War-wife, Refugee, Repatriate: A Needs Assessment of Women Repatriating to Laos. Washington, DC: Asia Resource Center, 1993; Cha, Dia, and Cathy A. Small. Policy Lessons from Lao and Hmong Women in Thai Refugee Camps. World Development, 22 (7) 1994: 1045–1059.

[34] Cha, Dia, and Jacquelyn Chagnon. Farmer, War-wife, Refugee, Repatriate: A Needs Assessment of Women Repatriating to Laos. Washington, DC: Asia Resource Center, 1993; Cha, Dia, and Cathy A. Small. Policy Lessons from Lao and Hmong Women in Thai Refugee Camps. World Development, 22 (7) 1994: 1045–1059.

[35] Cha, Dia, and Jacquelyn Chagnon. Farmer, War-wife, Refugee, Repatriate: A Needs Assessment of Women Repatriating to Laos. Washington, DC: Asia Resource Center, 1993; Cha, Dia, and Cathy A. Small. Policy Lessons from Lao and Hmong Women in Thai Refugee Camps. World Development, 22 (7) 1994: 1045–1059.

[36] Cha, Dia, and Jacquelyn Chagnon. Farmer, War-wife, Refugee, Repatriate: A Needs Assessment of Women Repatriating to Laos. Washington, DC: Asia Resource Center, 1993; Cha, Dia, and Cathy A. Small. Policy Lessons from Lao and Hmong Women in Thai Refugee Camps. World Development, 22 (7) 1994: 1045–1059.

[37] Cha, Dia, and Jacquelyn Chagnon. Farmer, War-wife, Refugee, Repatriate: A Needs Assessment of Women Repatriating to Laos. Washington, DC: Asia Resource Center, 1993; Cha, Dia, and Cathy A. Small. Policy Lessons from Lao and Hmong Women in Thai Refugee Camps. World Development, 22 (7) 1994: 1045–1059.

[38] Cha, Dia, and Jacquelyn Chagnon. Farmer, War-wife, Refugee, Repatriate: A Needs Assessment of Women Repatriating to Laos. Washington, DC: Asia Resource Center, 1993; Cha, Dia, and Cathy A. Small. Policy Lessons from Lao and Hmong Women in Thai Refugee Camps. World Development, 22 (7) 1994: 1045–1059.

[39] Cha, Dia, and Cathy A. Small. *Policy Lessons from Lao and Hmong Women in Thai Refugee Camps.* World Development, 22 (7) 1994: 1045–1059.

[40] Uba, Laura. *Asian Americans: Personality Patterns, Identity, and Mental Health.* New York: The Guilford Press, 1994; Westermeyer, Joseph. *Folk Medicine in Laos: A Comparison Between Two Ethnic Groups.* Social Science Medicine, 27 (8) 1988: 769–778; Westermeyer, Joseph, T. Lyfoung, K. Wahmanholm, and M. Westermeyer. *Delusions of Fatal Contagion Among Refugee Patients.* Psychosomatics, 30 (4) 1989(a): 374–382; Westermeyer, Joseph, J. Neider, and A. Callies. *Psychosocial Adjustment of Hmong Refugees during Their First Decade in the United States. A Longitudinal Study.* Journal of Nervous Mental Diseases, 177 (3) 1989(b): 132–9; Westermeyer, Joseph, T. F. Vang, and J. Neider. *Refugees Who Do and Do Not Seek Psychiatric Care. An Analysis of Premigratory and Postmigratory Characteristics.* Journal of Nervous Mental Diseases, 171 (2) 1983: 86–91.

[41] Uba, Laura. *Asian Americans: Personality Patterns, Identity, and Mental Health*. New York: The Guilford Press, 1994; Westermeyer, Joseph. *Folk Medicine in Laos: A Comparison Between Two Ethnic Groups*. Social Science Medicine, 27 (8) 1988: 769–778.

[42] Cooper, Robert, ed., *The Hmong*. Bangkok: Artasia Press Co. Ltd., 1991; Geddes, William Robert. *Migrants of the Mountains: The Cultural Ecology of the Blue Miao (Hmong Njua) of Thailand*. Oxford: Clarendon Press, 1976; Schein, Louisa. *Minority Rules: The Miao and The Feminine in China's Culture Politics*. Durham & London: Duke University Press, 2000; Tapp, Nicholas. *Sovereignty and Rebellion: The White Hmong of Northern Thailand*. Oxford: Oxford University Press, 1989; Uba, Laura. *Asian Americans: Personality Patterns, Identity, and Mental Health*. New York: The Guilford Press, 1994; Westermeyer, Joseph. *Folk Medicine in Laos: A Comparison Between Two Ethnic Groups*. Social Science Medicine, 27 (8) 1988: 769–778.

[43] Chan, Sucheng. *Hmong Means Free: Life in Laos and America*. Philadelphia: Temple University Press, 1994; Warner, Miriam E., and Marilyn Mochel. *The Hmong and Health Care in Merced, California*. Hmong Studies Journal, Spring, 1998, 2 (2); Uba, Laura. *Asian Americans: Personality Patterns, Identity, and Mental Health*. New York: The Guilford Press, 1994; Westermeyer, Joseph. *Hmong Drinking Practices in the United States: The Influence of Migration*. In *The American Experience with Alcohol: Contrasting Cultural Perspectives*. Linda A. Bennett and Genevieve M. Ames, eds. New York and London: Plenum Press, 1985.

[44] Ikeda, Noel R. *Who Are the Hmong?* A term paper submitted to the Hmong In America class, Department of Ethnic Studies. Boulder: University of Colorado, 1998. In the spring of 1998, Noel Ryuichi Ikeda, a student at the University of Colorado at Boulder, Colorado, conducted a telephone survey in the Denver/Boulder metropolitan area to determine what percentage of the American public knew of the existence of the Hmong. The results of this survey indicated that only ten percent of mainstream Americans had heard of or read about the Hmong. Ninety percent of the people surveyed either had no information about or had never heard of the Hmong. Ikeda's sample was fifty people; twenty-five from Denver, Colorado, and twenty-five from Boulder, Colorado.

[45] Warner, Miriam E., and Marilyn Mochel. *The Hmong and Health Care in Merced, California*. Hmong Studies Journal, Spring, 1998, 2 (2); Adler, Shelley R. *Refugee Stress and Folk Belief: Hmong Sudden Deaths*. Social Science Medicine, 40 (12) 1995: 1623–1629; Faderman, Lillian. *I Begin My Life All Over: The Hmong and the American Immigrant Experience*. Boston: Beacon Press, 1998; Bennett, Jane A., and Daniel F. Detzner. *Loneliness in Cultural Context, A Look at the Life History Narratives of Older Southeast Asian Refugee Women*. In *The Narrative Study of Lives*. A. Lieblich and R. Josselson, eds., 113–146. Thousand Oaks, CA: Sage, 1997; Westermeyer, Joseph. *A Matched Pairs Study of Depression Among Hmong Refugees with Particular Reference to Predisposing Factors and Treatment Outcome*. Social Psychiatry and Psychiatric Epidemiology, 23 (1) 1986: 64–67; Irby, Charles C., and Ernest M. Pon. *Confronting New Mountains: Mental Health Problems Among Male Hmong and Mien Refugees*. Amerasia Journal, 14 (1) 1988: 109–118; Chan, Sucheng. *Hmong Means Free: Life in Laos and America*. Philadelphia: Temple University Press, 1994; Fadiman, Anne. *The Spirit Catches*

You and You Fall Down: A Hmong Child, Her American Doctors, and the Collision of Two Cultures. New York: Farrar, Straus and Giroux, 1997; Quincy, Keith. Hmong: History of A People. Cheney, WA: Eastern Washington University Press, 1995; Kraub, Alan M. Healers and Strangers: Immigrant Attitudes Toward the Physician in America—A Relationship in Historical Perspective. Journal of the American Medical Association, 263 (13) 1990: 1807 – 1811; Uba, Laura. Asian Americans: Personality Patterns, Identity, and Mental Health. New York: The Guilford Press, 1994.

⁴⁶ Fadiman, Anne. The Spirit Catches You and You Fall Down: A Hmong Child, Her American Doctors, and the Collision of Two Cultures. New York: Farrar, Straus and Giroux, 1997.

⁴⁷ Uba, Laura. Asian Americans: Personality Patterns, Identity, and Mental Health. New York: The Guilford Press, 1994; Westermeyer, Joseph. Folk Medicine in Laos: A Comparison Between Two Ethnic Groups. Social Science Medicine, 27 (8) 1988: 769–778; Westermeyer, Joseph, T. F. Vang, and J. Neider. Refugees Who Do and Do Not Seek Psychiatric Care. An Analysis of Premigratory and Postmigratory Characteristics. Journal of Nervous Mental Diseases, 171 (2) 1983: 86–91; Westermeyer, Joseph, T. Lyfoung, K. Wahmanholm, and M. Westermeyer. Delusions of Fatal Contagion Among Refugee Patients. Psychosomatics, 30 (4) 1989(a): 374–382.

⁴⁸ Quincy, Keith. Hmong: History of A People. Cheney, WA: Eastern Washington University Press, 1995; Uba, Laura. Asian Americans: Personality Patterns, Identity, and Mental Health. New York: The Guilford Press, 1994; Warner, Miriam E., and Marilyn Mochel. The Hmong and Health Care in Merced, California. Hmong Studies Journal, Spring, 1998, 2 (2); Westermeyer, Joseph. Folk Medicine in Laos: A Comparison Between Two Ethnic Groups. Social Science Medicine, 27 (8) 1988: 769–778; Westermeyer, Joseph, T. Lyfoung, K. Wahmanholm, and M. Westermeyer. Delusions of Fatal Contagion Among Refugee Patients. Psychosomatics, 30 (4) 1989(a): 374–382;

Westermeyer, Joseph, J. Neider, and A. Callies. Psychosocial Adjustment of Hmong Refugees during Their First Decade in the United States. A Longitudinal Study. Journal of Nervous Mental Diseases, 177 (3) 1989(b): 132–9; Westermeyer, Joseph, T. F. Vang, and J. Neider. Refugees Who Do and Do Not Seek Psychiatric Care. An Analysis of Premigratory and Postmigratory Characteristics. Journal of Nervous Mental Diseases, 171 (2) 1983: 86–91.

⁴⁹ Westermeyer, Joseph, T. Lyfoung, K. Wahmanholm, and M. Westermeyer. Delusions of Fatal Contagion Among Refugee Patients. Psychosomatics, 30 (4) 1989(a): 374–382.

⁵⁰ Hirayama, Kasumi, and Hisashi Hirayama. Stress, Social Supports, and Adaptational Patterns in Hmong Refugee Families. Amerasia Journal, 14 (1) 1987: 93–108; Chan, Sucheng. Hmong Means Free: Life in Laos and America. Philadelphia: Temple University Press, 1994; Uba, Laura. Asian Americans: Personality Patterns, Identity, and Mental Health. New York: The Guilford Press, 1994; Waters, David A., Rama B. Rao, and Helen E. Petracchi. Providing Health Care for the Hmong. Wisconsin Medical Journal, 91 (11) 1992: 642–651; Westermeyer, Joseph, J. Neider, and A. Callies. Psychosocial Adjustment of Hmong Refugees during Their First Decade in the United States. A Longitudinal Study.

Journal of Nervous Mental Diseases, 177 (3) 1989(b): 132–9; Westermeyer, Joseph, T. F. Vang, and J. Neider. *Refugees Who Do and Do Not Seek Psychiatric Care. An Analysis of Premigratory and Postmigratory Characteristics.* Journal of Nervous Mental Diseases, 171 (2) 1983: 86–91; Tobin, J. J., and J. Friedman. *Spirits, Shamans, and Nightmare Death: Survivor Stress in a Hmong Refugee.* American Journal of Orthopsychiatry, 53 (3) 1983: 439–48.

    51 Uba, Laura. *Asian Americans: Personality Patterns, Identity, and Mental Health.* New York: The Guilford Press, 1994; Westermeyer, Joseph. *Folk Medicine in Laos: A Comparison Between Two Ethnic Groups.* Social Science Medicine, 27 (8) 1988: 769–778; Westermeyer, Joseph, T. Lyfoung, K. Wahmanholm, and M. Westermeyer. *Delusions of Fatal Contagion Among Refugee Patients.* Psychosomatics, 30 (4) 1989(a): 374–382; Westermeyer, Joseph, J. Neider, and A. Callies. *Psychosocial Adjustment of Hmong Refugees during Their First Decade in the United States. A Longitudinal Study.* Journal of Nervous Mental Diseases, 177 (3) 1989(b): 132–9; Westermeyer, Joseph, T. F. Vang, and J. Neider. *Refugees Who Do and Do Not Seek Psychiatric Care. An Analysis of Premigratory and Postmigratory Characteristics.* Journal of Nervous Mental Diseases, 171 (2) 1983: 86–91.

    52 Fadiman, Anne. The Spirit Catches You and You Fall Down: A Hmong Child, Her American Doctors, and the Collision of Two Cultures. New York: Farrar, Straus and Giroux, 1997; Irby, Charles C., and Ernest M. Pon. Confronting New Mountains: Mental Health Problems Among Male Hmong and Mien Refugees. Amerasia Journal, 14 (1) 1988: 109–118; Westermeyer, Joseph. Folk Medicine in Laos: A Comparison Between Two Ethnic Groups. Social Science Medicine, 27 (8) 1988: 769–778.

    53 Gong-Guy 1987 cited in Uba, Laura. *Asian Americans: Personality Patterns, Identity, and Mental Health.* New York: The Guilford Press, 1994.

    54 Westermeyer, Joseph, J. Neider, and A. Callies. *Psychosocial Adjustment of Hmong Refugees during Their First Decade in the United States. A Longitudinal Study.* Journal of Nervous Mental Diseases, 177 (3) 1989(b): 132–9.

    55 Waters, David A., Rama B. Rao, and Helen E. Petracchi. *Providing Health Care for the Hmong.* Wisconsin Medical Journal, 91 (11) 1992: 642–651.

    56 Mills, P. K., and R. Yang. *Cancer Incidence in the Hmong of Central California, United States, 1987–94.* Cancer Causes Control, 8 (5) 1997: 705–12.

    57 Mills, P. K., and R. Yang. *Cancer Incidence in the Hmong of Central California, United States, 1987–94.* Cancer Causes Control, 8 (5) 1997: 705–12.

    58 Yang, Pai, and Nora Murphy. *Hmong in the '90s: Stepping Towards the Future.* St. Paul: Hmong American Partnership, Inc., 1994.

    59 Wheeler, Sheba R. *Hmong Parents Strive to Connect: Cultural Rift Divide Adults from Children.* The Denver Post, Nov. 15, 1998, pp. B1, B5.

    60 Westermeyer, Joseph, T. F. Vang, and J. Neider. *Refugees Who Do and Do Not Seek Psychiatric Care. An Analysis of Premigratory and Postmigratory Characteristics.* Journal of Nervous Mental Diseases, 171 (2) 1983: 86–91.

    61 Fadiman, Anne. The Spirit Catches You and You Fall Down: A Hmong Child, Her American Doctors, and the Collision of Two Cultures. New York: Farrar, Straus and Giroux, 1997; Westermeyer, Joseph, J. Neider, and A. Callies. Psychosocial Adjustment of Hmong Refugees during Their First Decade in the

United States. A Longitudinal Study. Journal of Nervous Mental Diseases, 177 (3) 1989(b): 132–9.

[62] Moon and Tashima 1982, Gong-Guy 1987, cited in Uba, Laura. *Asian Americans: Personality Patterns, Identity, and Mental Health*. New York: The Guilford Press, 1994.

[63] Yang, Pai, and Nora Murphy. *Hmong in the '90s: Stepping Towards the Future*. St. Paul: Hmong American Partnership, Inc., 1994.

[64] Yang, Pai, and Nora Murphy. *Hmong in the '90s: Stepping Towards the Future*. St. Paul: Hmong American Partnership, Inc., 1994.

[65] Mills, P. K., and R. Yang. *Cancer Incidence in the Hmong of Central California, United States, 1987–94*. Cancer Causes Control, 8 (5) 1997: 705–12.

[66] Tobin, J. J., and J. Friedman. Spirits, Shamans, and Nightmare Death: Survivor Stress in a Hmong Refugee. American Journal of Orthopsychiatry, 53 (3) 1983: 439–48; Fadiman, Anne. The Spirit Catches You and You Fall Down: A Hmong Child, Her American Doctors, and the Collision of Two Cultures. New York: Farrar, Straus and Giroux, 1997; Uba, Laura. Asian Americans: Personality Patterns, Identity, and Mental Health. New York: The Guilford Press, 1994; Westermeyer, Joseph, T. F. Vang, and J. Neider. Refugees Who Do and Do Not Seek Psychiatric Care. An Analysis of Premigratory and Postmigratory Characteristics. Journal of Nervous Mental Diseases, 171 (2) 1983: 86–91; Westermeyer, Joseph, J. Neider, and A. Callies. Psychosocial Adjustment of Hmong Refugees during Their First Decade in the United States. A Longitudinal Study. Journal of Nervous Mental Diseases, 177 (3) 1989(b): 132–9; Westermeyer, Joseph. Folk Medicine in Laos: A Comparison Between Two Ethnic Groups. Social Science Medicine, 27 (8) 1988: 769–778.

[67] Barret, Bruce, et al. Hmong/Medicine Interactions: Improving Cross-cultural Health Care. Family Medicine Journal, 30 (3) 1998: 179–184; Fadiman, Anne. The Spirit Catches You and You Fall Down: A Hmong Child, Her American Doctors, and the Collision of Two Cultures. New York: Farrar, Straus and Giroux, 1997; Faderman, Lillian. I Begin My Life All Over: The Hmong and the American Immigrant Experience. Boston: Beacon Press, 1998; Waters, David A., Rama B. Rao, and Helen E. Petracchi. Providing Health Care for the Hmong. Wisconsin Medical Journal, 91 (11) 1992: 642–651.

[68] Fadiman, Anne. The Spirit Catches You and You Fall Down: A Hmong Child, Her American Doctors, and the Collision of Two Cultures. New York: Farrar, Straus and Giroux, 1997; Uba, Laura. Asian Americans: Personality Patterns, Identity, and Mental Health. New York: The Guilford Press, 1994.

[69] Gong-Guy, Elizabeth. *California Southeast Asian Mental Health Needs Assessment*. Oakland, CA: Asian Community Mental Health Services, 1987; Uba, Laura. *Asian Americans: Personality Patterns, Identity, and Mental Health*. New York: The Guilford Press, 1994; Westermeyer, Joseph, T. F. Vang, and J. Neider. *Refugees Who Do and Do Not Seek Psychiatric Care. An Analysis of Premigratory and Postmigratory Characteristics*. Journal of Nervous Mental Diseases, 171 (2) 1983: 86–91.

[70] Gong-Guy 1987 cited in Uba, Laura. *Asian Americans: Personality Patterns, Identity, and Mental Health*. New York: The Guilford Press, 1994.

[71] Gong-Guy, Elizabeth. *California Southeast Asian Mental Health Needs Assessment.* Oakland, CA: Asian Community Mental Health Services, 1987.

[72] Westermeyer, Joseph. *Folk Medicine in Laos: A Comparison Between Two Ethnic Groups.* Social Science Medicine, 27 (8) 1988: 769–778.

[73] Westermeyer, Joseph. *Folk Medicine in Laos: A Comparison Between Two Ethnic Groups.* Social Science Medicine, 27 (8) 1988: 769–778.

[74] Westermeyer, Joseph. *Folk Medicine in Laos: A Comparison Between Two Ethnic Groups.* Social Science Medicine, 27 (8) 1988: 769–778.

[75] Fadiman, Anne. The Spirit Catches You and You Fall Down: A Hmong Child, Her American Doctors, and the Collision of Two Cultures. New York: Farrar, Straus and Giroux, 1997; Uba, Laura. Asian Americans: Personality Patterns, Identity, and Mental Health. New York: The Guilford Press, 1994; Westermeyer, Joseph. Folk Medicine in Laos: A Comparison Between Two Ethnic Groups. Social Science Medicine, 27 (8) 1988: 769–778; Westermeyer, Joseph, T. F. Vang, and J. Neider. Refugees Who Do and Do Not Seek Psychiatric Care. An Analysis of Premigratory and Postmigratory Characteristics. Journal of Nervous Mental Diseases, 171 (2) 1983: 86–91; Westermeyer, Joseph, J. Neider, and A. Callies. Psychosocial Adjustment of Hmong Refugees during Their First Decade in the United States. A Longitudinal Study. Journal of Nervous Mental Diseases, 177 (3) 1989(b): 132–9; Tobin, J. J., and J. Friedman. Spirits, Shamans, and Nightmare Death: Survivor Stress in a Hmong Refugee. American Journal of Orthopsychiatry, 53 (3) 1983: 439–48.

[76] Westermeyer, Joseph. *Folk Medicine in Laos: A Comparison Between Two Ethnic Groups.* Social Science Medicine, 27 (8) 1988: 769–778; Uba, Laura. *Asian Americans: Personality Patterns, Identity, and Mental Health.* New York: The Guilford Press, 1994.

[77] Westermeyer, Joseph. *Folk Medicine in Laos: A Comparison Between Two Ethnic Groups.* Social Science Medicine, 27 (8) 1988: 769–778.

[78] Westermeyer, Joseph. *Folk Medicine in Laos: A Comparison Between Two Ethnic Groups.* Social Science Medicine, 27 (8) 1988: 769–778; Uba, Laura. *Asian Americans: Personality Patterns, Identity, and Mental Health.* New York: The Guilford Press, 1994.

NOTES TO CHAPTER II

[1] Lemoine, Jacques. *Shamanism in the Context of Hmong Resettlement.* In *The Hmong In Transition.* Hendricks, Glenn L. et al, eds. New York: Center for Migration Studies, 1986.

[2] Bliatout, Bruce Thowpaou. *Guidelines for Mental Health Professionals to Help Hmong Clients Seek Traditional Healing Treatment.* In *The Hmong In Transition.* Glenn L. Hendricks et al., eds., 349–363. New York: Center for Migration Studies, 1986.

[3] Cooper, Robert, ed., *The Hmong.* Bangkok: Artasia Press Co. Ltd., 1991.

[4] Chindarsi, Nusit. *The Religion of the Hmong Njua.* Bangkok: The Siam Society, 1976.

[5] Fadiman, Anne. The Spirit Catches You and You Fall Down: A Hmong Child, Her American Doctors, and the Collision of Two Cultures. New York: Farrar, Straus and Giroux, 1997.

[6] Rice, Pranee L., Blia Ly, and J. Lumley. Childbirth and Soul Loss: the Case of a Hmong Woman. Medical Journal of Australia, 160 (9) 1994: 577–8; Rice, Pranee L. The Hmong Way: Hmong Women and Reproduction. Westport, CT: Bergin & Garvey, 2000.

[7] Thao, Xoua. Southeast Asian Refugees of Rhode Island: The Hmong Perception of Illness. Rhode Island Medical Journal, 67 1984: 323–329; Thao, Xoua. Hmong Perception of Illness and Traditional Ways of Healing. In The Hmong In Transition. Glenn L. Hendricks et al., eds. pp. 365–378. New York: Center for Migration Studies, 1986.

[8] Adler, Shelley R. Sudden Unexpected Nocturnal Death Syndrome among Hmong Immigrants: Examining the Role of the "Nightmare." Journal of American Folklore, 104 1991: 54–70; Adler, Shelley R. Ethnomedical Pathogenesis and Hmong Immigrants' Sudden Nocturnal Deaths. Culture, Medicine, and Psychiatry, 18 (1) 1994: 23–59; Adler, Shelley R. Refugee Stress and Folk Belief: Hmong Sudden Deaths. Social Science Medicine, 40 (12) 1995: 1623–1629.

[9] Ensign, John. Traditional Healing in the Hmong Refugee Community of the California Central Valley. Ph.D. Dissertation. Fresno: California School of Professional Psychology, 1994.

[10] Long, Lynellyn D. Ban Vinai: The Refugee Camp. New York: Columbia University Press, 1993.

[11] O'Connor, Bonnie Blair. Healing Traditions: Alternative Medicine and the Health Professions. Philadelphia: University of Pennsylvania Press, 1995.

[12] Quincy, Keith. Hmong: History of A People. Cheney, WA: Eastern Washington University Press, 1995.

[13] Her, Koua. Hmong Medicine. In A Free People: Our Stories, Our Voices, Our Dreams. Minneapolis: The Hmong Youth Cultural Awareness Project, 1994.

[14] Henry, Rebecca Rose. Sweet Blood, Dry Liver: Diabetes and Hmong Embodiment in a Foreign Land. Ph.D. Dissertation. Chapel Hill: University of North Carolina, 1996.

[15] Spring, M. A. Ethnopharmacologic Analysis of Medicinal Plants used by Laotian Hmong Refugees in Minnesota. Journal of Ethnopharmacology, 26 1989: 65–91.

[16] Waters, David A., Rama B. Rao, and Helen E. Petracchi. Providing Health Care for the Hmong. Wisconsin Medical Journal, 91 (11) 1992: 642–651.

[17] Nuttall, P., and F. C. Flores. Hmong Healing Practices Used for Common Childhood Illnesses. Pediatric Nursing, 23 (3) 1997: 247–251.

[18] Barret, Bruce, et al. Hmong/Medicine Interactions: Improving Cross-cultural Health Care. Family Medicine Journal, 30 (3) 1998: 179–184.

[19] Warner, Miriam E., and Marilyn Mochel. The Hmong and Health Care in Merced, California. Hmong Studies Journal, Spring, 1998, 2 (2).

[20] Westermeyer, Joseph. Folk Medicine in Laos: A Comparison Between Two Ethnic Groups. Social Science Medicine, 27 (8) 1988: 769–778.

[21] Yang, Yeng. Practicing Modern Medicine: "A little medicine, a little neeb." Hmong Studies Journal, Spring, 1995, 2 (2).

[22] Bliatout, Bruce Thowpaou. *Guidelines for Mental Health Professionals to Help Hmong Clients Seek Traditional Healing Treatment.* In *The Hmong In Transition.* Glenn L. Hendricks et al., eds., 349–363. New York: Center for Migration Studies, 1986; Henry, Rebecca Rose. *Sweet Blood, Dry Liver: Diabetes and Hmong Embodiment in a Foreign Land.* Ph.D. Dissertation. Chapel Hill: University of North Carolina, 1996.

[23] Bliatout, Bruce Thowpaou. *Guidelines for Mental Health Professionals to Help Hmong Clients Seek Traditional Healing Treatment.* In *The Hmong In Transition.* Glenn L. Hendricks et al., eds., 349–363. New York: Center for Migration Studies, 1986.

[24] Chindarsi, Nusit. *The Religion of the Hmong Njua.* Bangkok: The Siam Society, 1976; Cooper, Robert, ed., *The Hmong.* Bangkok: Artasia Press Co. Ltd., 1991; Ensign, John. *Traditional Healing in the Hmong Refugee Community of the California Central Valley.* Ph.D. Dissertation. Fresno: California School of Professional Psychology, 1994; Rice, Pranee L., Blia Ly, and J. Lumley. *Childbirth and Soul Loss: the Case of a Hmong Woman.* Medical Journal of Australia, 160 (9) 1994: 577–8; Thao, Xoua. *Hmong Perception of Illness and Traditional Ways of Healing.* In *The Hmong In Transition.* Glenn L. Hendricks et al., eds. pp. 365–378. New York: Center for Migration Studies, 1986.

[25] Cooper, Robert, ed., *The Hmong.* Bangkok: Artasia Press Co. Ltd., 1991.

[26] Symonds, Patricia V. Cosmology and the Cycle of Life: Hmong View of Birth, Death, and Gender in a Mountain Village in Northern Thailand. Ph.D. Dissertation. Providence, Rhode Island: Brown University, 1991; Rice, Pranee L. The Hmong Way: Hmong Women and Reproduction. Westport, CT: Bergin & Garvey, 2000.

[27] Cooper, Robert, ed., *The Hmong.* Bangkok: Artasia Press Co. Ltd., 1991.

[28] Symonds, Patricia V. Cosmology and the Cycle of Life: Hmong View of Birth, Death, and Gender in a Mountain Village in Northern Thailand. Ph.D. Dissertation. Providence, Rhode Island: Brown University, 1991; Rice, Pranee L. The Hmong Way: Hmong Women and Reproduction. Westport, CT: Bergin & Garvey, 2000.

[29] Rice, Pranee L., Blia Ly, and J. Lumley. *Childbirth and Soul Loss: the Case of a Hmong Woman.* Medical Journal of Australia, 160 (9) 1994: 577–8; Rice, Pranee L. *The Hmong Way: Hmong Women and Reproduction.* Westport, CT: Bergin & Garvey, 2000.

[30] Rice, Pranee L. *The Hmong Way: Hmong Women and Reproduction.* Westport, CT: Bergin & Garvey, 2000.

[31] Cooper, Robert, ed., *The Hmong.* Bangkok: Artasia Press Co. Ltd., 1991: 54.

[32] Cooper, Robert, ed., *The Hmong.* Bangkok: Artasia Press Co. Ltd., 1991; Rice, Pranee L. *The Hmong Way: Hmong Women and Reproduction.* Westport, CT: Bergin & Garvey, 2000.

[33] Symonds, Patricia V. *Cosmology and the Cycle of Life: Hmong View of Birth, Death, and Gender in a Mountain Village in Northern Thailand.* Ph.D. Dissertation. Providence, Rhode Island: Brown University, 1991.

[34] Cooper, Robert, ed., *The Hmong.* Bangkok: Artasia Press Co. Ltd., 1991.

³⁵ Cooper, Robert, ed., *The Hmong*. Bangkok: Artasia Press Co. Ltd., 1991: 54.

³⁶ Cooper, Robert, ed., *The Hmong*. Bangkok: Artasia Press Co. Ltd., 1991; Rice, Pranee L. *The Hmong Way: Hmong Women and Reproduction*. Westport, CT: Bergin & Garvey, 2000.

³⁷ Cooper, Robert, ed., *The Hmong*. Bangkok: Artasia Press Co. Ltd., 1991: 54.

³⁸ Cooper, Robert, ed., *The Hmong*. Bangkok: Artasia Press Co. Ltd., 1991.

³⁹ Ovesen, Jan. A Minority Enters The Nation State: A Case Study of a Hmong Community in Vientiane Province, Laos. Sweden: Uppsala University, 1995.

⁴⁰ Cooper, Robert, ed., *The Hmong*. Bangkok: Artasia Press Co. Ltd., 1991.

⁴¹ Cooper, Robert, ed., *The Hmong*. Bangkok: Artasia Press Co. Ltd., 1991; Ovesen, Jan. *A Minority Enters The Nation State: A Case Study of a Hmong Community in Vientiane Province, Laos*. Sweden: Uppsala University, 1995.

⁴² Cooper, Robert, ed., *The Hmong*. Bangkok: Artasia Press Co. Ltd., 1991; Ovesen, Jan. *A Minority Enters The Nation State: A Case Study of a Hmong Community in Vientiane Province, Laos*. Sweden: Uppsala University, 1995.

⁴³ Cooper, Robert, ed., *The Hmong*. Bangkok: Artasia Press Co. Ltd., 1991; Ovesen, Jan. *A Minority Enters The Nation State: A Case Study of a Hmong Community in Vientiane Province, Laos*. Sweden: Uppsala University, 1995.

⁴⁴ Ovesen, Jan. A Minority Enters The Nation State: A Case Study of a Hmong Community in Vientiane Province, Laos. Sweden: Uppsala University, 1995.

⁴⁵ id.

⁴⁶ Bliatout, Bruce Thowpaou. *Guidelines for Mental Health Professionals to Help Hmong Clients Seek Traditional Healing Treatment*. In *The Hmong In Transition*. Glenn L. Hendricks et al., eds., 349–363. New York: Center for Migration Studies, 1986; Rice, Pranee L., Blia Ly, and J. Lumley. *Childbirth and Soul Loss: the Case of a Hmong Woman*. Medical Journal of Australia, 160 (9) 1994: 577–8.

⁴⁷ Chindarsi, Nusit. The Religion of the Hmong Njua. Bangkok: The Siam Society, 1976; Fadiman, Anne. The Spirit Catches You and You Fall Down: A Hmong Child, Her American Doctors, and the Collision of Two Cultures. New York: Farrar, Straus and Giroux, 1997; Westermeyer, Joseph. Folk Medicine in Laos: A Comparison Between Two Ethnic Groups. Social Science Medicine, 27 (8) 1988: 769–778; Quincy, Keith. Hmong: History of A People. Cheney, WA: Eastern Washington University Press, 1995.

⁴⁸ Bliatout, Bruce Thowpaou. *Guidelines for Mental Health Professionals to Help Hmong Clients Seek Traditional Healing Treatment*. In *The Hmong In Transition*. Glenn L. Hendricks et al., eds., 349–363. New York: Center for Migration Studies, 1986; Chindarsi, Nusit. *The Religion of the Hmong Njua*. Bangkok: The Siam Society, 1976; Cooper, Robert, ed., *The Hmong*. Bangkok: Artasia Press Co. Ltd., 1991; Ensign, John. *Traditional Healing in the Hmong Refugee Community of the California Central Valley*. Ph.D. Dissertation. Fresno: California School of Professional Psychology, 1994; Fadiman, Anne. *The Spirit Catches You and You Fall Down: A Hmong Child, Her American Doctors, and the Collision of Two Cultures*. New York: Farrar, Straus and Giroux, 1997; Nuttall, P., and F. C. Flores. *Hmong Healing Practices Used for Common Childhood Illnesses*.

Pediatric Nursing, 23 (3) 1997: 247–251; Quincy, Keith. *Hmong: History of A People*. Cheney, WA: Eastern Washington University Press, 1995; Rice, Pranee L. *The Hmong Way: Hmong Women and Reproduction*. Westport, CT: Bergin & Garvey, 2000; Thao, Xoua. *Hmong Perception of Illness and Traditional Ways of Healing*. In *The Hmong In Transition*. Glenn L. Hendricks et al., eds. pp. 365–378. New York: Center for Migration Studies, 1986; Rice, Pranee L., Blia Ly, and J. Lumley. *Childbirth and Soul Loss: the Case of a Hmong Woman*. Medical Journal of Australia, 160 (9) 1994: 577–8; Westermeyer, Joseph. *Folk Medicine in Laos: A Comparison Between Two Ethnic Groups*. Social Science Medicine, 27 (8) 1988: 769–778.

Yang, Dao. *The Hmong: Enduring Traditions*. In *Minority Cultures of Laos: Kammu, Lua', Lahu, Hmong, and Iu-Mien*. Judy Lewis, ed. Sacramento, CA: Southeast Asia Community Resource Center, 1991.

[49] Chindarsi, Nusit. *The Religion of the Hmong Njua*. Bangkok: The Siam Society, 1976; Cooper, Robert, ed., *The Hmong*. Bangkok: Artasia Press Co. Ltd., 1991; Fadiman, Anne. *The Spirit Catches You and You Fall Down: A Hmong Child, Her American Doctors, and the Collision of Two Cultures*. New York: Farrar, Straus and Giroux, 1997; Lemoine, Jacques. *Shamanism in the Context of Hmong Resettlement*. In *The Hmong In Transition*. Hendricks, Glenn L. et al, eds. New York: Center for Migration Studies, 1986; Nuttall, P., and F. C. Flores. *Hmong Healing Practices Used for Common Childhood Illnesses*. Pediatric Nursing, 23 (3) 1997: 247–251; O'Connor, Bonnie Blair. *Healing Traditions: Alternative Medicine and the Health Professions*. Philadelphia: University of Pennsylvania Press, 1995; Quincy, Keith. *Hmong: History of A People*. Cheney, WA: Eastern Washington University Press, 1995; Thao, Xoua. *Hmong Perception of Illness and Traditional Ways of Healing*. In *The Hmong In Transition*. Glenn L. Hendricks et al., eds. pp. 365–378. New York: Center for Migration Studies, 1986; Westermeyer, Joseph. *Folk Medicine in Laos: A Comparison Between Two Ethnic Groups*. Social Science Medicine, 27 (8) 1988: 769–778; Rice, Pranee L., Blia Ly, and J. Lumley. *Childbirth and Soul Loss: the Case of a Hmong Woman*. Medical Journal of Australia, 160 (9) 1994: 577–8.

[50] Bliatout, Bruce Thowpaou. *Guidelines for Mental Health Professionals to Help Hmong Clients Seek Traditional Healing Treatment*. In *The Hmong In Transition*. Glenn L. Hendricks et al., eds., 349–363. New York: Center for Migration Studies, 1986; Chindarsi, Nusit. *The Religion of the Hmong Njua*. Bangkok: The Siam Society, 1976; Cooper, Robert, ed., *The Hmong*. Bangkok: Artasia Press Co. Ltd., 1991; Westermeyer, Joseph. *Folk Medicine in Laos: A Comparison Between Two Ethnic Groups*. Social Science Medicine, 27 (8) 1988: 769–778; Nuttall, P., and F. C. Flores. *Hmong Healing Practices Used for Common Childhood Illnesses*. Pediatric Nursing, 23 (3) 1997: 247–251; Thao, Xoua. *Southeast Asian Refugees of Rhode Island: The Hmong Perception of Illness*. Rhode Island Medical Journal, 67 1984: 323–329.

[51] Chindarsi, Nusit. *The Religion of the Hmong Njua*. Bangkok: The Siam Society, 1976; Cooper, Robert, ed., *The Hmong*. Bangkok: Artasia Press Co. Ltd., 1991; Thao, Xoua. *Southeast Asian Refugees of Rhode Island: The Hmong Perception of Illness*. Rhode Island Medical Journal, 67 1984: 323–329; Thao, Xoua. *Hmong Perception of Illness and Traditional Ways of Healing*. In *The*

Hmong In Transition. Glenn L. Hendricks et al., eds. pp. 365–378. New York: Center for Migration Studies, 1986.

⁵² Bliatout, Bruce Thowpaou. *Guidelines for Mental Health Professionals to Help Hmong Clients Seek Traditional Healing Treatment.* In *The Hmong In Transition.* Glenn L. Hendricks et al., eds., 349–363. New York: Center for Migration Studies, 1986; Chindarsi, Nusit. *The Religion of the Hmong Njua.* Bangkok: The Siam Society, 1976; Cooper, Robert, ed., *The Hmong.* Bangkok: Artasia Press Co. Ltd., 1991; Ensign, John. *Traditional Healing in the Hmong Refugee Community of the California Central Valley.* Ph.D. Dissertation. Fresno: California School of Professional Psychology, 1994; Thao, Xoua. *Southeast Asian Refugees of Rhode Island: The Hmong Perception of Illness.* Rhode Island Medical Journal, 67 1984: 323–329.

⁵³ Chindarsi, Nusit. *The Religion of the Hmong Njua.* Bangkok: The Siam Society, 1976.

Cooper, Robert, ed., The Hmong. Bangkok: Artasia Press Co. Ltd., 1991; Ovesen, Jan. A Minority Enters The Nation State: A Case Study of a Hmong Community in Vientiane Province, Laos. Sweden: Uppsala University, 1995; Thao, Xoua. Hmong Perception of Illness and Traditional Ways of Healing. In The Hmong In Transition. Glenn L. Hendricks et al., eds. pp. 365–378. New York: Center for Migration Studies, 1986.

⁵⁴ Cooper, Robert, ed., *The Hmong.* Bangkok: Artasia Press Co. Ltd., 1991.

⁵⁵ Cooper, Robert, ed., *The Hmong.* Bangkok: Artasia Press Co. Ltd., 1991; Lemoine, Jacques. *Shamanism in the Context of Hmong Resettlement.* In *The Hmong In Transition.* Hendricks, Glenn L. et al, eds. New York: Center for Migration Studies, 1986; Rice, Pranee L. *The Hmong Way: Hmong Women and Reproduction.* Westport, CT: Bergin & Garvey, 2000; Symonds, Patricia V. *Cosmology and the Cycle of Life: Hmong View of Birth, Death, and Gender in a Mountain Village in Northern Thailand.* Ph.D. Dissertation. Providence, Rhode Island: Brown University, 1991.

⁵⁶ Chindarsi, Nusit. *The Religion of the Hmong Njua.* Bangkok: The Siam Society, 1976; Cooper, Robert, ed., *The Hmong.* Bangkok: Artasia Press Co. Ltd., 1991; Lemoine, Jacques. *Shamanism in the Context of Hmong Resettlement.* In *The Hmong In Transition.* Hendricks, Glenn L. et al, eds. New York: Center for Migration Studies, 1986; O'Connor, Bonnie Blair. *Healing Traditions: Alternative Medicine and the Health Professions.* Philadelphia: University of Pennsylvania Press, 1995; Thao, Xoua. *Hmong Perception of Illness and Traditional Ways of Healing.* In *The Hmong In Transition.* Glenn L. Hendricks et al., eds. pp. 365–378. New York: Center for Migration Studies, 1986; Waters, David A., Rama B. Rao, and Helen E. Petracchi. *Providing Health Care for the Hmong.* Wisconsin Medical Journal, 91 (11) 1992: 642–651.

⁵⁷ Lemoine, Jacques. *Shamanism in the Context of Hmong Resettlement.* In *The Hmong In Transition.* Hendricks, Glenn L. et al, eds. New York: Center for Migration Studies, 1986; Long, Lynellyn D. *Ban Vinai: The Refugee Camp.* New York: Columbia University Press, 1993; Thao, Xoua. *Hmong Perception of Illness and Traditional Ways of Healing.* In *The Hmong In Transition.* Glenn L. Hendricks et al., eds. pp. 365–378. New York: Center for Migration Studies, 1986.

⁵⁸ Lemoine, Jacques. *Shamanism in the Context of Hmong Resettlement.* In *The Hmong In Transition.* Hendricks, Glenn L. et al, eds. New York: Center for Migration Studies, 1986.

⁵⁹ Bliatout, Bruce Thowpaou. *Guidelines for Mental Health Professionals to Help Hmong Clients Seek Traditional Healing Treatment.* In *The Hmong In Transition.* Glenn L. Hendricks et al., eds., 349–363. New York: Center for Migration Studies, 1986; Chindarsi, Nusit. *The Religion of the Hmong Njua.* Bangkok: The Siam Society, 1976; Cooper, Robert, ed., *The Hmong.* Bangkok: Artasia Press Co. Ltd., 1991; Lemoine, Jacques. *Shamanism in the Context of Hmong Resettlement.* In *The Hmong In Transition.* Hendricks, Glenn L. et al, eds. New York: Center for Migration Studies, 1986; Long, Lynellyn D. *Ban Vinai: The Refugee Camp.* New York: Columbia University Press, 1993; O'Connor, Bonnie Blair. *Healing Traditions: Alternative Medicine and the Health Professions.* Philadelphia: University of Pennsylvania Press, 1995; Quincy, Keith. *Hmong: History of A People.* Cheney, WA: Eastern Washington University Press, 1995; Thao, Xoua. *Hmong Perception of Illness and Traditional Ways of Healing.* In *The Hmong In Transition.* Glenn L. Hendricks et al., eds. pp. 365–378. New York: Center for Migration Studies, 1986; Westermeyer, Joseph. *Folk Medicine in Laos: A Comparison Between Two Ethnic Groups.* Social Science Medicine, 27 (8) 1988: 769–778; Yang, Dao. *The Hmong: Enduring Traditions.* In *Minority Cultures of Laos: Kammu, Lua', Lahu, Hmong, and Iu-Mien.* Judy Lewis, ed. Sacramento, CA: Southeast Asia Community Resource Center, 1991.

⁶⁰ Long, Lynellyn D. *Ban Vinai: The Refugee Camp.* New York: Columbia University Press, 1993.

⁶¹ Fadiman, Anne. The Spirit Catches You and You Fall Down: A Hmong Child, Her American Doctors, and the Collision of Two Cultures. New York: Farrar, Straus and Giroux, 1997.

⁶² Chindarsi, Nusit. *The Religion of the Hmong Njua.* Bangkok: The Siam Society, 1976; Cooper, Robert, ed., *The Hmong.* Bangkok: Artasia Press Co. Ltd., 1991; Lemoine, Jacques. *Shamanism in the Context of Hmong Resettlement.* In *The Hmong In Transition.* Hendricks, Glenn L. et al, eds. New York: Center for Migration Studies, 1986; Long, Lynellyn D. *Ban Vinai: The Refugee Camp.* New York: Columbia University Press, 1993; O'Connor, Bonnie Blair. *Healing Traditions: Alternative Medicine and the Health Professions.* Philadelphia: University of Pennsylvania Press, 1995; Quincy, Keith. *Hmong: History of A People.* Cheney, WA: Eastern Washington University Press, 1995; Thao, Xoua. *Hmong Perception of Illness and Traditional Ways of Healing.* In *The Hmong In Transition.* Glenn L. Hendricks et al., eds. pp. 365–378. New York: Center for Migration Studies, 1986.

⁶³ Long, Lynellyn D. *Ban Vinai: The Refugee Camp.* New York: Columbia University Press, 1993.

⁶⁴ Lemoine, Jacques. *Shamanism in the Context of Hmong Resettlement.* In *The Hmong In Transition.* Hendricks, Glenn L. et al, eds. New York: Center for Migration Studies, 1986; Cheon-Klessig, Y., D. D. Camilleri, B. J. McElmurry, and V. M. Ohlson. *Folk Medicine in the Health Practice of Hmong Refugees.* Western Journal of Nursing Research, 10 (5) 1988: 647–60; Nuttall, P., and F. C. Flores.

Hmong Healing Practices Used for Common Childhood Illnesses. Pediatric Nursing, 23 (3) 1997: 247–251.

[65] Lemoine, Jacques. *Shamanism in the Context of Hmong Resettlement.* In *The Hmong In Transition.* Hendricks, Glenn L. et al, eds. New York: Center for Migration Studies, 1986; Long, Lynellyn D. *Ban Vinai: The Refugee Camp.* New York: Columbia University Press, 1993: 127–128.

[66] Irby, Charles C., and Ernest M. Pon. *Confronting New Mountains: Mental Health Problems Among Male Hmong and Mien Refugees.* Amerasia Journal, 14 (1) 1988: 109–118; Westermeyer, Joseph. *A Matched Pairs Study of Depression Among Hmong Refugees with Particular Reference to Predisposing Factors and Treatment Outcome.* Social Psychiatry and Psychiatric Epidemiology, 23 (1) 1986: 64–67.

Cooper, Robert, ed., *The Hmong.* Bangkok: Artasia Press Co. Ltd., 1991; Lemoine, Jacques. *Shamanism in the Context of Hmong Resettlement.* In *The Hmong In Transition.* Hendricks, Glenn L. et al, eds. New York: Center for Migration Studies, 1986; Long, Lynellyn D. *Ban Vinai: The Refugee Camp.* New York: Columbia University Press, 1993.

[67] Cooper, Robert, ed., *The Hmong.* Bangkok: Artasia Press Co. Ltd., 1991; Cheon-Klessig, Y., D. D. Camilleri, B. J. McElmurry, and V. M. Ohlson. *Folk Medicine in the Health Practice of Hmong Refugees.* Western Journal of Nursing Research, 10 (5) 1988: 647–60; Fadiman, Anne. *The Spirit Catches You and You Fall Down: A Hmong Child, Her American Doctors, and the Collision of Two Cultures.* New York: Farrar, Straus and Giroux, 1997.

[68] Lemoine, Jacques. *Shamanism in the Context of Hmong Resettlement.* In *The Hmong In Transition.* Hendricks, Glenn L. et al, eds. New York: Center for Migration Studies, 1986; Adler, Shelley R. *Refugee Stress and Folk Belief: Hmong Sudden Deaths.* Social Science Medicine, 40 (12) 1995: 1623–1629; Tapp, Nicholas. *Sovereignty and Rebellion: The White Hmong of Northern Thailand.* Oxford: Oxford University Press, 1989; Westermeyer, Joseph. *Folk Medicine in Laos: A Comparison Between Two Ethnic Groups.* Social Science Medicine, 27 (8) 1988: 769–778.

[69] Chindarsi, Nusit. *The Religion of the Hmong Njua.* Bangkok: The Siam Society, 1976.

Cooper, Robert, ed., *The Hmong.* Bangkok: Artasia Press Co. Ltd., 1991; Lemoine, Jacques. *Shamanism in the Context of Hmong Resettlement.* In *The Hmong In Transition.* Hendricks, Glenn L. et al, eds. New York: Center for Migration Studies, 1986; Thao, Xoua. *Hmong Perception of Illness and Traditional Ways of Healing.* In *The Hmong In Transition.* Glenn L. Hendricks et al., eds. pp. 365–378. New York: Center for Migration Studies, 1986; Thao, Xoua. *Southeast Asian Refugees of Rhode Island: The Hmong Perception of Illness.* Rhode Island Medical Journal, 67 1984: 323–329; Westermeyer, Joseph. *Folk Medicine in Laos: A Comparison Between Two Ethnic Groups.* Social Science Medicine, 27 (8) 1988: 769–778.

[70] Chindarsi, Nusit. *The Religion of the Hmong Njua.* Bangkok: The Siam Society, 1976; Cooper, Robert, ed., *The Hmong.* Bangkok: Artasia Press Co. Ltd., 1991; Lemoine, Jacques. *Shamanism in the Context of Hmong Resettlement.* In *The Hmong In Transition.* Hendricks, Glenn L. et al, eds. New York: Center for

Migration Studies, 1986; Thao, Xoua. *Southeast Asian Refugees of Rhode Island: The Hmong Perception of Illness.* Rhode Island Medical Journal, 67 1984: 323–329; Westermeyer, Joseph. *Folk Medicine in Laos: A Comparison Between Two Ethnic Groups.* Social Science Medicine, 27 (8) 1988: 769–778. The distinction between shaman and ritualist may seem finucane, but it is significant. Hmong become shamans because they are called upon by the spirit helpers of the shaman's realm, and, generally speaking, they do not have any choice in the matter. Hmong become ritualists, on the other hand, because, 1) they are interested in the profession; 2) they have a desire to help others; and, 3) they wish to maintain their cultural traditions. For the most part, they must inherit the associated practices.

[71] Lemoine, Jacques. *Shamanism in the Context of Hmong Resettlement.* In *The Hmong In Transition.* Hendricks, Glenn L. et al, eds. New York: Center for Migration Studies, 1986: 339–340.

[72] Bliatout, Bruce Thowpaou. *Guidelines for Mental Health Professionals to Help Hmong Clients Seek Traditional Healing Treatment.* In *The Hmong In Transition.* Glenn L. Hendricks et al., eds., 349–363. New York: Center for Migration Studies, 1986; Chindarsi, Nusit. *The Religion of the Hmong Njua.* Bangkok: The Siam Society, 1976; Cooper, Robert, ed., *The Hmong.* Bangkok: Artasia Press Co. Ltd., 1991; Lemoine, Jacques. *Shamanism in the Context of Hmong Resettlement.* In *The Hmong In Transition.* Hendricks, Glenn L. et al, eds. New York: Center for Migration Studies, 1986; Long, Lynellyn D. *Ban Vinai: The Refugee Camp.* New York: Columbia University Press, 1993; Ovesen, Jan. *A Minority Enters The Nation State: A Case Study of a Hmong Community in Vientiane Province, Laos.* Sweden: Uppsala University, 1995; Thao, Xoua. *Southeast Asian Refugees of Rhode Island: The Hmong Perception of Illness.* Rhode Island Medical Journal, 67 1984: 323–329.

[73] Cooper, Robert, ed., *The Hmong.* Bangkok: Artasia Press Co. Ltd., 1991; Lemoine, Jacques. *Shamanism in the Context of Hmong Resettlement.* In *The Hmong In Transition.* Hendricks, Glenn L. et al, eds. New York: Center for Migration Studies, 1986; Long, Lynellyn D. *Ban Vinai: The Refugee Camp.* New York: Columbia University Press, 1993; O'Connor, Bonnie Blair. *Healing Traditions: Alternative Medicine and the Health Professions.* Philadelphia: University of Pennsylvania Press, 1995; Thao, Xoua. *Southeast Asian Refugees of Rhode Island: The Hmong Perception of Illness.* Rhode Island Medical Journal, 67 1984: 323–329; Yang, Dao. *The Hmong: Enduring Traditions.* In *Minority Cultures of Laos: Kammu, Lua', Lahu, Hmong, and Iu-Mien.* Judy Lewis, ed. Sacramento, CA: Southeast Asia Community Resource Center, 1991.

[74] Lemoine, Jacques. *Shamanism in the Context of Hmong Resettlement.* In *The Hmong In Transition.* Hendricks, Glenn L. et al, eds. New York: Center for Migration Studies, 1986: 340.

[75] Chindarsi, Nusit. *The Religion of the Hmong Njua.* Bangkok: The Siam Society, 1976.

Cooper, Robert, ed., *The Hmong.* Bangkok: Artasia Press Co. Ltd., 1991; Lemoine, Jacques. *Shamanism in the Context of Hmong Resettlement.* In *The Hmong In Transition.* Hendricks, Glenn L. et al, eds. New York: Center for Migration Studies, 1986; Long, Lynellyn D. *Ban Vinai: The Refugee Camp.* New York: Columbia University Press, 1993; Thao, Xoua. *Southeast Asian Refugees of*

Rhode Island: The Hmong Perception of Illness. Rhode Island Medical Journal, 67 1984: 323–329.

⁷⁶ Chindarsi, Nusit. *The Religion of the Hmong Njua*. Bangkok: The Siam Society, 1976; Cooper, Robert, ed., *The Hmong*. Bangkok: Artasia Press Co. Ltd., 1991; Lemoine, Jacques. *Shamanism in the Context of Hmong Resettlement*. In *The Hmong In Transition*. Hendricks, Glenn L. et al, eds. New York: Center for Migration Studies, 1986; Long, Lynellyn D. *Ban Vinai: The Refugee Camp*. New York: Columbia University Press, 1993; O'Connor, Bonnie Blair. *Healing Traditions: Alternative Medicine and the Health Professions*. Philadelphia: University of Pennsylvania Press, 1995; Thao, Xoua. *Southeast Asian Refugees of Rhode Island: The Hmong Perception of Illness*. Rhode Island Medical Journal, 67 1984: 323–329.

⁷⁷ Lemoine, Jacques. *Shamanism in the Context of Hmong Resettlement*. In *The Hmong In Transition*. Hendricks, Glenn L. et al, eds. New York: Center for Migration Studies, 1986.

⁷⁸ Lemoine, Jacques. *Shamanism in the Context of Hmong Resettlement*. In *The Hmong In Transition*. Hendricks, Glenn L. et al, eds. New York: Center for Migration Studies, 1986: 341.

⁷⁹ Chindarsi, Nusit. *The Religion of the Hmong Njua*. Bangkok: The Siam Society, 1976.

Cooper, Robert, ed., *The Hmong*. Bangkok: Artasia Press Co. Ltd., 1991; Lemoine, Jacques. *Shamanism in the Context of Hmong Resettlement*. In *The Hmong In Transition*. Hendricks, Glenn L. et al, eds. New York: Center for Migration Studies, 1986.

⁸⁰ Chindarsi, Nusit. *The Religion of the Hmong Njua*. Bangkok: The Siam Society, 1976.

Cooper, Robert, ed., *The Hmong*. Bangkok: Artasia Press Co. Ltd., 1991; Lemoine, Jacques. *Shamanism in the Context of Hmong Resettlement*. In *The Hmong In Transition*. Hendricks, Glenn L. et al, eds. New York: Center for Migration Studies, 1986; Thao, Xoua. *Southeast Asian Refugees of Rhode Island: The Hmong Perception of Illness*. Rhode Island Medical Journal, 67 1984: 323–329.

⁸¹ Lemoine, Jacques. *Shamanism in the Context of Hmong Resettlement*. In *The Hmong In Transition*. Hendricks, Glenn L. et al, eds. New York: Center for Migration Studies, 1986.

⁸² Chindarsi, Nusit. *The Religion of the Hmong Njua*. Bangkok: The Siam Society, 1976; Cooper, Robert, ed., *The Hmong*. Bangkok: Artasia Press Co. Ltd., 1991; Lemoine, Jacques. *Shamanism in the Context of Hmong Resettlement*. In *The Hmong In Transition*. Hendricks, Glenn L. et al, eds. New York: Center for Migration Studies, 1986; Long, Lynellyn D. *Ban Vinai: The Refugee Camp*. New York: Columbia University Press, 1993; Thao, Xoua. *Southeast Asian Refugees of Rhode Island: The Hmong Perception of Illness*. Rhode Island Medical Journal, 67 1984: 323–329.

⁸³ Cooper, Robert, ed., *The Hmong*. Bangkok: Artasia Press Co. Ltd., 1991; Lemoine, Jacques. *Shamanism in the Context of Hmong Resettlement*. In *The Hmong In Transition*. Hendricks, Glenn L. et al, eds. New York: Center for Migration Studies, 1986; Thao, Xoua. *Southeast Asian Refugees of Rhode Island:*

The Hmong Perception of Illness. Rhode Island Medical Journal, 67 1984: 323–329; Westermeyer, Joseph. *Folk Medicine in Laos: A Comparison Between Two Ethnic Groups*. Social Science Medicine, 27 (8) 1988: 769–778.

[84] Lemoine, Jacques. *Shamanism in the Context of Hmong Resettlement*. In *The Hmong In Transition*. Hendricks, Glenn L. et al, eds. New York: Center for Migration Studies, 1986: 342.

[85] Bliatout, Bruce Thowpaou. *Guidelines for Mental Health Professionals to Help Hmong Clients Seek Traditional Healing Treatment*. In *The Hmong In Transition*. Glenn L. Hendricks et al., eds., 349–363. New York: Center for Migration Studies, 1986; Cooper, Robert, ed., *The Hmong*. Bangkok: Artasia Press Co. Ltd., 1991; Thao, Xoua. *Hmong Perception of Illness and Traditional Ways of Healing*. In *The Hmong In Transition*. Glenn L. Hendricks et al., eds. pp. 365–378. New York: Center for Migration Studies, 1986.

[86] Lemoine, Jacques. *Shamanism in the Context of Hmong Resettlement*. In *The Hmong In Transition*. Hendricks, Glenn L. et al, eds. New York: Center for Migration Studies, 1986; Chindarsi, Nusit. *The Religion of the Hmong Njua*. Bangkok: The Siam Society, 1976; Cooper, Robert, ed., *The Hmong*. Bangkok: Artasia Press Co. Ltd., 1991; Bliatout, Bruce Thowpaou. *Guidelines for Mental Health Professionals to Help Hmong Clients Seek Traditional Healing Treatment*. In *The Hmong In Transition*. Glenn L. Hendricks et al., eds., 349–363. New York: Center for Migration Studies, 1986; Thao, Xoua. *Southeast Asian Refugees of Rhode Island: The Hmong Perception of Illness*. Rhode Island Medical Journal, 67 1984: 323–329.

[87] Cooper, Robert, ed., *The Hmong*. Bangkok: Artasia Press Co. Ltd., 1991; Lemoine, Jacques. *Shamanism in the Context of Hmong Resettlement*. In *The Hmong In Transition*. Hendricks, Glenn L. et al, eds. New York: Center for Migration Studies, 1986; Thao, Xoua. *Southeast Asian Refugees of Rhode Island: The Hmong Perception of Illness*. Rhode Island Medical Journal, 67 1984: 323–329.

[88] Thao, Xoua. *Hmong Perception of Illness and Traditional Ways of Healing*. In *The Hmong In Transition*. Glenn L. Hendricks et al., eds. pp. 365–378. New York: Center for Migration Studies, 1986.

[89] Cooper, Robert, ed., *The Hmong*. Bangkok: Artasia Press Co. Ltd., 1991; Lemoine, Jacques. *Shamanism in the Context of Hmong Resettlement*. In *The Hmong In Transition*. Hendricks, Glenn L. et al, eds. New York: Center for Migration Studies, 1986; Thao, Xoua. *Hmong Perception of Illness and Traditional Ways of Healing*. In *The Hmong In Transition*. Glenn L. Hendricks et al., eds. pp. 365–378. New York: Center for Migration Studies, 1986; Rice, Pranee L. *The Hmong Way: Hmong Women and Reproduction*. Westport, CT: Bergin & Garvey, 2000.

[90] Cooper, Robert, ed., *The Hmong*. Bangkok: Artasia Press Co. Ltd., 1991; Lemoine, Jacques. *Shamanism in the Context of Hmong Resettlement*. In *The Hmong In Transition*. Hendricks, Glenn L. et al, eds. New York: Center for Migration Studies, 1986; Long, Lynellyn D. *Ban Vinai: The Refugee Camp*. New York: Columbia University Press, 1993; Quincy, Keith. *Hmong: History of A People*. Cheney, WA: Eastern Washington University Press, 1995; Thao, Xoua. *Southeast Asian Refugees of Rhode Island: The Hmong Perception of Illness*.

Rhode Island Medical Journal, 67 1984: 323–329; Westermeyer, Joseph. *Folk Medicine in Laos: A Comparison Between Two Ethnic Groups.* Social Science Medicine, 27 (8) 1988: 769–778; Yang, Dao. *The Hmong: Enduring Traditions.* In *Minority Cultures of Laos: Kammu, Lua', Lahu, Hmong, and Iu-Mien.* Judy Lewis, ed. Sacramento, CA: Southeast Asia Community Resource Center, 1991.

    [91] Cooper, Robert, ed., *The Hmong.* Bangkok: Artasia Press Co. Ltd., 1991; Ensign, John. *Traditional Healing in the Hmong Refugee Community of the California Central Valley.* Ph.D. Dissertation. Fresno: California School of Professional Psychology, 1994; Lemoine, Jacques. *Shamanism in the Context of Hmong Resettlement.* In *The Hmong In Transition.* Hendricks, Glenn L. et al, eds. New York: Center for Migration Studies, 1986; Thao, Xoua. *Southeast Asian Refugees of Rhode Island: The Hmong Perception of Illness.* Rhode Island Medical Journal, 67 1984: 323–329.

    [92] O'Connor, Bonnie Blair. Healing Traditions: Alternative Medicine and the Health Professions. Philadelphia: University of Pennsylvania Press, 1995; Lemoine, Jacques. Shamanism in the Context of Hmong Resettlement. In The Hmong In Transition. Hendricks, Glenn L. et al, eds. New York: Center for Migration Studies, 1986; Thao, Xoua. Southeast Asian Refugees of Rhode Island: The Hmong Perception of Illness. Rhode Island Medical Journal, 67 1984: 323–329.

    [93] Lemoine, Jacques. *Shamanism in the Context of Hmong Resettlement.* In *The Hmong In Transition.* Hendricks, Glenn L. et al, eds. New York: Center for Migration Studies, 1986: 344.

    [94] Lemoine, Jacques. Shamanism in the Context of Hmong Resettlement. In The Hmong In Transition. Hendricks, Glenn L. et al, eds. New York: Center for Migration Studies, 1986; Thao, Xoua. Southeast Asian Refugees of Rhode Island: The Hmong Perception of Illness. Rhode Island Medical Journal, 67 1984: 323–329.

    [95] Chindarsi, Nusit. *The Religion of the Hmong Njua.* Bangkok: The Siam Society, 1976; Cooper, Robert, ed., *The Hmong.* Bangkok: Artasia Press Co. Ltd., 1991; Lemoine, Jacques. *Shamanism in the Context of Hmong Resettlement.* In *The Hmong In Transition.* Hendricks, Glenn L. et al, eds. New York: Center for Migration Studies, 1986; Rice, Pranee L. *The Hmong Way: Hmong Women and Reproduction.* Westport, CT: Bergin & Garvey, 2000.

    [96] Chindarsi, Nusit. *The Religion of the Hmong Njua.* Bangkok: The Siam Society, 1976; Cooper, Robert, ed., *The Hmong.* Bangkok: Artasia Press Co. Ltd., 1991; Lemoine, Jacques. *Shamanism in the Context of Hmong Resettlement.* In *The Hmong In Transition.* Hendricks, Glenn L. et al, eds. New York: Center for Migration Studies, 1986; Bliatout, Bruce Thowpaou. *Guidelines for Mental Health Professionals to Help Hmong Clients Seek Traditional Healing Treatment.* In *The Hmong In Transition.* Glenn L. Hendricks et al., eds., 349–363. New York: Center for Migration Studies, 1986; Thao, Xoua. *Hmong Perception of Illness and Traditional Ways of Healing.* In *The Hmong In Transition.* Glenn L. Hendricks et al., eds. pp. 365–378. New York: Center for Migration Studies, 1986.

    [97] Chindarsi, Nusit. *The Religion of the Hmong Njua.* Bangkok: The Siam Society, 1976.

    Cooper, Robert, ed., *The Hmong.* Bangkok: Artasia Press Co. Ltd., 1991; Lemoine, Jacques. *Shamanism in the Context of Hmong Resettlement.* In *The*

Hmong In Transition. Hendricks, Glenn L. et al, eds. New York: Center for Migration Studies, 1986.

[98] Lemoine, Jacques. *Shamanism in the Context of Hmong Resettlement*. In *The Hmong In Transition*. Hendricks, Glenn L. et al, eds. New York: Center for Migration Studies, 1986.

[99] Thao, Xoua. *Southeast Asian Refugees of Rhode Island: The Hmong Perception of Illness*. Rhode Island Medical Journal, 67 1984: 323–329.

[100] Cooper, Robert, ed., *The Hmong*. Bangkok: Artasia Press Co. Ltd., 1991; Lemoine, Jacques. *Shamanism in the Context of Hmong Resettlement*. In *The Hmong In Transition*. Hendricks, Glenn L. et al, eds. New York: Center for Migration Studies, 1986.

[101] Her, Koua. Hmong Medicine. In A Free People: Our Stories, Our Voices, Our Dreams. Minneapolis: The Hmong Youth Cultural Awareness Project, 1994; Thao, Xoua. Southeast Asian Refugees of Rhode Island: The Hmong Perception of Illness. Rhode Island Medical Journal, 67 1984: 323–329.

[102] Bliatout, Bruce Thowpaou. *Guidelines for Mental Health Professionals to Help Hmong Clients Seek Traditional Healing Treatment*. In *The Hmong In Transition*. Glenn L. Hendricks et al., eds., 349–363. New York: Center for Migration Studies, 1986; Chindarsi, Nusit. *The Religion of the Hmong Njua*. Bangkok: The Siam Society, 1976; Cooper, Robert, ed., *The Hmong*. Bangkok: Artasia Press Co. Ltd., 1991; Fadiman, Anne. *The Spirit Catches You and You Fall Down: A Hmong Child, Her American Doctors, and the Collision of Two Cultures*. New York: Farrar, Straus and Giroux, 1997; Lemoine, Jacques. *Shamanism in the Context of Hmong Resettlement*. In *The Hmong In Transition*. Hendricks, Glenn L. et al, eds. New York: Center for Migration Studies, 1986; O'Connor, Bonnie Blair. *Healing Traditions: Alternative Medicine and the Health Professions*. Philadelphia: University of Pennsylvania Press, 1995; Thao, Xoua. *Hmong Perception of Illness and Traditional Ways of Healing*. In *The Hmong In Transition*. Glenn L. Hendricks et al., eds. pp. 365–378. New York: Center for Migration Studies, 1986.

[103] Cooper, Robert, ed., *The Hmong*. Bangkok: Artasia Press Co. Ltd., 1991; Thao, Xoua. *Hmong Perception of Illness and Traditional Ways of Healing*. In *The Hmong In Transition*. Glenn L. Hendricks et al., eds. pp. 365–378. New York: Center for Migration Studies, 1986.

[104] Thao, Xoua. Southeast Asian Refugees of Rhode Island: The Hmong Perception of Illness. Rhode Island Medical Journal, 67 1984: 323–329.

[105] Cooper, Robert, ed., *The Hmong*. Bangkok: Artasia Press Co. Ltd., 1991; Thao, Xoua. *Hmong Perception of Illness and Traditional Ways of Healing*. In *The Hmong In Transition*. Glenn L. Hendricks et al., eds. pp. 365–378. New York: Center for Migration Studies, 1986; Thao, Xoua. *Southeast Asian Refugees of Rhode Island: The Hmong Perception of Illness*. Rhode Island Medical Journal, 67 1984: 323–329.

[106] Fackelmann, Kathy A. *Food, Drug, or Poison?* (Toxic Plants Used by Tribal Cultures as Food or Medicine). Science News, 143 (20) 1993: 312–314; Thao, Xoua. *Southeast Asian Refugees of Rhode Island: The Hmong Perception of Illness*. Rhode Island Medical Journal, 67 1984: 323–329; Warner, Miriam E., and

Marilyn Mochel. *The Hmong and Health Care in Merced, California*. Hmong Studies Journal, Spring, 1998, 2 (2).

[107] Fackelmann, Kathy A. *Food, Drug, or Poison?* (Toxic Plants Used by Tribal Cultures as Food or Medicine). Science News, 143 (20) 1993: 312–314.

[108] Spring, M. A. Ethnopharmacologic Analysis of Medicinal Plants used by Laotian Hmong Refugees in Minnesota. Journal of Ethnopharmacology, 26 1989: 65–91.

[109] id.

[110] Bliatout, Bruce Thowpaou. *Guidelines for Mental Health Professionals to Help Hmong Clients Seek Traditional Healing Treatment*. In *The Hmong In Transition*. Glenn L. Hendricks et al., eds., 349–363. New York: Center for Migration Studies, 1986; Chindarsi, Nusit. *The Religion of the Hmong Njua*. Bangkok: The Siam Society, 1976; Cooper, Robert, ed., *The Hmong*. Bangkok: Artasia Press Co. Ltd., 1991; Thao, Xoua. *Southeast Asian Refugees of Rhode Island: The Hmong Perception of Illness*. Rhode Island Medical Journal, 67 1984: 323–329.

[111] Buchwald, D., Thomas M. Hooton, and Sanjiv Panwala. *Use of Traditional Health Practices by Southeast Asian Refugees in a Primary Care Clinic*. The Western Journal of Medicine, 156 (5) 1992: 507–511; Fadiman, Anne. *The Spirit Catches You and You Fall Down: A Hmong Child, Her American Doctors, and the Collision of Two Cultures*. New York: Farrar, Straus and Giroux, 1997; Waters, David A., Rama B. Rao, and Helen E. Petracchi. *Providing Health Care for the Hmong*. Wisconsin Medical Journal, 91 (11) 1992: 642–651.

[112] Waters, David A., Rama B. Rao, and Helen E. Petracchi. *Providing Health Care for the Hmong*. Wisconsin Medical Journal, 91 (11) 1992: 642–651.

[113] Bliatout, Bruce Thowpaou. *Guidelines for Mental Health Professionals to Help Hmong Clients Seek Traditional Healing Treatment*. In *The Hmong In Transition*. Glenn L. Hendricks et al., eds., 349–363. New York: Center for Migration Studies, 1986; Cooper, Robert, ed., *The Hmong*. Bangkok: Artasia Press Co. Ltd., 1991; Fadiman, Anne. *The Spirit Catches You and You Fall Down: A Hmong Child, Her American Doctors, and the Collision of Two Cultures*. New York: Farrar, Straus and Giroux, 1997; Thao, Xoua. *Southeast Asian Refugees of Rhode Island: The Hmong Perception of Illness*. Rhode Island Medical Journal, 67 1984: 323–329; Waters, David A., Rama B. Rao, and Helen E. Petracchi. *Providing Health Care for the Hmong*. Wisconsin Medical Journal, 91 (11) 1992: 642–651.

[114] Fadiman, Anne. *The Spirit Catches You and You Fall Down: A Hmong Child, Her American Doctors, and the Collision of Two Cultures*. New York: Farrar, Straus and Giroux, 1997; Warner, Miriam E., and Marilyn Mochel. *The Hmong and Health Care in Merced, California*. Hmong Studies Journal, Spring, 1998, 2 (2); Waters, David A., Rama B. Rao, and Helen E. Petracchi. *Providing Health Care for the Hmong*. Wisconsin Medical Journal, 91 (11) 1992: 642–651.

[115] Arax, Mark. Hmong's Sacrifice of Puppy Reopens Cultural Wounds: Immigrant Shaman's Act Stirs Outrage in Fresno, But He Believes It Was Only Way To Cure His Ill Wife. (Chia Thai Moua's sacrifice incurs racism and dislike of Southeast Asians in Fresno). Los Angeles Times, Dec 16, 1995, v114, pA1, Col 5 (40 col in); Fadiman, Anne. The Spirit Catches You and You Fall Down: A Hmong

Child, Her American Doctors, and the Collision of Two Cultures. New York: Farrar, Straus and Giroux, 1997.

[116] Arax, Mark. *Cancer Case Ignites Culture Clash; Hmong Parents Refuse To Agree To Court Ordered Chemotherapy For Teenage Daughter.* (Case in Fresno, California Highlights Parents' Fear That Ovarian Cancer Treatment Will Render Daughter Infertile And Thus Unmarriageable). Los Angeles Times, Nov 21, 1994, v113, pA3, Col 1 (35 col in); Fadiman, Anne. *The Spirit Catches You and You Fall Down: A Hmong Child, Her American Doctors, and the Collision of Two Cultures.* New York: Farrar, Straus and Giroux, 1997; True, Gala. *My Soul Will Come Back to Trouble You: Cultural and Ethical Issues in the Coerced Treatment of a Hmong Adolescent.* (Cultural diversity in medical education). Southern Folklore, 54 (2) 1995: 101–114; Waters, David A., Rama B. Rao, and Helen E. Petracchi. *Providing Health Care for the Hmong.* Wisconsin Medical Journal, 91 (11) 1992: 642–651.

[117] Fadiman, Anne. The Spirit Catches You and You Fall Down: A Hmong Child, Her American Doctors, and the Collision of Two Cultures. New York: Farrar, Straus and Giroux, 1997.

[118] id.

[119] Waters, David A., Rama B. Rao, and Helen E. Petracchi. *Providing Health Care for the Hmong.* Wisconsin Medical Journal, 91 (11) 1992: 642–651.

[120] Barret, Bruce, et al. Hmong/Medicine Interactions: Improving Cross-cultural Health Care. Family Medicine Journal, 30 (3) 1998: 179–184; Fadiman, Anne. The Spirit Catches You and You Fall Down: A Hmong Child, Her American Doctors, and the Collision of Two Cultures. New York: Farrar, Straus and Giroux, 1997; Gervais, Karen G. Providing Culturally Competent Health Care to Hmong Patients. Minnesota Medicine, 79 (5) 1996: 49–51; O'Connor, Bonnie Blair. Healing Traditions: Alternative Medicine and the Health Professions. Philadelphia: University of Pennsylvania Press, 1995; Thao, Xoua. Hmong Perception of Illness and Traditional Ways of Healing. In The Hmong In Transition. Glenn L. Hendricks et al., eds. pp. 365–378. New York: Center for Migration Studies, 1986; Waters, David A., Rama B. Rao, and Helen E. Petracchi. Providing Health Care for the Hmong. Wisconsin Medical Journal, 91 (11) 1992: 642–651.

[121] Engebretson, Joan. Folk Healing and Biomedicine: Culture Clash or Complimentary Approach? Journal of Holistic Nursing, 12 (3) 1994: 240–250; Pachter, Lee M. Culture and Clinical Care: Folk Illness Beliefs and Behaviors and Their Implications for Health Care Delivery. Journal of the American Medical Association, 271 (9) 1994: 690–694; Waters, David A., Rama B. Rao, and Helen E. Petracchi. Providing Health Care for the Hmong. Wisconsin Medical Journal, 91 (11) 1992: 642–651.

[122] Waters, David A., Rama B. Rao, and Helen E. Petracchi. *Providing Health Care for the Hmong.* Wisconsin Medical Journal, 91 (11) 1992: 642–651.

[123] Barret, Bruce, et al. *Hmong/Medicine Interactions: Improving Cross-cultural Health Care.* Family Medicine Journal, 30 (3) 1998: 179–184; Waters, David A., Rama B. Rao, and Helen E. Petracchi. *Providing Health Care for the Hmong.* Wisconsin Medical Journal, 91 (11) 1992: 642–651.

[124] Waters, David A., Rama B. Rao, and Helen E. Petracchi. *Providing Health Care for the Hmong.* Wisconsin Medical Journal, 91 (11) 1992: 642–651; Fadiman, Anne. *The Spirit Catches You and You Fall Down: A Hmong Child, Her*

American Doctors, and the Collision of Two Cultures. New York: Farrar, Straus and Giroux, 1997.

125 Gervais, Karen G. Providing Culturally Competent Health Care to Hmong Patients. Minnesota Medicine, 79 (5) 1996: 49–51.

126 Cheon-Klessig, Y., D. D. Camilleri, B. J. McElmurry, and V. M. Ohlson. Folk Medicine in the Health Practice of Hmong Refugees. Western Journal of Nursing Research, 10 (5) 1988: 647–60; Fadiman, Anne. The Spirit Catches You and You Fall Down: A Hmong Child, Her American Doctors, and the Collision of Two Cultures. New York: Farrar, Straus and Giroux, 1997; Gervais, Karen G. Providing Culturally Competent Health Care to Hmong Patients. Minnesota Medicine, 79 (5) 1996: 49–51.

127 Barret, Bruce, et al. Hmong/Medicine Interactions: Improving Cross-cultural Health Care. Family Medicine Journal, 30 (3) 1998: 179–184; Fadiman, Anne. The Spirit Catches You and You Fall Down: A Hmong Child, Her American Doctors, and the Collision of Two Cultures. New York: Farrar, Straus and Giroux, 1997; Waters, David A., Rama B. Rao, and Helen E. Petracchi. Providing Health Care for the Hmong. Wisconsin Medical Journal, 91 (11) 1992: 642–651.

128 Waters, David A., Rama B. Rao, and Helen E. Petracchi. Providing Health Care for the Hmong. Wisconsin Medical Journal, 91 (11) 1992: 642–651.

129 Fadiman, Anne. The Spirit Catches You and You Fall Down: A Hmong Child, Her American Doctors, and the Collision of Two Cultures. New York: Farrar, Straus and Giroux, 1997; Waters, David A., Rama B. Rao, and Helen E. Petracchi. Providing Health Care for the Hmong. Wisconsin Medical Journal, 91 (11) 1992: 642–651.

130 Hamilton-Merritt, Jane. Tragic Mountains: The Hmong, the Americans, and the Secret Wars for Laos, 1942–1992. Bloomington and Indianapolis: Indiana University Press, 1993; Ranard, Donald A. The Last Bus; The Hmong are Reluctant to Come to America: That is Their Tragedy and Thailand's Trouble. The Atlantic, 260 (6) 1987: 26; Waters, David A., Rama B. Rao, and Helen E. Petracchi. Providing Health Care for the Hmong. Wisconsin Medical Journal, 91 (11) 1992: 642–651.

131 Waters, David A., Rama B. Rao, and Helen E. Petracchi. Providing Health Care for the Hmong. Wisconsin Medical Journal, 91 (11) 1992: 642–651.

132 Thao, Xoua. Southeast Asian Refugees of Rhode Island: The Hmong Perception of Illness. Rhode Island Medical Journal, 67 1984: 323–329.

133 Barret, Bruce, et al. Hmong/Medicine Interactions: Improving Cross-cultural Health Care. Family Medicine Journal, 30 (3) 1998: 179–184.

134 Fadiman, Anne. The Spirit Catches You and You Fall Down: A Hmong Child, Her American Doctors, and the Collision of Two Cultures. New York: Farrar, Straus and Giroux, 1997; Waters, David A., Rama B. Rao, and Helen E. Petracchi. Providing Health Care for the Hmong. Wisconsin Medical Journal, 91 (11) 1992: 642–651.

135 Barret, Bruce, et al. Hmong/Medicine Interactions: Improving Cross-cultural Health Care. Family Medicine Journal, 30 (3) 1998: 179–184; Fadiman, Anne. The Spirit Catches You and You Fall Down: A Hmong Child, Her American Doctors, and the Collision of Two Cultures. New York: Farrar, Straus and Giroux, 1997.

[136] Kirton, Elizabeth S. *The Locked Medicine Cabinet: Hmong Health Care in America.* Ph. D. Dissertation. Santa Barbara: University of California, 1985; Waters, David A., Rama B. Rao, and Helen E. Petracchi. *Providing Health Care for the Hmong.* Wisconsin Medical Journal, 91 (11) 1992: 642–651.

[137] Barret, Bruce, et al. Hmong/Medicine Interactions: Improving Cross-cultural Health Care. Family Medicine Journal, 30 (3) 1998: 179–184; Fadiman, Anne. The Spirit Catches You and You Fall Down: A Hmong Child, Her American Doctors, and the Collision of Two Cultures. New York: Farrar, Straus and Giroux, 1997; Waters, David A., Rama B. Rao, and Helen E. Petracchi. Providing Health Care for the Hmong. Wisconsin Medical Journal, 91 (11) 1992: 642–651.

[138] Barret, Bruce, et al. *Hmong/Medicine Interactions: Improving Cross-cultural Health Care.* Family Medicine Journal, 30 (3) 1998: 179–184.

[139] Barret, Bruce, et al. Hmong/Medicine Interactions: Improving Cross-cultural Health Care. Family Medicine Journal, 30 (3) 1998: 179–184; Faller, H. S. Perinatal Needs of Immigrant Hmong Women: Surveys of Women and Health Care Providers. Public Health Report, 100 (3) 1985: 340–343; Waters, David A., Rama B. Rao, and Helen E. Petracchi. Providing Health Care for the Hmong. Wisconsin Medical Journal, 91 (11) 1992: 642–651.

[140] Barret, Bruce, et al. Hmong/Medicine Interactions: Improving Cross-cultural Health Care. Family Medicine Journal, 30 (3) 1998: 179–184; Fadiman, Anne. The Spirit Catches You and You Fall Down: A Hmong Child, Her American Doctors, and the Collision of Two Cultures. New York: Farrar, Straus and Giroux, 1997; Waters, David A., Rama B. Rao, and Helen E. Petracchi. Providing Health Care for the Hmong. Wisconsin Medical Journal, 91 (11) 1992: 642–651.

[141] Gervais, Karen G. Providing Culturally Competent Health Care to Hmong Patients. Minnesota Medicine, 79 (5) 1996: 49; Engebretson, Joan. Folk Healing and Biomedicine: Culture Clash or Complimentary Approach? Journal of Holistic Nursing, 12 (3) 1994: 240–250.

[142] Barret, Bruce, et al. Hmong/Medicine Interactions: Improving Cross-cultural Health Care. Family Medicine Journal, 30 (3) 1998: 179–184; Fadiman, Anne. The Spirit Catches You and You Fall Down: A Hmong Child, Her American Doctors, and the Collision of Two Cultures. New York: Farrar, Straus and Giroux, 1997; Gervais, Karen G. Providing Culturally Competent Health Care to Hmong Patients. Minnesota Medicine, 79 (5) 1996: 49–51; O'Connor, Bonnie Blair. Healing Traditions: Alternative Medicine and the Health Professions. Philadelphia: University of Pennsylvania Press, 1995; Thao, Xoua. Southeast Asian Refugees of Rhode Island: The Hmong Perception of Illness. Rhode Island Medical Journal, 67 1984: 323–329; Warner, Miriam E., and Marilyn Mochel. The Hmong and Health Care in Merced, California. Hmong Studies Journal, Spring, 1998, 2 (2); Waters, David A., Rama B. Rao, and Helen E. Petracchi. Providing Health Care for the Hmong. Wisconsin Medical Journal, 91 (11) 1992: 642–651.

[143] Gervais, Karen G. *Providing Culturally Competent Health Care to Hmong Patients.* Minnesota Medicine, 79 (5) 1996: 49–51.

[144] Barret, Bruce, et al. Hmong/Medicine Interactions: Improving Cross-cultural Health Care. Family Medicine Journal, 30 (3) 1998: 179–184; Bliatout, Bruce Thowpaou. Guidelines for Mental Health Professionals to Help Hmong Clients Seek Traditional Healing Treatment. In The Hmong In Transition. Glenn L.

Hendricks et al., eds., 349–363. New York: Center for Migration Studies, 1986; Engebretson, Joan. Folk Healing and Biomedicine: Culture Clash or Complimentary Approach? Journal of Holistic Nursing, 12 (3) 1994: 240–250; Gervais, Karen G. Providing Culturally Competent Health Care to Hmong Patients. Minnesota Medicine, 79 (5) 1996: 49–51; O'Connor, Bonnie Blair. Healing Traditions: Alternative Medicine and the Health Professions. Philadelphia: University of Pennsylvania Press, 1995; Thao, Xoua. Hmong Perception of Illness and Traditional Ways of Healing. In The Hmong In Transition. Glenn L. Hendricks et al., eds. pp. 365–378. New York: Center for Migration Studies, 1986; Waters, David A., Rama B. Rao, and Helen E. Petracchi. Providing Health Care for the Hmong. Wisconsin Medical Journal, 91 (11) 1992: 642–651.

[145] Barret, Bruce, et al. Hmong/Medicine Interactions: Improving Cross-cultural Health Care. Family Medicine Journal, 30 (3) 1998: 179–184; Fadiman, Anne. The Spirit Catches You and You Fall Down: A Hmong Child, Her American Doctors, and the Collision of Two Cultures. New York: Farrar, Straus and Giroux, 1997; Gervais, Karen G. Providing Culturally Competent Health Care to Hmong Patients. Minnesota Medicine, 79 (5) 1996: 49–51; O'Connor, Bonnie Blair. Healing Traditions: Alternative Medicine and the Health Professions. Philadelphia: University of Pennsylvania Press, 1995; Waters, David A., Rama B. Rao, and Helen E. Petracchi. Providing Health Care for the Hmong. Wisconsin Medical Journal, 91 (11) 1992: 642–651.

[146] Bliatout, Bruce Thowpaou. *Guidelines for Mental Health Professionals to Help Hmong Clients Seek Traditional Healing Treatment.* In *The Hmong In Transition.* Glenn L. Hendricks et al., eds., 349–363. New York: Center for Migration Studies, 1986; Cheon-Klessig, Y., D. D. Camilleri, B. J. McElmurry, and V. M. Ohlson. *Folk Medicine in the Health Practice of Hmong Refugees.* Western Journal of Nursing Research, 10 (5) 1988: 647–60; Thao, Xoua. *Hmong Perception of Illness and Traditional Ways of Healing.* In *The Hmong In Transition.* Glenn L. Hendricks et al., eds. pp. 365–378. New York: Center for Migration Studies, 1986; Waters, David A., Rama B. Rao, and Helen E. Petracchi. *Providing Health Care for the Hmong.* Wisconsin Medical Journal, 91 (11) 1992: 642–651.

[147] Barret, Bruce, et al. Hmong/Medicine Interactions: Improving Cross-cultural Health Care. Family Medicine Journal, 30 (3) 1998: 179–184; Fadiman, Anne. The Spirit Catches You and You Fall Down: A Hmong Child, Her American Doctors, and the Collision of Two Cultures. New York: Farrar, Straus and Giroux, 1997; Waters, David A., Rama B. Rao, and Helen E. Petracchi. Providing Health Care for the Hmong. Wisconsin Medical Journal, 91 (11) 1992: 642–651.

[148] Barret, Bruce, et al. *Hmong/Medicine Interactions: Improving Cross-cultural Health Care.* Family Medicine Journal, 30 (3) 1998: 179–184.

[149] Ohnuki-Tierney, Emiko. *Illness and Culture in Contemporary Japan.* New York: Cambridge University Press, 1984.

[150] Kleinman, Arthur. *Neurasthenia and Depression: A Study of Somatization and Culture in China.* Culture, Medicine, and Psychiatry, 6 1992:177–190.

[151] Cooper, Robert, ed., *The Hmong.* Bangkok: Artasia Press Co. Ltd., 1991; Fadiman, Anne. *The Spirit Catches You and You Fall Down: A Hmong Child, Her American Doctors, and the Collision of Two Cultures.* New York: Farrar, Straus

and Giroux, 1997; Mottin, Jean. *History of the Hmong.* Bangkok: Odeon Store, 1980; O'Connor, Bonnie Blair. *Healing Traditions: Alternative Medicine and the Health Professions.* Philadelphia: University of Pennsylvania Press, 1995; Tapp, Nicholas. *Sovereignty and Rebellion: The White Hmong of Northern Thailand.* Oxford: Oxford University Press, 1989; Waters, David A., Rama B. Rao, and Helen E. Petracchi. *Providing Health Care for the Hmong.* Wisconsin Medical Journal, 91 (11) 1992: 642–651.

[152] Fadiman, Anne. The Spirit Catches You and You Fall Down: A Hmong Child, Her American Doctors, and the Collision of Two Cultures. New York: Farrar, Straus and Giroux, 1997; O'Connor, Bonnie Blair. Healing Traditions: Alternative Medicine and the Health Professions. Philadelphia: University of Pennsylvania Press, 1995; Waters, David A., Rama B. Rao, and Helen E. Petracchi. Providing Health Care for the Hmong. Wisconsin Medical Journal, 91 (11) 1992: 642–651.

[153] Barret, Bruce, et al. Hmong/Medicine Interactions: Improving Cross-cultural Health Care. Family Medicine Journal, 30 (3) 1998: 179–184; Fadiman, Anne. The Spirit Catches You and You Fall Down: A Hmong Child, Her American Doctors, and the Collision of Two Cultures. New York: Farrar, Straus and Giroux, 1997; O'Connor, Bonnie Blair. Healing Traditions: Alternative Medicine and the Health Professions. Philadelphia: University of Pennsylvania Press, 1995.

[154] Barret, Bruce, et al. *Hmong/Medicine Interactions: Improving Cross-cultural Health Care.* Family Medicine Journal, 30 (3) 1998: 179–184.

[155] Fadiman, Anne. The Spirit Catches You and You Fall Down: A Hmong Child, Her American Doctors, and the Collision of Two Cultures. New York: Farrar, Straus and Giroux, 1997; Waters, David A., Rama B. Rao, and Helen E. Petracchi. Providing Health Care for the Hmong. Wisconsin Medical Journal, 91 (11) 1992: 642–651.

[156] Gervais, Karen G. Providing Culturally Competent Health Care to Hmong Patients. Minnesota Medicine, 79 (5) 1996: 49–51; Lee, Gary Yia. Cultural Identity In Post-Modern Society: Reflections on What is aHmong? Hmong Studies Journal, 1 (1) 1996.

[157] Gervais, Karen G. *Providing Culturally Competent Health Care to Hmong Patients.* Minnesota Medicine, 79 (5) 1996: 49.

[158] Bliatout, Bruce Thowpaou. *Hmong Attitudes Towards Surgery: How It Affects Patient Prognosis.* Migration World, XVI (1) 1988: 25–27; Waters, David A., Rama B. Rao, and Helen E. Petracchi. *Providing Health Care for theHmong.* Wisconsin Medical Journal, 91 (11) 1992: 642–651.

[159] Bliatout, Bruce Thowpaou. *Hmong Attitudes Towards Surgery: How It Affects Patient Prognosis.* Migration World, XVI (1) 1988: 25–27.

[160] id.

[161] Cheon-Klessig, Y., D. D. Camilleri, B. J. McElmurry, and V. M. Ohlson. *Folk Medicine in the Health Practice of Hmong Refugees.* Western Journal of Nursing Research, 10 (5) 1988: 647–60; Fadiman, Anne. *The Spirit Catches You and You Fall Down: A Hmong Child, HerAmerican Doctors, and the Collision of Two Cultures.* New York: Farrar, Straus and Giroux, 1997; Waters, David A., Rama B. Rao, and Helen E. Petracchi. *Providing Health Care for the Hmong.* Wisconsin Medical Journal, 91 (11) 1992: 642–651.

[162] Waters, David A., Rama B. Rao, and Helen E. Petracchi. *Providing Health Care for the Hmong*. Wisconsin Medical Journal, 91 (11) 1992: 642–651.

[163] Lonsdorf, Nancy, Veronica Butler, and Melanie Brown. *A Woman's Best Medicine: Health, Happiness, and Long Life through Maharishi Ayur-Veda*. New York: Jeremy Tarcher, 1993.

[164] Lonsdorf, Nancy, Veronica Butler, and Melanie Brown. *A Woman's Best Medicine: Health, Happiness, and Long Life through Maharishi Ayur-Veda*. New York: Jeremy Tarcher, 1993.

[165] Lonsdorf, Nancy, Veronica Butler, and Melanie Brown. *A Woman's Best Medicine: Health, Happiness, and Long Life through Maharishi Ayur-Veda*. New York: Jeremy Tarcher, 1993: 31.

[166] Lonsdorf, Nancy, Veronica Butler, and Melanie Brown. *A Woman's Best Medicine: Health, Happiness, and Long Life through Maharishi Ayur-Veda*. New York: Jeremy Tarcher, 1993.

[167] Cheon-Klessig, Y., D. D. Camilleri, B. J. McElmurry, and V. M. Ohlson. *Folk Medicine in the Health Practice of Hmong Refugees*. Western Journal of Nursing Research, 10 (5) 1988: 647–60.

[168] Waters, David A., Rama B. Rao, and Helen E. Petracchi. *Providing Health Care for the Hmong*. Wisconsin Medical Journal, 91 (11) 1992: 642–651; Bliatout, Bruce Thowpaou. *Hmong Attitudes Towards Surgery: How It Affects PatientPrognosis*. Migration World, XVI (1) 1988: 25–27.

[169] Cheon-Klessig, Y., D. D. Camilleri, B. J. McElmurry, and V. M. Ohlson. *Folk Medicine in the Health Practice of Hmong Refugees*. Western Journal of Nursing Research, 10 (5) 1988: 647–60.

[170] Fadiman, Anne. The Spirit Catches You and You Fall Down: A Hmong Child, Her American Doctors, and the Collision of Two Cultures. New York: Farrar, Straus and Giroux, 1997; Waters, David A., Rama B. Rao, and Helen E. Petracchi. Providing Health Care for the Hmong. Wisconsin Medical Journal, 91 (11) 1992: 642–651.

[171] Fadiman, Anne. The Spirit Catches You and You Fall Down: A Hmong Child, Her American Doctors, and the Collision of Two Cultures. New York: Farrar, Straus and Giroux, 1997; Uba, Laura. Cultural Barriers to Health Care for Southeast Asian Refugees. Public Health Reports, v107 n5 p544 (5). Sept-Oct, 1992; Waters, David A., Rama B. Rao, and Helen E. Petracchi. Providing Health Care for theHmong. Wisconsin Medical Journal, 91 (11) 1992: 642–651.

[172] Barret, Bruce, et al. Hmong/Medicine Interactions: Improving Cross-cultural Health Care. Family Medicine Journal, 30 (3) 1998: 179–184; Fadiman, Anne. The Spirit Catches You and You Fall Down: A Hmong Child, Her American Doctors, and the Collision of Two Cultures. New York: Farrar, Straus and Giroux, 1997; Waters, David A., Rama B. Rao, and Helen E. Petracchi. Providing Health Care for the Hmong. Wisconsin Medical Journal, 91 (11) 1992: 642–651.

[173] Vawter, Dorothy E, and Barbara Babbitt. *Hospice Care for Terminally Ill Hmong Patients. A Good Cultural Fit?* Minnesota Medicine, 80 (11) 1997: 42–44; Cheon-Klessig, Y., D. D. Camilleri, B. J. McElmurry, and V. M. Ohlson. *Folk Medicine in the Health Practice of Hmong Refugees*. Western Journal of Nursing Research, 10 (5) 1988: 647–60; Fadiman, Anne. *The Spirit Catches You and You*

Fall Down: A Hmong Child, Her American Doctors, and the Collision of Two Cultures. New York: Farrar, Straus and Giroux, 1997.

[174] Uba, Laura. *Cultural Barriers to Health Care for Southeast Asian Refugees.* Public Health Reports, v107 n5 p544 (5). Sept-Oct, 1992: 546.

[175] Lonsdorf, Nancy, Veronica Butler, and Melanie Brown. *A Woman's Best Medicine: Health, Happiness, and Long Life through Maharishi Ayur-Veda.* New York: Jeremy Tarcher, 1993.

[176] Lonsdorf, Nancy, Veronica Butler, and Melanie Brown. *A Woman's Best Medicine: Health, Happiness, and Long Life through Maharishi Ayur-Veda.* New York: Jeremy Tarcher, 1993: 31.

[177] Lonsdorf, Nancy, Veronica Butler, and Melanie Brown. *A Woman's Best Medicine: Health, Happiness, and Long Life through Maharishi Ayur-Veda.* New York: Jeremy Tarcher, 1993: 31.

[178] Gallin, Bernard. Comments on Contemporary Sociocultural Studies of Medicine in Chinese Societies. In Culture and Healing In Asian Societies. Arthur Kleinman, et al. eds., Cambridge, Mass: Schenkman Publishing Company, 1978.

[179] Waters, David A., Rama B. Rao, and Helen E. Petracchi. *Providing Health Care for theHmong.* Wisconsin Medical Journal, 91 (11) 1992: 642–651; O'Connor, Bonnie Blair. *Healing Traditions: Alternative Medicine and the HealthProfessions.* Philadelphia: University of Pennsylvania Press, 1995; Ohnuki-Tierney, Emiko. *Illness and Culture in Contemporary Japan.* New York: Cambridge University Press, 1984; Lonsdorf, Nancy, Veronica Butler, and Melanie Brown. *A Woman's Best Medicine: Health, Happiness, and Long Life through Maharishi Ayur-Veda.* New York: Jeremy Tarcher, 1993; Fadiman, Anne. *The Spirit Catches You and You Fall Down: A Hmong Child, Her American Doctors, and the Collision of Two Cultures.* New York: Farrar, Straus and Giroux, 1997.

[180] Barrett, Bruce, et al. *Hmong/Medicine Interactions: Improving Cross-cultural Health*
Care. Family Medicine Journal, 30 (3) 1998: 179–184; Fadiman, Anne. The Spirit Catches You and You Fall Down: A Hmong Child, Her American Doctors, and the Collision of Two Cultures. New York: Farrar, Straus and Giroux, 1997; Kraub, Alan M. Healers and Strangers: Immigrant Attitudes Toward the Physician in America—A Relationship in Historical Perspective. Journal of the American Medical Association, 263 (13) 1990: 1807 – 1811; Waters, David A., Rama B. Rao, and Helen E. Petracchi. Providing Health Care for the Hmong. Wisconsin Medical Journal, 91 (11) 1992: 642–651.

[181] Smith, L. Critical Thinking, Health Policy, and the Hmong Culture Group, Part I. Journal of Cultural Diversity, 4 (2) 1995: 59–67; Fadiman, Anne. The Spirit Catches You and You Fall Down: A Hmong Child, Her American Doctors, and the Collision of Two Cultures. New York: Farrar, Straus and Giroux, 1997; Waters, David A., Rama B. Rao, and Helen E. Petracchi. Providing Health Care for the Hmong. Wisconsin Medical Journal, 91 (11) 1992: 642–651.

[182] Barrett, Bruce, et al. Hmong/Medicine Interactions: Improving Cross-cultural Health Care. Family Medicine Journal, 30 (3) 1998: 179–184; Fadiman, Anne. The Spirit Catches You and You Fall Down: A Hmong Child, Her American Doctors, and the Collision of Two Cultures. New York: Farrar, Straus and Giroux, 1997; Kraub, Alan M. Healers and Strangers: Immigrant Attitudes Toward the

Physician in America—A Relationship in Historical Perspective. *Journal of the American Medical Association*, 263 (13) 1990: 1807 – 1811; Waters, David A., Rama B. Rao, and Helen E. Petracchi. *Providing Health Care for the Hmong.* Wisconsin Medical Journal, 91 (11) 1992: 642–651.

¹⁸³ Cheon-Klessig, Y., D. D. Camilleri, B. J. McElmurry, and V. M. Ohlson. *Folk Medicine in the Health Practice of Hmong Refugees.* Western Journal of Nursing Research, 10 (5) 1988: 647–60; Kraub, Alan M. *Healers and Strangers: Immigrant Attitudes Toward the Physician in America—A Relationship in Historical Perspective.* Journal of the American Medical Association, 263 (13) 1990: 1807 – 1811; Waters, David A., Rama B. Rao, and Helen E. Petracchi. *Providing Health Care for the Hmong.* Wisconsin Medical Journal, 91 (11) 1992: 642–651.

¹⁸⁴ Smith, L. *Critical Thinking, Health Policy, and the Hmong Culture Group, Part I.* Journal of Cultural Diversity, 4 (2) 1995: 59–67; Waters, David A., Rama B. Rao, and Helen E. Petracchi. *Providing Health Care for the Hmong.* Wisconsin Medical Journal, 91 (11) 1992: 642–651.

¹⁸⁵ Waters, David A., Rama B. Rao, and Helen E. Petracchi. *Providing Health Care for the Hmong.* Wisconsin Medical Journal, 91 (11) 1992: 646.

¹⁸⁶ Barrett, Bruce, et al. *Hmong/Medicine Interactions: Improving Cross-cultural Health Care.* Family Medicine Journal, 30 (3) 1998: 183.

¹⁸⁷ Barrett, Bruce, et al. *Hmong/Medicine Interactions: Improving Cross-cultural Health Care.* Family Medicine Journal, 30 (3) 1998: 179–184; Fadiman, Anne. *The Spirit Catches You and You Fall Down: A Hmong Child, Her American Doctors, and the Collision of Two Cultures.* New York: Farrar, Straus and Giroux, 1997; Waters, David A., Rama B. Rao, and Helen E. Petracchi. *Providing Health Care for the Hmong.* Wisconsin Medical Journal, 91 (11) 1992: 642–651.

¹⁸⁸ Waters, David A., Rama B. Rao, and Helen E. Petracchi. *Providing Health Care for the Hmong.* Wisconsin Medical Journal, 91 (11) 1992: 646.

¹⁸⁹ Barrett, Bruce, et al. *Hmong/Medicine Interactions: Improving Cross-cultural Health Care.* Family Medicine Journal, 30 (3) 1998: 179–184; Fadiman, Anne. *The Spirit Catches You and You Fall Down: A Hmong Child, Her American Doctors, and the Collision of Two Cultures.* New York: Farrar, Straus and Giroux, 1997.

¹⁹⁰ O'Connor, Bonnie Blair. *Healing Traditions: Alternative Medicine and the Health Professions.* Philadelphia: University of Pennsylvania Press, 1995.

¹⁹¹ Waters, David A., Rama B. Rao, and Helen E. Petracchi. *Providing Health Care for the Hmong.* Wisconsin Medical Journal, 91 (11) 1992: 642–651.

¹⁹² Barrett, Bruce, et al. *Hmong/Medicine Interactions: Improving Cross-cultural Health Care.* Family Medicine Journal, 30 (3) 1998: 179–184; O'Connor, Bonnie Blair. *Healing Traditions: Alternative Medicine and the Health Professions.* Philadelphia: University of Pennsylvania Press, 1995; Waters, David A., Rama B. Rao, and Helen E. Petracchi. *Providing Health Care for the Hmong.* Wisconsin Medical Journal, 91 (11) 1992: 642–651.

¹⁹³ Barrett, Bruce, et al. *Hmong/Medicine Interactions: Improving Cross-cultural Health Care.* Family Medicine Journal, 30 (3) 1998: 179–184; Gervais, Karen G. *Providing Culturally Competent Health Care to Hmong Patients.* Minnesota Medicine, 79 (5) 1996: 49–51.

[194] Fadiman, Anne. *The Spirit Catches You and You Fall Down: A Hmong Child, Her American Doctors, and the Collision of Two Cultures.* New York: Farrar, Straus and Giroux, 1997; Waters, David A., Rama B. Rao, and Helen E. Petracchi. *Providing Health Care for the Hmong.* Wisconsin Medical Journal, 91 (11) 1992: 642–651.

[195] Waters, David A., Rama B. Rao, and Helen E. Petracchi. *Providing Health Care for the Hmong.* Wisconsin Medical Journal, 91 (11) 1992: 642–651.

[196] Cheon-Klessig, Y., D. D. Camilleri, B. J. McElmurry, and V. M. Ohlson. *Folk Medicine in the Health Practice of Hmong Refugees.* Western Journal of Nursing Research, 10 (5) 1988: 647–60; Fadiman, Anne. *The Spirit Catches You and You Fall Down: A Hmong Child, Her American Doctors, and the Collision of Two Cultures.* New York: Farrar, Straus and Giroux, 1997; Waters, David A., Rama B. Rao, and Helen E. Petracchi. *Providing Health Care for the Hmong.* Wisconsin Medical Journal, 91 (11) 1992: 642–651.

[197] Fadiman, Anne. *The Spirit Catches You and You Fall Down: A Hmong Child, Her American Doctors, and the Collision of Two Cultures.* New York: Farrar, Straus and Giroux, 1997; Waters, David A., Rama B. Rao, and Helen E. Petracchi. *Providing Health Care for the Hmong.* Wisconsin Medical Journal, 91 (11) 1992: 642–651.

[198] Barrett, Bruce, et al. *Hmong/Medicine Interactions: Improving Cross-cultural Health Care.* Family Medicine Journal, 30 (3) 1998: 179–184; Bliatout, Bruce Thowpaou. *Hmong Attitudes Towards Surgery: How It Affects Patient Prognosis.* Migration World, XVI (1) 1988: 25–27; Fadiman, Anne. *The Spirit Catches You and You Fall Down: A Hmong Child, Her American Doctors, and the Collision of Two Cultures.* New York: Farrar, Straus and Giroux, 1997; Waters, David A., Rama B. Rao, and Helen E. Petracchi. Providing Health Care for the Hmong. Wisconsin Medical Journal, 91 (11) 1992: 642–651.

[199] Cheon-Klessig, Y., D. D. Camilleri, B. J. McElmurry, and V. M. Ohlson. *Folk Medicine in the Health Practice of Hmong Refugees.* Western Journal of Nursing Research, 10 (5) 1988: 647–60.

[200] id.

[201] Bliatout, Bruce Thowpaou. *Hmong Attitudes Towards Surgery: How It Affects Patient Prognosis.* Migration World, XVI (1) 1988: 25–27.

[202] Barrett, Bruce, et al. *Hmong/Medicine Interactions: Improving Cross-cultural Health Care.* Family Medicine Journal, 30 (3) 1998: 179–184; Fadiman, Anne. *The Spirit Catches You and You Fall Down: A Hmong Child, Her American Doctors, and the Collision of Two Cultures.* New York: Farrar, Straus and Giroux, 1997; Long, Lynellyn D. *Ban Vinai: The Refugee Camp.* New York: Columbia University Press, 1993; Munger, Ronald G. *Sleep Disturbances and Sudden Death of Hmong Refugees: A Report on Fieldwork Conducted in the Ban Vinai Refugee Camp.* In *The Hmong In Transition.* Glenn L. Hendricks et al., eds. New York: Center for Migration Studies, 1986; O'Connor, Bonnie Blair. *Healing Traditions: Alternative Medicine and the Health Professions.* Philadelphia: University of Pennsylvania Press, 1995; Waters, David A., Rama B. Rao, and Helen E. Petracchi. *Providing Health Care for the Hmong.* Wisconsin Medical Journal, 91 (11) 1992: 642–651.

203 Fadiman, Anne. *The Spirit Catches You and You Fall Down: A Hmong Child, Her American Doctors, and the Collision of Two Cultures.* New York: Farrar, Straus and Giroux, 1997; Waters, David A., Rama B. Rao, and Helen E. Petracchi. *Providing Health Care for the Hmong.* Wisconsin Medical Journal, 91 (11) 1992: 642–651.

204 Barrett, Bruce, et al. *Hmong/Medicine Interactions: Improving Cross-cultural Health Care.* Family Medicine Journal, 30 (3) 1998: 179–184; Fadiman, Anne. *The Spirit Catches You and You Fall Down: A Hmong Child, Her American Doctors, and the Collision of Two Cultures.* New York: Farrar, Straus and Giroux, 1997; Waters, David A., Rama B. Rao, and Helen E. Petracchi. *Providing Health Care for the Hmong.* Wisconsin Medical Journal, 91 (11) 1992: 642–651.

205 Barrett, Bruce, et al. *Hmong/Medicine Interactions: Improving Cross-cultural Health Care.* Family Medicine Journal, 30 (3) 1998: 179–184; Fadiman, Anne. *The Spirit Catches You and You Fall Down: A Hmong Child, Her American Doctors, and the Collision of Two Cultures.* New York: Farrar, Straus and Giroux, 1997; Velasco, Joyce D. *Exploration of Employment Possibilities for Hmong Women with Psychiatric Disorders.* The Journal of Rehabilitation 62 (4) 1996: 33–38; Waters, David A., Rama B. Rao, and Helen E. Petracchi. *Providing Health Care for the Hmong.* Wisconsin Medical Journal, 91 (11) 1992: 642–651.

206 Waters, David A., Rama B. Rao, and Helen E. Petracchi. *Providing Health Care for the Hmong.* Wisconsin Medical Journal, 91 (11) 1992: 642–651.

207 Barrett, Bruce, et al. *Hmong/Medicine Interactions: Improving Cross-cultural Health Care.* Family Medicine Journal, 30 (3) 1998: 179–184; Fadiman, Anne. *The Spirit Catches You and You Fall Down: A Hmong Child, Her American Doctors, and the Collision of Two Cultures.* New York: Farrar, Straus and Giroux, 1997; Waters, David A., Rama B. Rao, and Helen E. Petracchi. *Providing Health Care for the Hmong.* Wisconsin Medical Journal, 91 (11) 1992: 642–651.

208 Fadiman, Anne. *The Spirit Catches You and You Fall Down: A Hmong Child, Her American Doctors, and the Collision of Two Cultures.* New York: Farrar, Straus and Giroux, 1997; Mielke, H. W., B. Blake, S. Burroughs, and N. Hassinger. *Urban Lead Levels in Minneapolis: the Case of the Hmong Children.* Environmental Research, 34 (1) 1984: 64–76; Waters, David A., Rama B. Rao, and Helen E. Petracchi. *Providing Health Care for the Hmong.* Wisconsin Medical Journal, 91 (11) 1992: 642–651..

209 Waters, David A., Rama B. Rao, and Helen E. Petracchi. *Providing Health Care for the Hmong.* Wisconsin Medical Journal, 91 (11) 1992: 642–651.

210 Bliatout, Bruce Thowpaou. *Hmong Attitudes Towards Surgery: How It Affects Patient Prognosis.* Migration World, XVI (1) 1988: 25–27.

211 Waters, David A., Rama B. Rao, and Helen E. Petracchi. *Providing Health Care for the Hmong.* Wisconsin Medical Journal, 91 (11) 1992: 642–651; Westermeyer, Joseph. *Folk Medicine in Laos: A Comparison Between Two Ethnic Groups.* Social Science Medicine, 27 (8) 1988: 769–778; Barrett, Bruce, et al. *Hmong/Medicine Interactions: Improving Cross-cultural Health Care.* Family Medicine Journal, 30 (3) 1998: 179–184; Bliatout, Bruce Thowpaou. *Hmong Attitudes Towards Surgery: How It Affects Patient Prognosis.* Migration World, XVI (1) 1988: 25–27.

212 Waters, David A., Rama B. Rao, and Helen E. Petracchi. *Providing Health Care for the Hmong*. Wisconsin Medical Journal, 91 (11) 1992: 642–651; Bliatout, Bruce Thowpaou. *Hmong Attitudes Towards Surgery: How It Affects Patient Prognosis*. Migration World, XVI (1) 1988: 25–27.

213 Long, Lynellyn D. *Ban Vinai: The Refugee Camp*. New York: Columbia University Press, 1993; Fadiman, Anne. *The Spirit Catches You and You Fall Down: A Hmong Child, Her American Doctors, and the Collision of Two Cultures*. New York: Farrar, Straus and Giroux, 1997; Waters, David A., Rama B. Rao, and Helen E. Petracchi. *Providing Health Care for the Hmong*. Wisconsin Medical Journal, 91 (11) 1992: 642–651.

214 Bliatout, Bruce Thowpaou. *Hmong Attitudes Towards Surgery: How It Affects Patient Prognosis*. Migration World, XVI (1) 1988: 25–27; Fadiman, Anne. *The Spirit Catches You and You Fall Down: A Hmong Child, Her American Doctors, and the Collision of Two Cultures*. New York: Farrar, Straus and Giroux, 1997; Waters, David A., Rama B. Rao, and Helen E. Petracchi. *Providing Health Care for the Hmong*. Wisconsin Medical Journal, 91 (11) 1992: 642–651.

215 Barrett, Bruce, et al. *Hmong/Medicine Interactions: Improving Cross-cultural Health Care*. Family Medicine Journal, 30 (3) 1998: 179–184; Fadiman, Anne. *The Spirit Catches You and You Fall Down: A Hmong Child, Her American Doctors, and the Collision of Two Cultures*. New York: Farrar, Straus and Giroux, 1997; Gervais, Karen G. *Providing Culturally Competent Health Care to Hmong Patients*. Minnesota Medicine, 79 (5) 1996: 49–51; Spring, M. A., P. J. Ross, N. L. Etkin, and A. S. Deinard. *Sociocultural Factors in the Use of Prenatal Care by Hmong Women in Minneapolis*. American Journal of Public Health, 85 (7) 1995: 1015–7; Waters, David A., Rama B. Rao, and Helen E. Petracchi. *Providing Health Care for the Hmong*. Wisconsin Medical Journal, 91 (11) 1992: 642–651.

216 Waters, David A., Rama B. Rao, and Helen E. Petracchi. *Providing Health Care for the Hmong*. Wisconsin Medical Journal, 91 (11) 1992: 642–651.

217 Cooper, Robert, ed., *The Hmong*. Bangkok: Artasia Press Co. Ltd., 1991; Chindarsi, Nusit. *The Religion of the Hmong Njua*. Bangkok: The Siam Society, 1976; Fadiman, Anne. *The Spirit Catches You and You Fall Down: A Hmong Child, Her American Doctors, and the Collision of Two Cultures*. New York: Farrar, Straus and Giroux, 1997; Tapp, Nicholas. *Sovereignty and Rebellion: The White Hmong of Northern Thailand*. Oxford: Oxford University Press, 1989; Thao, Xoua. *Hmong Perception of Illness and Traditional Ways of Healing*. In *The Hmong In Transition*. Glenn L. Hendricks et al., eds. pp. 365–378. New York: Center for Migration Studies, 1986; Waters, David A., Rama B. Rao, and Helen E. Petracchi. *Providing Health Care for the Hmong*. Wisconsin Medical Journal, 91 (11) 1992: 642–651.

218 Cooper, Robert, ed., *The Hmong*. Bangkok: Artasia Press Co. Ltd., 1991; Waters, David A., Rama B. Rao, and Helen E. Petracchi. *Providing Health Care for the Hmong*. Wisconsin Medical Journal, 91 (11) 1992: 642–651.

219 Waters, David A., Rama B. Rao, and Helen E. Petracchi. *Providing Health Care for the Hmong*. Wisconsin Medical Journal, 91 (11) 1992: 642–651.

220 Chindarsi, Nusit. *The Religion of the Hmong Njua*. Bangkok: The Siam Society, 1976; Cooper, Robert, ed., *The Hmong*. Bangkok: Artasia Press Co. Ltd., 1991; Fadiman, Anne. *The Spirit Catches You and You Fall Down: A Hmong*

Child, Her American Doctors, and the Collision of Two Cultures. New York: Farrar, Straus and Giroux, 1997; Waters, David A., Rama B. Rao, and Helen E. Petracchi. *Providing Health Care for the Hmong.* Wisconsin Medical Journal, 91 (11) 1992: 642–651.

[221] Fadiman, Anne. *The Spirit Catches You and You Fall Down: A Hmong Child, Her American Doctors, and the Collision of Two Cultures.* New York: Farrar, Straus and Giroux, 1997; Waters, David A., Rama B. Rao, and Helen E. Petracchi. *Providing Health Care for the Hmong.* Wisconsin Medical Journal, 91 (11) 1992: 642–651.

[222] Thao, Xoua. *Southeast Asian Refugees of Rhode Island: The Hmong Perception of Illness.* Rhode Island Medical Journal, 67 1984: 323–329; Cheon-Klessig, Y., D. D. Camilleri, B. J. McElmurry, and V. M. Ohlson. *Folk Medicine in the Health Practice of Hmong Refugees.* Western Journal of Nursing Research, 10 (5) 1988: 647–60; Chindarsi, Nusit. *The Religion of the Hmong Njua.* Bangkok: The Siam Society, 1976.

[223] Cooper, Robert, ed., *The Hmong.* Bangkok: Artasia Press Co. Ltd., 1991; Waters, David A., Rama B. Rao, and Helen E. Petracchi. *Providing Health Care for the Hmong.* Wisconsin Medical Journal, 91 (11) 1992: 642–651.

[224] Chindarsi, Nusit. *The Religion of the Hmong Njua.* Bangkok: The Siam Society, 1976; Fadiman, Anne. *The Spirit Catches You and You Fall Down: A Hmong Child, Her American Doctors, and the Collision of Two Cultures.* New York: Farrar, Straus and Giroux, 1997; Waters, David A., Rama B. Rao, and Helen E. Petracchi. *Providing Health Care for the Hmong.* Wisconsin Medical Journal, 91 (11) 1992: 642–651.

[225] Waters, David A., Rama B. Rao, and Helen E. Petracchi. *Providing Health Care for the Hmong.* Wisconsin Medical Journal, 91 (11) 1992: 642–651.

[226] Thao, Xoua. *Hmong Perception of Illness and Traditional Ways of Healing.* In *The Hmong In Transition.* Glenn L. Hendricks et al., eds. pp. 365–378. New York: Center for Migration Studies, 1986; Waters, David A., Rama B. Rao, and Helen E. Petracchi. *Providing Health Care for the Hmong.* Wisconsin Medical Journal, 91 (11) 1992: 642–651.

[227] Catanzaro, A., and R. J. Moser. *Health Status of Refugees From Vietnam, Laos, and Cambodia.* Journal of the American Medical Association, 247 (9) 1982: 1303–8; Edwards L. E., C. J. Rautio, and E. Y. Hakanson. *Pregnancy in Hmong Refugee Women.* Minnesota Medicine, 70 (11) 1986: 633–7, 655; Richman, D., and S. Dixon. *Comparative Study of Cambodian, Hmong, and Caucasian Infant and Maternal Perinatal Profiles.* Journal of Nurse Midwifery, 30 (6) 1985: 313–9; Smith, L. *Critical Thinking, Health Policy, and the Hmong Culture Group, Part I.* Journal of Cultural Diversity, 4 (2) 1995: 59–67; Fadiman, Anne. *The Spirit Catches You and You Fall Down: A Hmong Child, Her American Doctors, and the Collision of Two Cultures.* New York: Farrar, Straus and Giroux, 1997; Uba, Laura. *Cultural Barriers to Health Care for Southeast Asian Refugees.* Public Health Reports, v107 n5 p544 (5). Sept-Oct, 1992; Waters, David A., Rama B. Rao, and Helen E. Petracchi. *Providing Health Care for the Hmong.* Wisconsin Medical Journal, 91 (11) 1992: 642–651.

[228] Edwards L. E., C. J. Rautio, and E. Y. Hakanson. *Pregnancy in Hmong Refugee Women.* Minnesota Medicine, 70 (11) 1986: 633–7, 655.

²²⁹ Smith, L. Critical Thinking, Health Policy, and the Hmong Culture Group, Part I. Journal of Cultural Diversity, 4 (2) 1995: 59–67.

²³⁰ Gjerdingen, D. K., and V. Lor. *Hepatitis B Status of Hmong Patients.* Journal of the American Board of Family Practice, 10(5) 1997: 322–328.

²³¹ Gjerdingen, D. K., and V. Lor. *Hepatitis B Status of Hmong Patients.* Journal of the American Board of Family Practice, 10(5) 1997: 322–328; Hurie M. B., E. E. Mast, and J. P. Davis. *Horizontal Transmission of Hepatitis B Virus Infection to United States-Born Children of Hmong Refugees.* Pediatrics, 89 (2) 1990: 269–73.

²³² Gjerdingen, D. K., and V. Lor. *Hepatitis B Status of Hmong Patients.* Journal of the American Board of Family Practice, 10(5) 1997: 322–328.

²³³ Gjerdingen, D. K., and V. Lor. *Hepatitis B Status of Hmong Patients.* Journal of the American Board of Family Practice, 10(5) 1997: 325.

²³⁴ Kleinman, Arthur. *Neurasthenia and Depression: A Study of Somatization and Culture in China.* Culture, Medicine, and Psychiatry, 6 1992:177–190; cited in Lin, Elizabeth H. B., William B. Carter; and Arthur M. Kleinman. *An Exploration of Somatization among Asian Refugees and Immigrants in Primary Care.* American Journal of Public Health, 75 (9) 1985: 1080.

²³⁵ Bliatout, Bruce Thowpaou. *Guidelines for Mental Health Professionals to Help Hmong Clients Seek Traditional Healing Treatment.* In *The Hmong In Transition.* Glenn L. Hendricks et al., eds., 349–363. New York: Center for Migration Studies, 1986.

²³⁶ id.

²³⁷ Barrett, Bruce, et al. *Hmong/Medicine Interactions: Improving Cross-cultural Health Care.* Family Medicine Journal, 30 (3) 1998: 179–184; Gurung, Carolyn Ruth. *The Reported Symptoms of Depression by Hmong Refugee Women.* M.S. Thesis. Oshkosh: University of Wisconsin, 1996; Jacobson, M. L., and T. W. Crowson. *Screening for Depression in Hmong Refugees.* Minnesota Medicine, 66 (9) 1983: 573–4; Smith, L. *Critical Thinking, Health Policy, and the Hmong Culture Group, Part I.* Journal of Cultural Diversity, 4 (2) 1995: 59–67; Weeks, John R., and Ruben G. Rumbaut. *Infant Mortality Among Ethnic Immigrant Groups.* Social Science Medicine, 33 (3) 1991: 327–334; Westermeyer, Joseph. *Folk Medicine in Laos: A Comparison Between Two Ethnic Groups.* Social Science Medicine, 27 (8) 1988: 769–778; Westermeyer, Joseph. *A Matched Pairs Study of Depression Among Hmong Refugees with Particular Reference to Predisposing Factors and Treatment Outcome.* Social Psychiatry and Psychiatric Epidemiology, 23 (1) 1986: 64–67; Westermeyer, Joseph, J. Neider, and A. Callies. *Psychosocial Adjustment of Hmong Refugees During Their First Decade in the United States. A Longitudinal Study.* Journal of Nervous Mental Diseases, 177 (3) 1989(b): 132–9; Westermeyer, Joseph, T. F. Vang, and J. Neider. *Refugees Who Do and Do Not Seek Psychiatric Care. An Analysis of Premigratory and Postmigratory Characteristics.* Journal of Nervous Mental Diseases, 171 (2) 1983: 86–91.

²³⁸ Barrett, Bruce, et al. *Hmong/Medicine Interactions: Improving Cross-cultural Health Care.* Family Medicine Journal, 30 (3) 1998: 179–184; Gurung, Carolyn Ruth. *The Reported Symptoms of Depression by Hmong Refugee Women.* M.S. Thesis. Oshkosh: University of Wisconsin, 1996; Jacobson, M. L., and T. W. Crowson. *Screening for Depression in Hmong Refugees.* Minnesota Medicine, 66

(9) 1983: 573–4; Smith, L. *Critical Thinking, Health Policy, and the Hmong Culture Group, Part I.* Journal of Cultural Diversity, 4 (2) 1995: 59–67; Waters, David A., Rama B. Rao, and Helen E. Petracchi. *Providing Health Care for the Hmong.* Wisconsin Medical Journal, 91 (11) 1992: 642–651; Westermeyer, Joseph. *Folk Medicine in Laos: A Comparison Between Two Ethnic Groups.* Social Science Medicine, 27 (8) 1988: 769–778; Westermeyer, Joseph. *A Matched Pairs Study of Depression Among Hmong Refugees with Particular Reference to Predisposing Factors and Treatment Outcome.* Social Psychiatry and Psychiatric Epidemiology, 23 (1) 1986: 64–67; Westermeyer, Joseph, J. Neider, and A. Callies. *Psychosocial Adjustment of Hmong Refugees During Their First Decade in the United States. A Longitudinal Study.* Journal of Nervous Mental Diseases, 177 (3) 1989(b): 132–9; Westermeyer, Joseph, T. F. Vang, and J. Neider. *Refugees Who Do and Do Not Seek Psychiatric Care. An Analysis of Premigratory and Postmigratory Characteristics.* Journal of Nervous Mental Diseases, 171 (2) 1983: 86–91.

[239] Mouanoutoua, V. L., L. G. Brown, G. G. Cappelletty, and R. V. Levine. *A Hmong Adaptation of the Beck Depression Inventory.* Journal of Personality Assessment, 57 (2) 1991: 309–22.

[240] Jacobson, M. L., and T. W. Crowson. *Screening for Depression in Hmong Refugees.* Minnesota Medicine, 66 (9) 1983: 573–4.

[241] id.

[242] id.

[243] Barrett, Bruce, et al. *Hmong/Medicine Interactions: Improving Cross-cultural Health Care.* Family Medicine Journal, 30 (3) 1998: 179–184; Smith, L. *Critical Thinking, Health Policy, and the Hmong Culture Group, Part I.* Journal of Cultural Diversity, 4 (2) 1995: 59–67; Waters, David A., Rama B. Rao, and Helen E. Petracchi. *Providing Health Care for the Hmong.* Wisconsin Medical Journal, 91 (11) 1992: 642–651; Westermeyer, Joseph, T. F. Vang, and J. Neider. *Refugees Who Do and Do Not Seek Psychiatric Care. An Analysis of Premigratory and Postmigratory Characteristics.* Journal of Nervous Mental Diseases, 171 (2) 1983: 86–91; Westermeyer, Joseph, T. Lyfoung, K. Wahmanholm, and M. Westermeyer. *Delusions of Fatal Contagion Among Refugee Patients.* Psychosomatics, 30 (4) 1989(a): 374–382; Westermeyer, Joseph, J. Neider, and A. Callies. *Psychosocial Adjustment of Hmong Refugees During Their First Decade in the United States. A Longitudinal Study.* Journal of Nervous Mental Diseases, 177 (3) 1989(b): 132–9.

[244] Barrett, Bruce, et al. *Hmong/Medicine Interactions: Improving Cross-cultural Health Care.* Family Medicine Journal, 30 (3) 1998: 179–184; Bliatout, Bruce Thowpaou. *Guidelines for Mental Health Professionals to Help Hmong Clients Seek Traditional Healing Treatment.* In *The Hmong In Transition.* Glenn L. Hendricks et al., eds., 349–363. New York: Center for Migration Studies, 1986; Fadiman, Anne. *The Spirit Catches You and You Fall Down: A Hmong Child, Her American Doctors, and the Collision of Two Cultures.* New York: Farrar, Straus and Giroux, 1997; Westermeyer, Joseph. *Folk Medicine in Laos: A Comparison Between Two Ethnic Groups.* Social Science Medicine, 27 (8) 1988: 769–778; Westermeyer, Joseph. *A Matched Pairs Study of Depression Among Hmong Refugees with Particular Reference to Predisposing Factors and Treatment Outcome.* Social Psychiatry and Psychiatric Epidemiology, 23 (1) 1986: 64–67.

²⁴⁵ Barrett, Bruce, et al. *Hmong/Medicine Interactions: Improving Cross-cultural Health Care.* Family Medicine Journal, 30 (3) 1998: 179–184.

²⁴⁶ Westermeyer, Joseph. *Folk Medicine in Laos: A Comparison Between Two Ethnic Groups.* Social Science Medicine, 27 (8) 1988: 769–778; Smith, L. Critical Thinking, Health Policy, and the Hmong Culture Group, Part I. Journal of Cultural Diversity, 4 (2) 1995: 59–67.

²⁴⁷ Smith, L. *Critical Thinking, Health Policy, and the Hmong Culture Group, Part I.* Journal of Cultural Diversity, 4 (2) 1995: 59–67; Westermeyer, Joseph. *Folk Medicine in Laos: A Comparison Between Two Ethnic Groups.* Social Science Medicine, 27 (8) 1988: 769–778; Westermeyer, Joseph, T. F. Vang, and J. Neider. *Refugees Who Do and Do Not Seek Psychiatric Care. An Analysis of Premigratory and Postmigratory Characteristics.* Journal of Nervous Mental Diseases, 171 (2) 1983: 86–91; Westermeyer, Joseph, T. Lyfoung, K. Wahmanholm, and M. Westermeyer. *Delusions of Fatal Contagion Among Refugee Patients.* Psychosomatics, 30 (4) 1989(a): 374–382; Westermeyer, Joseph, J. Neider, and A. Callies. *Psychosocial Adjustment of Hmong Refugees During Their First Decade in the United States. A Longitudinal Study.* Journal of Nervous Mental Diseases, 177 (3) 1989(b): 132–9.

²⁴⁸ Cooper, Robert, ed., *The Hmong.* Bangkok: Artasia Press Co. Ltd., 1991; Fadiman, Anne. *The Spirit Catches You and You Fall Down: A Hmong Child, Her American Doctors, and the Collision of Two Cultures.* New York: Farrar, Straus and Giroux, 1997; Barrett, Bruce, et al. *Hmong/Medicine Interactions: Improving Cross-cultural Health Care.* Family Medicine Journal, 30 (3) 1998: 179–184.

²⁴⁹ Warner, Miriam E., and Marilyn Mochel. *The Hmong and Health Care in Merced, California.* Hmong Studies Journal, Spring, 1998, 2 (2); Barrett, Bruce, et al. *Hmong/Medicine Interactions: Improving Cross-cultural Health Care.* Family Medicine Journal, 30 (3) 1998: 179–184.

²⁵⁰ Fadiman, Anne. *The Spirit Catches You and You Fall Down: A Hmong Child, Her American Doctors, and the Collision of Two Cultures.* New York: Farrar, Straus and Giroux, 1997; Barrett, Bruce, et al. *Hmong/Medicine Interactions: Improving Cross-cultural Health Care.* Family Medicine Journal, 30 (3) 1998: 179–184.

²⁵¹ Barrett, Bruce, et al. *Hmong/Medicine Interactions: Improving Cross-cultural Health Care.* Family Medicine Journal, 30 (3) 1998: 179–184.

NOTES TO CHAPTER III

¹ For the remainder of this discussion, these cities will be referred to collectively as the Denver/Boulder metropolitan area.

² Wheeler, Sheba R. *Hmong Parents Strive to Connect: Cultural Rift Divide Adults from Children.* The Denver Post, Nov. 15, 1998, pp. B1, B5.

³ For example, a Hmong patient was diagnosed as having colon cancer in the early stage of development.

Her conventional health care doctor recommended surgery to remove the affected area, but she and her husband refused. Other Hmong advised them to use Hmong herbs and tablets sent from Asia, and they agreed. However, her health condition was found to be devastated six months later. She and her husband returned to her doctor, ready to have the surgery. By that time, however, the cancer had already spread throughout her internal organs and her doctor could not save her.

[4] Pasick, Rena J., Carol N. D'Onofrio, and Regina Otero-Sabogal. *Similarities and Differences Across Cultures: Questions to Inform a Third Generation for Health Promotion Research.* Health Education Quarterly, 23 (Supplement) 1996: S142 - S161.

[5] Pasick, Rena J., Carol N. D'Onofrio, and Regina Otero-Sabogal. *Similarities and Differences Across Cultures: Questions to Inform a Third Generation for Health Promotion Research.* Health Education Quarterly, 23 (Supplement) 1996: S143.

[6] Waters, David A., Rama B. Rao, and Helen E. Petracchi. *Providing Health Care for the Hmong.* Wisconsin Medical Journal, 91 (11) 1992: 642–651.

[7] id.

[8] id.

[9] Barret, Bruce, et al. *Hmong/Medicine Interactions: Improving Cross-cultural Health Care.* Family Medicine Journal, 30 (3) 1998: 179–184; Cheon-Klessig, Y., D. D. Camilleri, B. J. McElmurry, and V. M. Ohlson. *Folk Medicine in the Health Practice of Hmong Refugees.* Western Journal of Nursing Research, 10 (5) 1988: 647–60; Fadiman, Anne. *The Spirit Catches You and You Fall Down: A Hmong Child, Her American Doctors, and the Collision of Two Cultures.* New York: Farrar, Straus and Giroux, 1997; O'Connor, Bonnie Blair. *Healing Traditions: Alternative Medicine and the Health Professions.* Philadelphia: University of Pennsylvania Press, 1995; Thao, Xoua. *Hmong Perception of Illness and Traditional Ways of Healing.* In *The Hmong In Transition.* Glenn L. Hendricks et al., eds. pp. 365–378. New York: Center for Migration Studies, 1986; Waters, David A., Rama B. Rao, and Helen E. Petracchi. *Providing Health Care for the Hmong.* Wisconsin Medical Journal, 91 (11) 1992: 642–651.

[10] Bliatout, Bruce Thowpaou. *Guidelines for Mental Health Professionals to Help Hmong Clients Seek Traditional Healing Treatment.* In *The Hmong In Transition.* Glenn L. Hendricks et al., eds., 349–363. New York: Center for Migration Studies, 1986; Cheon-Klessig, Y., D. D. Camilleri, B. J. McElmurry, and V. M. Ohlson. *Folk Medicine in the Health Practice of Hmong Refugees.* Western Journal of Nursing Research, 10 (5) 1988: 647–60; Fadiman, Anne. *The Spirit Catches You and You Fall Down: A Hmong Child, Her American Doctors, and the Collision of Two Cultures.* New York: Farrar, Straus and Giroux, 1997; Waters, David A., Rama B. Rao, and Helen E. Petracchi. *Providing Health Care for the Hmong.* Wisconsin Medical Journal, 91 (11) 1992: 642–651.

[11] Cheon-Klessig, Y., D. D. Camilleri, B. J. McElmurry, and V. M. Ohlson. *Folk Medicine in the Health Practice of Hmong Refugees.* Western Journal of Nursing Research, 10 (5) 1988: 647–60; Fadiman, Anne. *The Spirit Catches You and You Fall Down: A Hmong Child, Her American Doctors, and the Collision of Two Cultures.* New York: Farrar, Straus and Giroux, 1997; Waters, David A., Rama B. Rao, and Helen E. Petracchi. *Providing Health Care for the Hmong.* Wisconsin Medical Journal, 91 (11) 1992: 642–651.

[12] Fadiman, Anne. *The Spirit Catches You and You Fall Down: A Hmong Child, Her American Doctors, and the Collision of Two Cultures.* New York: Farrar, Straus and Giroux, 1997.

[13] Uba, Laura. *Asian Americans: Personality Patterns, Identity, and Mental Health.* New York: The Guilford Press, 1994.

[14] Uba, Laura. *Asian Americans: Personality Patterns, Identity, and Mental Health.* New York: The Guilford Press, 1994: 240.

[15] Uba, Laura. *Asian Americans: Personality Patterns, Identity, and Mental Health.* New York: The Guilford Press, 1994.

[16] id.

[17] Barret, Bruce, et al. *Hmong/Medicine Interactions: Improving Cross-cultural Health Care.* Family Medicine Journal, 30 (3) 1998: 179–184; Fadiman, Anne. *The Spirit Catches You and You Fall Down: A Hmong Child, Her American Doctors, and the Collision of Two Cultures.* New York: Farrar, Straus and Giroux, 1997.

[18] Fadiman, Anne. *The Spirit Catches You and You Fall Down: A Hmong Child, Her American Doctors, and the Collision of Two Cultures.* New York: Farrar, Straus and Giroux, 1997; Waters, David A., Rama B. Rao, and Helen E. Petracchi. *Providing Health Care for the Hmong.* Wisconsin Medical Journal, 91 (11) 1992: 642–651.

[19] Uba, Laura. *Asian Americans: Personality Patterns, Identity, and Mental Health.* New York: The Guilford Press, 1994.

[20] id.

[21] id.

[22] Barrett, Bruce, et al. *Hmong/Medicine Interactions: Improving Cross-cultural Health Care.* Family Medicine Journal, 30 (3) 1998: 179–184; Fadiman, Anne. *The Spirit Catches You and You Fall Down: A Hmong Child, Her American Doctors, and the Collision of Two Cultures.* New York: Farrar, Straus and Giroux, 1997; Waters, David A., Rama B. Rao, and Helen E. Petracchi. *Providing Health Care for the Hmong.* Wisconsin Medical Journal, 91 (11) 1992: 642–651.

NOTES TO CHAPTER IV

[1] Cooper, Robert, ed., *The Hmong.* Bangkok: Artasia Press Co. Ltd., 1991.

[2] Livo, Norma J., and Dia Cha. *Folk Stories of the Hmong: Peoples of Laos, Thailand, and Vietnam.* Englewood, CO: Libraries Unlimited, 1991.

[3] Johnson, Charles. *Myths, Legends and Folk Tales from the Hmong of Laos.* St. Paul: Macalester College, 1985.

[4] Rice, Pranee L. *The Hmong Way: Hmong Women and Reproduction.* Westport, CT: Bergin & Garvey, 2000.

[5] Cooper, Robert, ed., *The Hmong.* Bangkok: Artasia Press Co. Ltd., 1991; Rice, Pranee L. *The Hmong Way: Hmong Women and Reproduction.* Westport, CT: Bergin & Garvey, 2000.

[6] Bliatout, Bruce Thowpaou. *Guidelines for Mental Health Professionals to Help Hmong Clients Seek Traditional Healing Treatment.* In *The Hmong In Transition.* Glenn L. Hendricks et al., eds., 349–363. New York: Center for Migration Studies, 1986; Thao, Xoua. *Southeast Asian Refugees of Rhode Island: The Hmong Perception of Illness.* Rhode Island Medical Journal, 67 1984: 323–329; Lemoine, Jacques. *Shamanism in the Context of Hmong Resettlement.* In *The Hmong In Transition.* Hendricks, Glenn L. et al, eds. New York: Center for

Migration Studies, 1986; Ovesen, Jan. *A Minority Enters The Nation State: A Case Study of a Hmong Community in Vientiane Province, Laos*. Sweden: Uppsala University, 1995; Cooper, Robert, ed., *The Hmong*. Bangkok: Artasia Press Co. Ltd., 1991; Rice, Pranee L. *The Hmong Way: Hmong Women and Reproduction*. Westport, CT: Bergin & Garvey, 2000.

[7] Cooper, Robert, ed., *The Hmong*. Bangkok: Artasia Press Co. Ltd., 1991.

[8] The majority of Hmong Americans still practice the wedding rites as described in this paper. However, if a Christian Hmong is marrying another Christian Hmong, then they may not observe all details of the rite as traditionally prescribed. They may not, for example, pack the lunch or stop half way for lunch. In addition to such details of the traditional formula as may be embraced, the newly wedded Christian Hmong couple usually holds a wedding ceremony at a Christian church.

[9] Chindarsi, Nusit. *The Religion of the Hmong Njua*. Bangkok: The Siam Society, 1976; Cooper, Robert, ed., *The Hmong*. Bangkok: Artasia Press Co. Ltd., 1991; Lemoine, Jacques. *Shamanism in the Context of Hmong Resettlement*. In *The Hmong In Transition*. Hendricks, Glenn L. et al, eds. New York: Center for Migration Studies, 1986; Thao, Xoua. *Southeast Asian Refugees of Rhode Island: The Hmong Perception of Illness*. Rhode Island Medical Journal, 67 1984: 323–329.

[10] From the earliest times to as recently as the 1970s, Hmong leaders in power made their own rules or laws to govern their people. Good leaders exercised restraint and pursued justice in dealing with the common people, but bad leaders occasionally came to power—and abused it.

[11] This has probably led to the development of a Hmong taboo on praise for anyone of beauty or talent. Ironically, this lack of praise and reluctance to pay appropriate compliments for achievement may have contributed to the social problems faced by many in the modern Hmong American community. Hmong youth and Hmong spouses who have become acculturated in the American mainstream will often experience difficulty in believing that their parents or partners love them, since, no matter how hard they may try, success is met so seldom with any positive verbal response. This despite the fact that, in the American culture portrayed daily in the media, praise is a routine expression both of affection and of merit.

[12] Despite its mythological overtones, the author was reassured that this was a true story, not a legend.

[13] The fee charged to apprentices varies among healers. Some charge more; others charge less—and depends upon the relationship of the healer to the apprentice and on the nature of the skills or knowledge being transferred. Fees for tutelage in the skills and knowledge necessary to the treatment of serious illness will be higher.

[14] Lonsdorf, Nancy, Veronica Butler, and Melanie Brown. *A Woman's Best Medicine: Health, Happiness, and Long Life through Maharishi Ayur-Veda*. New York: Jeremy Tarcher, 1993.

[15] Lonsdorf, Nancy, Veronica Butler, and Melanie Brown. *A Woman's Best Medicine: Health, Happiness, and Long Life through Maharishi Ayur-Veda*. New York: Jeremy Tarcher, 1993.

¹⁶ Moua, Yer. *Knowledge and Attitudes of Hmong Health Care Workers About Hmong Traditional Healing Practices: A Need Assessment*. M.A. Thesis. Division of Epidemiology, School of Public Health. Minneapolis: University of Minnesota, 1998.

17 At the time of writing, The Denver Post had recently run an article addressing the serious condition facing Denver metropolitan area hospitals. In summary, the story related a rationale which is no excuse: more patients, but fewer hospital beds and fewer nurses.

NOTES TO CHAPTER V

¹ O'Connor, Bonnie Blair. *Healing Traditions: Alternative Medicine and the Health Professions*. Philadelphia: University of Pennsylvania Press, 1995: 53.

² Leslie, Charles, and Allen Young. *Paths to Asian Medical Knowledge*. Berkeley: University of California Press, 1990: 6.

³ Cha, Dia, and Cathy A. Small. *Policy Lessons from Lao and Hmong Women in Thai Refugee Camps*. World Development, 22 (7) 1994: 1045–1059.

⁴ Bliatout, Bruce Thowpaou, Bruce T. Downing, Judy Lewis, and Dao Yang. *Handbook for Teaching Hmong-Speaking Students*. Sacramento, CA: Folsom Cordova Unified School District and Southeast Asia Community, 1988.

⁵ Ovesen, Jan. A Minority Enters The Nation State: A Case Study of a Hmong Community in Vientiane Province, Laos. Sweden: Uppsala University, 1995.

⁶ Cha, Dia, and Cathy A. Small. Policy Lessons from Lao and Hmong Women in Thai Refugee Camps. World Development, 22 (7) 1994: 1045–1059; Cha, Dia, and Jacquelyn Chagnon. Farmer, War-wife, Refugee, Repatriate: A Needs Assessment of Women Repatriating to Laos. Washington, DC: Asia Resource Center, 1993.

⁷ Cooper, Robert, ed., *The Hmong*. Bangkok: Artasia Press Co. Ltd., 1991; Ovesen, Jan. *A Minority Enters The Nation State: A Case Study of a Hmong Community in Vientiane Province, Laos*. Sweden: Uppsala University, 1995; Rice, Pranee L. *The Hmong Way: Hmong Women and Reproduction*. Westport, CT: Bergin & Garvey, 2000; Tapp, Nicholas. *Sovereignty and Rebellion: The White Hmong of Northern Thailand*. Oxford: Oxford University Press, 1989; Geddes, William Robert. *Migrants of the Mountains: The Cultural Ecology of the Blue Miao (Hmong Njua) of Thailand*. Oxford: Clarendon Press, 1976.

⁸ Westermeyer, Joseph, T. F. Vang, and J. Neider. *Refugees Who Do and Do Not Seek Psychiatric Care. An Analysis of Premigratory and Postmigratory Characteristics*. Journal of Nervous Mental Diseases, 171 (2) 1983: 86–91.

⁹ One informant stated that he had witnessed a case in which the patient wrapped the wrong herbs on her hand and, as a result. two of her fingers later fell off. Another inform- ant reported witnessing severe swelling after the application of what was later termed an excess of a particular herbal preparation to a wounded area.

¹⁰ Lonsdorf, Nancy, Veronica Butler, and Melanie Brown. *A Woman's Best Medicine: Health, Happiness, and Long Life through Maharishi Ayur-Veda*. New York: Jeremy Tarcher, 1993: 28.

¹¹ Tobin, J. J., and J. Friedman. *Spirits, Shamans, and Nightmare Death: Survivor Stress in a Hmong Refugee*. American Journal of Orthopsychiatry, 53 (3) 1983: 439–48; Fadiman, Anne. *The Spirit Catches You and You Fall Down: A Hmong Child, Her*

American Doctors, and the Collision of Two Cultures. New York: Farrar, Straus and Giroux, 1997; Uba, Laura. *Asian Americans: Personality Patterns, Identity, and Mental Health.* New York: The Guilford Press, 1994; Westermeyer, Joseph, T. F. Vang, and J. Neider. *Refugees Who Do and Do Not Seek Psychiatric Care. An Analysis of Premigratory and Postmigratory Characteristics.* Journal of Nervous Mental Diseases, 171 (2) 1983: 86–91; Westermeyer, Joseph, J. Neider, and A. Callies. *Psychosocial Adjustment of Hmong Refugees during Their First Decade in the United States. A Longitudinal Study.* Journal of Nervous Mental Diseases, 177 (3) 1989(b): 132–9.

Westermeyer, Joseph. *Folk Medicine in Laos: A Comparison Between Two Ethnic Groups.* Social Science Medicine, 27 (8) 1988: 769–778.

[12] Ohnuki-Tierney, Emiko. *Illness and Culture in Contemporary Japan.* New York: Cambridge University Press, 1984.

Bibliography

Adler, Shelley R. *Refugee Stress and Folk Belief: Hmong Sudden Deaths.* Social Science Medicine, 40 (12) 1995: 1623–1629.

Adler, Shelley R. *Ethnomedical Pathogenesis and Hmong Immigrants' Sudden Nocturnal Deaths.* Culture, Medicine, and Psychiatry, 18 (1) 1994: 23–59.

Adler, Shelley R. *Sudden Unexpected Nocturnal Death Syndrome among Hmong Immigrants: Examining the Role of the "Nightmare."* Journal of American Folklore, 104 1991: 54–70.

Arax, Mark. *Hmong's Sacrifice of Puppy Reopens Cultural Wounds: Immigrant Shaman's Act Stirs Outrage in Fresno, But He Believes It Was Only Way To Cure His Ill Wife.* (Chia Thai Moua's Sacrifice Incurs Racism and Dislike of Southeast Asians in Fresno). Los Angeles Times, Dec 16, 1995, v114, pA1, Col 5 (40 col in).

Arax, Mark. *Cancer Case Ignites Culture Clash; Hmong Parents Refuse To Agree To Court Ordered Chemotherapy For Teenage Daughter.* (Case in Fresno, California, Highlights Parents' Fear that Ovarian Cancer Treatment will Render Daughter Infertile and Thus Unmarriageable). Los Angeles Times, Nov 21, 1994, v113, pA3, Col 1 (35 col in).

Austin, Marsha. *Hospitals in Serious Condition.* The Denver Post, Aug. 27, 2000, pp. 1M, 5M.

Barney, G. Le. *Christianity and Innovation in Meo Culture: A Case Study in Missionization.* Unpublished M. A. thesis. Minneapolis: University of Minnesota, 1957.

Barrett, Bruce, et al. *Hmong/Medicine Interactions: Improving Cross-cultural Health Care.* Family Medicine Journal, 30 (3) 1998: 179–184.

Barsky, Arthur J., and Jonathan F. Borus. *Somatization and Medicalization in the Era of Managed Care*. Journal of the American Medical Association, 274 (24) 1995: 1931–1934.

Bennett, Jane A., and Daniel F. Detzner. *Loneliness in Cultural Context, A Look at the Life History Narratives of Older Southeast Asian Refugee Women*. In *The Narrative Study of Lives*. A. Lieblich and R. Josselson, eds., 113–146. Thousand Oaks, CA: Sage, 1997.

Bliatout, Bruce Thowpaou. *Guidelines for Mental Health Professionals to Help Hmong Clients Seek Traditional Healing Treatment*. In *The Hmong In Transition*. Glenn L. Hendricks et al., eds., 349–363. New York: Center for Migration Studies, 1986.

Bliatout, Bruce Thowpaou. *Hmong Attitudes Towards Surgery: How It Affects Patient Prognosis*. Migration World, XVI (1) 1988: 25–27.

Bliatout, Bruce Thowpaou, Bruce T. Downing, Judy Lewis, and Dao Yang. *Handbook for Teaching Hmong-Speaking Students*. Sacramento, CA: Folsom Cordova Unified School District and Southeast Asia Community, 1988.

Buchwald, D., Thomas M. Hooton, and Sanjiv Panwala. *Use of Traditional Health Practices by Southeast Asian Refugees in a Primary Care Clinic*. The Western Journal of Medicine, 156 (5) 1992: 507–511.

Catanzaro, A., and R. J. Moser. *Health Status of Refugees From Vietnam, Laos, and Cambodia*. Journal of the American Medical Association, 247 (9) 1982: 1303–8.

Cha, Dia, and Jacquelyn Chagnon. *Farmer, War-wife, Refugee, Repatriate: A Needs Assessment of Women Repatriating to Laos*. Washington, DC: Asia Resource Center, 1993.

Cha, Dia, and Cathy A. Small. *Policy Lessons from Lao and Hmong Women in Thai Refugee Camps*. World Development, 22 (7) 1994: 1045–1059.

Chan, Sucheng. *Hmong Means Free: Life in Laos and America*. Philadelphia: Temple University Press, 1994.

Cheon-Klessig, Y., D. D. Camilleri, B. J. McElmurry, and V. M. Ohlson. *Folk Medicine in the Health Practice of Hmong Refugees*. Western Journal of Nursing Research, 10 (5) 1988: 647–60.

Chindarsi, Nusit. *The Religion of the Hmong Njua*. Bangkok: The Siam Society, 1976.

Cooper, Robert, ed., *The Hmong*. Bangkok: Artasia Press Co. Ltd., 1991.

Cooper, Robert, ed. *Resource Scarcity and the Hmong Response: Patterns of Settlement and Economy in Transition*. National University of Singapore: Singapore University Press, 1984. Edwards L. E., C. J. Rautio, and E. Y. Hakanson. *Pregnancy in Hmong Refugee Women*. Minnesota Medicine, 70 (11) 1986: 633–7, 655.

Engebretson, Joan. *Folk Healing and Biomedicine: Culture Clash or Complimentary Approach?* Journal of Holistic Nursing, 12 (3) 1994: 240–250.

Ensign, John. *Traditional Healing in the Hmong Refugee Community of the California Central Valley.* Ph.D. Dissertation. Fresno: California School of Professional Psychology, 1994.

Estroff, Sue E. *Making it Crazy: An Ethnography of Psychiatric Clients in an American Community.* Berkeley: University of California Press, 1981.

Fackelmann, Kathy A. *Food, Drug, or Poison?* (Toxic Plants Used by Tribal Cultures as Food or Medicine). Science News, 143 (20) 1993: 312–314.

Faderman, Lillian. *I Begin My Life All Over: The Hmong and the American Immigrant Experience.* Boston: Beacon Press, 1998.

Fadiman, Anne. *The Spirit Catches You and You Fall Down: A Hmong Child, Her American Doctors, and the Collision of Two Cultures.* New York: Farrar, Straus and Giroux, 1997.

Faller, H. S. *Perinatal Needs of Immigrant Hmong Women: Surveys of Women and Health Care Providers.* Public Health Report, 100 (3) 1985: 340–343.

Gallin, Bernard. *Comments on Contemporary Sociocultural Studies of Medicine in Chinese Societies.* In *Culture and Healing In Asian Societies.* Arthur Kleinman, et al. eds., Cambridge, Mass: Schenkman Publishing Company, 1978.

Geddes, William Robert. *Migrants of the Mountains: The Cultural Ecology of the Blue Miao (Hmong Njua) of Thailand.* Oxford: Clarendon Press, 1976.

Gervais, Karen G. *Providing Culturally Competent Health Care to Hmong Patients.* Minnesota Medicine, 79 (5) 1996: 49–51.

Gjerdingen, D. K., and V. Lor. *Hepatitis B Status of Hmong Patients.* Journal of the American Board of Family Practice, 10(5) 1997: 322–328.

Gong-Guy, Elizabeth. *California Southeast Asian Mental Health Needs Assessment.* Oakland, CA: Asian Community Mental Health Services, 1987.

Gurung, Carolyn Ruth. *The Reported Symptoms of Depression by Hmong Refugee Women.* M.S. Thesis. Oshkosh: University of Wisconsin, 1996.

Hamilton-Merritt, Jane. *Tragic Mountains: The Hmong, the Americans, and the Secret Wars for Laos, 1942–1992.* Bloomington and Indianapolis: Indiana University Press, 1993.

Heimbach, M. *At Any Cost: The Story of Graham Ray Orpin.* London: Overseas Missionary Fellowship, 1976.

Henry, Rebecca Rose. *Sweet Blood, Dry Liver: Diabetes and Hmong Embodiment in a Foreign Land.* Ph.D. Dissertation. Chapel Hill: University of North Carolina, 1996.

Her, Koua. *Hmong Medicine.* In *A Free People: Our Stories, Our Voices, Our Dreams.* Minneapolis: The Hmong Youth Cultural Awareness Project, 1994.

Hirayama, Kasumi, and Hisashi Hirayama. *Stress, Social Supports, and Adaptational Patterns in Hmong Refugee Families.* Amerasia Journal, 14 (1) 1987: 93–108.

Hmong National Development, Inc. *Hmong American Population.* Washington, DC: Newsletter (Summer), 2000.

Hurie M. B., E. E. Mast, and J. P. Davis. *Horizontal Transmission of Hepatitis B Virus Infection to United States-Born Children of Hmong Refugees.* Pediatrics, 89 (2) 1990: 269–73.

Ikeda, Noel R. *Who Are the Hmong?* A Term Paper Submitted to the Hmong In America Class, Department of Ethnic Studies. Boulder: University of Colorado, 1998.

Kirby, Charles C., and Ernest M. Pon. *Confronting New Mountains: Mental Health Problems Among Male Hmong and Mien Refugees.* Amerasia Journal, 14 (1) 1988: 109–118.

Jacobson, M. L., and T. W. Crowson. *Screening for Depression in Hmong Refugees.* Minnesota Medicine, 66 (9) 1983: 573–4.

Jambunathan, J., and S. Stewart. *Hmong Women in Wisconsin: What Are Their Concerns in Pregnancy and Childbirth?* Birth, 22 (4) 1995: 204–10.

Janes, Craig R. *Migration, Social Change, and Health: A Samoan Community in Urban California.* Palo Alto: Stanford University Press, 1990.

Johnson, Charles. *Myths, Legends and Folk Tales from the Hmong of Laos.* St. Paul: Macalester College, 1985.

Kirton, Elizabeth S. *The Locked Medicine Cabinet: Hmong Health Care in America.* Ph.D. Dissertation. Santa Barbara: University of California, 1985.

Kleinman, Arthur. *Patients and Healers in the Context of Culture: An Exploration of the Borderland Between Anthropology, Medicine, and Psychiatry.* Berkeley: University of California Press, 1980.

Kleinman, Arthur. *Neurasthenia and Depression: A Study of Somatization and Culture in China.* Culture, Medicine, and Psychiatry, 6 1992:177–190.

Kraub, Alan M. *Healers and Strangers: Immigrant Attitudes Toward the Physician in America—A Relationship in Historical Perspective.* Journal of the American Medical Association, 263 (13) 1990: 1807 - 1811.

Kuhn, I. *Ascent to the Tribes: Pioneering in North Thailand.* London: Overseas Missionary Fellowship, 1956.

Kunstadter, Peter, S. L. Kunstadter, C. Podhisita, and P. Leepreecha. *Demographic Variables in Fetal and Child Mortality: Hmong in Thailand.* Social Science Medicine, 36 (9) 1993: 1109–20.

Lee, Gary Yia. *Cultural Identity In Post-Modern Society: Reflections on What is a Hmong?* Hmong Studies Journal, 1 (1) 1996.

Lemoine, Jacques. *Shamanism in the Context of Hmong Resettlement.* In *The Hmong In Transition.* Hendricks, Glenn L. et al, eds. New York: Center for Migration Studies, 1986.

Leslie, Charles, and Allen Young. *Paths to Asian Medical Knowledge*. Berkeley: University of California Press, 1990.

Lin, Elizabeth H. B., William B. Carter; and Arthur M. Kleinman. *An Exploration of Somatization among Asian Refugees and Immigrants in Primary Care*. American Journal of Public Health, 75 (9) 1985: 1080–1084.

Livo, Norma J., and Dia Cha. *Folk Stories of the Hmong: Peoples of Laos, Thailand, and Vietnam*. Englewood, CO: Libraries Unlimited, 1991.

Long, Lynellyn D. *Ban Vinai: The Refugee Camp*. New York: Columbia University Press, 1993.

Lonsdorf, Nancy, Veronica Butler, and Melanie Brown. *A Woman's Best Medicine: Health, Happiness, and Long Life through Maharishi Ayur-Veda*. New York: Jeremy Tarcher, 1993.

Mielke, H. W., B. Blake, S. Burroughs, and N. Hassinger. *Urban Lead Levels in Minneapolis: the Case of the Hmong Children*. Environmental Research, 34 (1) 1984: 64–76.

Mills, P. K., and R. Yang. *Cancer Incidence in the Hmong of Central California, United States, 1987–94*. Cancer Causes Control, 8 (5) 1997: 705–12.

Moon, Anson, and Nathaniel Tashima. *Help Seeking Behavior and Attitudes of Southeast Asian Refugees*. San Francisco: Pacific Asian Mental Health Research Project, 1982.

Morrow, Kathleen. *Transcultural Midwifery. Adapting to Hmong Birthing Customs in California*. Journal of Nurse Midwifery, 31 (6) 1986: 285–8.

Mottin, Jean. *History of the Hmong*. Bangkok: Odeon Store, 1980.

Moua, Yer. *Knowledge and Attitudes of Hmong Health Care Workers About Hmong Traditional Healing Practices: A Need Assessment*. M.A. Thesis. Division of Epidemiology, School of Public Health. Minneapolis: University of Minnesota, 1998.

Mouanoutoua, V. L., L. G. Brown, G. G. Cappelletty, and R. V. Levine. *A Hmong Adaptation of the Beck Depression Inventory*. Journal of Personality Assessment, 57 (2) 1991: 309–22.

Munger, Ronald G. *Sleep Disturbances and Sudden Death of Hmong Refugees: A Report on Fieldwork Conducted in the Ban Vinai Refugee Camp*. In *The Hmong In Transition*. Glenn L. Hendricks et al., eds. New York: Center for Migration Studies, 1986.

Nuland, Sherwin B. Review of *A Spirit Catches You and You Fall Down*, by Anne Fadiman. New Republic, 217 (15) 1997: 31–40.

Nuttall, P., and F. C. Flores. *Hmong Healing Practices Used for Common Childhood Illnesses*. Pediatric Nursing, 23 (3) 1997: 247–251.

O'Connor, Bonnie Blair. *Healing Traditions: Alternative Medicine and the Health Professions*. Philadelphia: University of Pennsylvania Press, 1995.

Ohnuki-Tierney, Emiko. *Illness and Culture in Contemporary Japan*. New York: Cambridge University Press, 1984.

Ovesen, Jan. *A Minority Enters The Nation State: A Case Study of a Hmong Community in Vientiane Province, Laos.* Sweden: Uppsala University, 1995.

Pachter, Lee M. *Culture and Clinical Care: Folk Illness Beliefs and Behaviors and Their Implications for Health Care Delivery.* Journal of the American Medical Association, 271 (9) 1994: 690–694.

Pasick, Rena J., Carol N. D'Onofrio, and Regina Otero-Sabogal. *Similarities and Differences Across Cultures: Questions to Inform a Third Generation for Health Promotion Research.* Health Education Quarterly, 23 (Supplement) 1996: S142 - S161.

Payer, Lynn. *Medicine and Culture.* New York: Penguin Books, 1987.

Quincy, Keith. *Hmong: History of A People.* Cheney, WA: Eastern Washington University Press, 1995.

Ranard, Donald A. *The Last Bus; The Hmong are Reluctant to Come to America: That is Their Tragedy and Thailand's Trouble.* The Atlantic, 260 (6) 1987: 26.

Rice, Pranee L. *The Hmong Way: Hmong Women and Reproduction.* Westport, CT: Bergin & Garvey, 2000.   Rice, Pranee L., Blia Ly, and J. Lumley. *Childbirth and Soul Loss: the Case of a Hmong Woman.* Medical Journal of Australia, 160 (9) 1994: 577–8.

Richman, D., and S. Dixon. *Comparative Study of Cambodian, Hmong, and Caucasian Infant and Maternal Perinatal Profiles.* Journal of Nurse Midwifery, 30 (6) 1985: 313–9.

Schein, Louisa. *Minority Rules: The Miao and The Feminine in China's Culture Politics.* Durham & London: Duke University Press, 2000.

Smalley, William A., Chia Koua Vang, and Gnia Yee Yang. *Mother of Writing: The Origin and Development of a Hmong Messianic Script.* Chicago: The University of Chicago Press, 1988.

Smith, L. *Critical Thinking, Health Policy, and the Hmong Culture Group, Part I.* Journal of Cultural Diversity, 4 (2) 1995: 59–67.

Spring, M. A. *Ethnopharmacologic Analysis of Medicinal Plants used by Laotian Hmong Refugees in Minnesota.* Journal of Ethnopharmacology, 26 1989: 65–91.

Spring, M. A., P. J. Ross, N. L. Etkin, and A. S. Deinard. *Sociocultural Factors in the Use of Prenatal Care by Hmong Women in Minneapolis.* American Journal of Public Health, 85 (7) 1995: 1015–7.

Symonds, Patricia V. *Cosmology and the Cycle of Life: Hmong View of Birth, Death, and Gender in a Mountain Village in Northern Thailand.* Ph.D. Dissertation. Providence, Rhode Island: Brown University, 1991.

Tapp, Nicholas. *Sovereignty and Rebellion: The White Hmong of Northern Thailand.* Oxford: Oxford University Press, 1989.

Thao, Xoua. *Hmong Perception of Illness and Traditional Ways of Healing.* In *The Hmong In Transition.* Glenn L. Hendricks et al., eds. pp. 365–378. New York: Center for Migration Studies, 1986.

Thao, Xoua. *Southeast Asian Refugees of Rhode Island: The Hmong Perception of Illness*. Rhode Island Medical Journal, 67 1984: 323–329.

Tobin, J. J., and J. Friedman. *Spirits, Shamans, and Nightmare Death: Survivor Stress in a Hmong Refugee*. American Journal of Orthopsychiatry, 53 (3) 1983: 439–48.

True, Gala. *My Soul Will Come Back to Trouble You: Cultural and Ethical Issues in the Coerced Treatment of a Hmong Adolescent*. (Cultural Diversity in Medical Education). Southern Folklore, 54 (2) 1995: 101–114.

Uba, Laura. *Asian Americans: Personality Patterns, Identity, and Mental Health*. New York: The Guilford Press, 1994.

Uba, Laura. *Cultural Barriers to Health Care for Southeast Asian Refugees*. Public Health Reports, v107 n5 p544 (5). Sept-Oct, 1992.

Vawter, Dorothy E, and Barbara Babbitt. *Hospice Care for Terminally Ill Hmong Patients. A Good Cultural Fit?* Minnesota Medicine, 80 (11) 1997: 42–44.

Velasco, Joyce D. *Exploration of Employment Possibilities for Hmong Women with Psychiatric Disorders*. The Journal of Rehabilitation 62 (4) 1996: 33–38.

Warner, Miriam E., and Marilyn Mochel. *The Hmong and Health Care in Merced, California*. Hmong Studies Journal, Spring, 1998, 2 (2).

Warner, Roger. *Back Fire: The CIA's Secret War in Laos and Its Link to the War in Vietnam*. New York: Simon & Schuster, 1995.

Warner, Roger. *Shooting at the Moon*. South Royalton, Vermont: Steerforth Press, 1996.

Waters, David A., Rama B. Rao, and Helen E. Petracchi. *Providing Health Care for the Hmong*. Wisconsin Medical Journal, 91 (11) 1992: 642–651.

Weeks, John R., and Ruben G. Rumbaut. *Infant Mortality Among Ethnic Immigrant Groups*. Social Science Medicine, 33 (3) 1991: 327–334.

Westermeyer, Joseph. *Folk Medicine in Laos: A Comparison Between Two Ethnic Groups*. Social Science Medicine, 27 (8) 1988: 769–778.

Westermeyer, Joseph. *A Matched Pairs Study of Depression Among Hmong Refugees with Particular Reference to Predisposing Factors and Treatment Outcome*. Social Psychiatry and Psychiatric Epidemiology, 23 (1) 1986: 64–67.

Westermeyer, Joseph. *Hmong Drinking Practices in the United States: The Influence of Migration*. In *The American Experience with Alcohol: Contrasting Cultural Perspectives*. Linda A. Bennett and Genevieve M. Ames, eds. New York and London: Plenum Press, 1985.

Westermeyer, Joseph, T. F. Vang, and J. Neider. *Refugees Who Do and Do Not Seek Psychiatric Care. An Analysis of Premigratory and Postmigratory Characteristics*. Journal of Nervous Mental Diseases, 171 (2) 1983: 86–91.

Westermeyer, Joseph, T. Lyfoung, K. Wahmanholm, and M. Westermeyer. *Delusions of Fatal Contagion Among Refugee Patients*. Psychosomatics, 30 (4) 1989(a): 374–382.

Westermeyer, Joseph, J. Neider, and A. Callies. *Psychosocial Adjustment of Hmong Refugees During Their First Decade in the United States. A Longitudinal Study.* Journal of Nervous Mental Diseases, 177 (3) 1989(b): 132–9.

Wheeler, Sheba R. *Hmong Parents Strive to Connect: Cultural Rift Divide Adults from Children.* The Denver Post, Nov. 15, 1998, pp. B1, B5.

Yang, Dao. *The Hmong: Enduring Traditions.* In *Minority Cultures of Laos: Kammu, Lua', Lahu, Hmong, and Iu-Mien.* Judy Lewis, ed. Sacramento, CA: Southeast Asia Community Resource Center, 1991.

Yang, Kaoly. *Problems in the Interpretation of Hmong Clan Surnames (Hais Txog Kev Nrhiav Hmoob Cov Xeem).* Paper presented at the First International Workshop on the Hmong/Miao in Asia at the Centre des Archives d'Outre-Mer, Aix-en-Provence, France, 1998.

Yang, Pai, and Nora Murphy. *Hmong in the '90s: Stepping Towards the Future.* St. Paul: Hmong American Partnership, Inc., 1994.

Yang, Yeng. *Practicing Modern Medicine: "A little medicine, a little neeb."* Hmong Studies Journal, Spring, 1995, 2 (2).

Index